Workbook

Textbook of
Radiographic Positioning
and Related Anatomy

Eighth edition

Kenneth L. Bontrager, MA

John P. Lampignano, MEd, RT(R)(CT)

Leslie E. Kendrick, MS, RT(R)(CT)(MR)

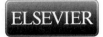
ELSEVIER

3251 Riverport Lane
St. Louis, Missouri 63043

WORKBOOK FOR TEXTBOOK OF RADIOGRAPHIC POSITIONING
AND RELATED ANATOMY, EIGHTH EDITION

ISBN: 978-0-323-08832-9

Notices

Knowledge and best practice in this field are constantly changing. As new research and experience broaden
our understanding, changes in research methods, professional practices, or medical treatment may become
necessary.
Practitioners and researchers must always rely on their own experience and knowledge in evaluating and
using any information, methods, compounds, or experiments described herein. In using such information or
methods they should be mindful of their own safety and the safety of others, including parties for whom
they have a professional responsibility.
With respect to any drug or pharmaceutical products identified, readers are advised to check the most current information provided (i) on procedures featured or (ii) by the manufacturer of each product to be administered, to verify the recommended dose or formula, the method and duration of administration, and
contraindications. It is the responsibility of practitioners, relying on their own experience and knowledge
of their patients, to make diagnoses, to determine dosages and the best treatment for each individual patient, and to take all appropriate safety precautions.
To the fullest extent of the law, neither the Publisher nor the authors, contributors, or editors, assume any
liability for any injury and/or damage to persons or property as a matter of products liability, negligence or
otherwise, or from any use or operation of any methods, products, instructions, or ideas contained in the
material herein.

ISBN: 978-0-323-08832-9

Executive Content Strategist: Jennifer Janson
Content Development Specialist: Andrea Hunolt
Publishing Services Manager: Catherine Jackson
Senior Production Editor: Carol O'Connell

Printed in United States of America

Last digit is the print number: 9 8 7 6 5 4 3 2

Acknowledgments

I would like to thank **Ken Bontrager** for his patience and mentorship in developing my skills as a writer. I've been honored to work with him over the past five editions. Ken has poured his heart and expertise into this text. Through his hard work and vision he has created a tremendous resource for students. **Mary Lou Bontrager** continues to provide the energy, technical support, and encouragement behind the scenes. Thank you, Mary Lou, for being there for both of us.

Ms. Leslie Kendrick, of Boise State University, joined us as co-author for the eighth edition of the workbook. Leslie is a dedicated educator and talented writer who has brought a high degree of quality and currency to this edition. Her attention to detail and quality is reflected in this new edition. I look forward to our collaboration for future editions. Thank you, Leslie.

Ms. Andrea Hunolt, our developmental editor, deserves praise for her dedication and vision in coordinating this project. **Ms. Anne Simon,** developmental editor, was instrumental in assisting Leslie and me with the first drafts of the workbook. Special thanks also to **Ms. Jennifer Janson,** Executive Content Strategist, for her leadership on the text and related ancillaries. **Ms. Lori A. Christensson,** GateWay Community College, and **Ms. Kaylee Hirst,** from Boise State University, reviewed every exercise and assessment for this edition of the workbook. Both did a stellar job in their attention to detail and ensuring the accuracy of every exercise and assessment. They will be outstanding radiologic technologists. Special thanks to **Ms. Carol O'Connell,** the Production Project Manager, for her attention to detail and her professionalism during the editing phase of the text and workbooks. Also, thanks to **Ms. Lois Schubert** with Top Graphics for her work on the art.

This edition is dedicated to the students and faculty who continue to provide us valuable feedback on how we can improve the text and workbook materials. A special thanks to **Michele L. Murphy BSRS, R.T.(R)(M),** faculty at Allen College in Waterloo, Iowa. Michele and her students have been a valuable resource in providing feedback on how we can make the text and workbook more meaningful and accurate.

Finally, the faculty who dedicated their careers in preparing future generations of health care professions. My colleagues at GateWay Community College are always willing to assist me with all aspect of the text and materials. Thank you.

JPL

Thank you to **Mr. John P. Lampignano** and **Mr. Kenneth Bontrager** for granting me the opportunity to be a part of this workbook edition. The project has been an amazing experience and such a privilege. I cannot sufficiently express the gratitude felt to have been given the chance to contribute to the profession in this manner. It is my hope that this workbook be a valued teaching tool for the enhancement of student success. Thank you again for trusting in me.

LEK

Preface

The success of the first seven editions of this workbook and laboratory manual, the accompanying textbook, along with the associated ancillary materials, has been adopted by the many schools of radiologic technology throughout the United States, Canada, and other countries that have been using all or parts of these instructional media for more than 34 years.

NEW TO THIS EDITION

The eighth edition workbook is a single volume as opposed to the two-volume sets of past editions. The elimination of outdated content and the consolidation of material made this possible. With a reorganization of similar content, the number of chapters in the eighth edition of the text and workbook was reduced from 23 to 20.

New illustrations, photographs, and expanded questions have been added to reflect all of the new content added to the eighth edition of *Textbook of Radiographic Positioning and Related Anatomy*. The use of visuals in these review exercises not only increases comprehension but also increases retention because most individuals retain information most effectively through visual images.

The detailed laboratory activities have been updated and the positioning question and answer exercises have been expanded, with less emphasis on rote memory recall. More situational questions involving clinical applications have been added. These questions assist in the application of positioning principles and critical evaluation of images. The clinical situational questions added to each chapter require students to analyze and apply this positioning information to specific clinical examples.

Pathology and clinical indication questions have been expanded to help students understand why they are performing specific exams and how exposure factors or positioning may be affected.

As in the textbook, updated information and concepts in digital imaging have been added in this edition. The bone densitometry section has also been expanded and included with other advanced modalities found in Chapter 20. Introductions to CT, MRI, nuclear medicine, PET, radiation oncology, ultrasound imaging, and MRI have also been updated and expanded.

BONTRAGER POCKET ATLAS HANDBOOK

The new eighth edition of the expanded *Bontrager's Handbook of Radiographic Positioning and Techniques* is now available from Elsevier as part of this comprehensive learning package on radiographic positioning and imaging. The new eighth edition of this handbook includes the unique added feature of a printed radiographic image of the position being described along with a basic critique checklist alongside each image. These primary critique checklist items are grouped in a consistent manner for all projections and are listed in more detail in the positioning pages of the textbook in the Evaluation Criteria section.

This unique handbook provides a guide for students to carry with them in the clinical setting as they learn what to look for when they evaluate each radiograph after it has been taken and processed. This critique checklist also provides a system for the clinical instructors to use in which they can check off each critique item for that radiograph and sign off that exam as a completed competency for that student.

INFORMATION FOR FACULTY

Instructor Resources
Electronic instructor resources are available on the Evolve website at http://evolve.elsevier.com/Bontrager and consist of the following four components:

- **Self-Test Answer Key:** Each chapter in the workbook has a self-test that the students can complete following the review exercises. Based on feedback from educators prior to this edition, the answer keys have been removed from the student workbook and placed on the **Evolve website under Instructor Resources.** Instructors can chose to share the answer keys with their students beforehand or keep them for instructor access only, based on the level and immediacy of feedback they wish to provide.
- **Computerized Test Bank:** This test bank features more than 2000 questions divided into the 20 chapters. It has been updated, expanded, and revised into more registry-level questions that can be used as final evaluation exams for each chapter. The questions and related answers have been reviewed by the authors and a second-year imaging

student. They can be used to produce paper-based exams, or they can be integrated into a Learning Management System (LMS) such as BlackBoard, Angel, or WebCT. Answer keys are provided for each examination and can be found on the Evolve Educator's website. These questions can be downloaded to use for any assessment, and you will be able to delete or add questions to create your own personal test bank.

- **Electronic Image Collection:** Also available is an updated and expanded electronic image collection of images from all 20 chapters of the eighth edition of the textbook. These non-annotated images can be used by instructors to create PowerPoint presentations or for other web-based applications.
- **Electronic Instructional Presentation in PowerPoint:** Now included is an updated and expanded electronic image PowerPoint program that is fully coordinated with all 20 chapters of the eighth edition textbook and workbook. These electronic images include text slides, some of which contain embedded anatomy and radiographic images, resulting in a visually led instructional narrative. This can then be used as a complete chapter-by-chapter PowerPoint lecture guide. Sections from the more advanced chapters can also be used for in-service training or with postgraduate presentations. They can be downloaded to your desktop to personalize with your own content.

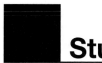

Student Instructions

The following information will describe how to effectively use this workbook and the accompanying textbook to help you master radiographic anatomy and positioning.

Because this course becomes the core of all your studies and your work as a radiologic technologist, it is one that you must master. You cannot become a proficient technologist by marginally passing this course. Therefore, please read these instructions carefully before beginning Chapter 1.

OBJECTIVES

Gain a clear understanding of your competency goals by reading the lists of objectives found at the beginning of each chapter.

TEXTBOOK AND WORKBOOK

Chapter 1 includes a comprehensive introduction that prepares you for the remaining chapters of this positioning course. This chapter contains basic positioning and technical principles that will apply to the remainder of the text and workbook exercises. Your instructor may assign all or specific sections of these chapters at various times during your study of radiographic positioning or procedures.

Chapters 2-14 are specific positioning chapters that include the anatomy, positioning, and related procedures for all parts of the body.

Chapters 15-20 are more specialized procedures and modalities that are commonly studied later in a medical radiography program.

LEARNING EXERCISES

These exercises are the focal point of this workbook. Using them correctly will help you learn and remember the important information presented in each chapter of the textbook. To maximize the benefits from each exercise, follow the correct six-step order of activities as outlined below.

ANATOMY ACTIVITIES

Step 1 (Textbook)
Carefully read and learn the radiographic anatomy section of each of these chapters. Include the anatomic reviews on labeled radiographs provided in the textbook. Pay particular attention to those items in bold type and to the summary review boxes, where provided.

Step 2 (Workbook, Part I)
Complete Part I of the review exercises on radiographic anatomy. Do not look up the answers in the textbook or look at the answer sheet until you have answered as many of the questions as you can. Then refer to the textbook or the answer sheet and correct or complete those questions you missed. Reread those sections of the textbook in which you could not answer questions. Textbook page numbers are provided next to each review exercise in this workbook.

POSITIONING ACTIVITIES

Step 3 (Textbook)
Carefully read and study Part II on all of the parts on radiographic positioning. Note the general positioning considerations, alternate modalities, and clinical indications for each chapter. Information from these sections will be seen on workbook review exercises and self-tests. Learn the specific positioning steps, the central ray location and angle, and the five-part radiographic criteria for each projection or position.

Step 4 (Workbook, Part II)

Complete Part II of the review exercises, which include technical considerations and positioning. Also included is a section on problem solving for technical and positioning errors. As before, complete as many of the questions as you can before looking up the answers in the textbook or checking the answers on the answer sheet.

The last review exercise in each positioning chapter covers radiographic critique questions in the workbook. These questions may involve radiographic evaluation of images from the text. These important exercises will help you make the transition from factual knowledge to application and will help you prepare for clinical experience. Compare each critique radiograph that demonstrates errors with the correctly positioned radiographs in that chapter of the textbook and see if you can determine which radiographic criteria points could be improved and which are repeatable errors.

With digital imaging, you will learn that in some cases postprocessing adjustments can be made to improve the exposures and the diagnostic value of the images rather than repeating the exam. Positioning errors, however, would still need to be repeated as they would with analog (film-screen) imaging and processing. Students who successfully complete these exercises will be ahead of those students who do not attempt them before coming to the classroom. The instructor will then explain and clarify the repeatable and nonrepeatable errors on each radiograph.

LABORATORY ACTIVITY

Step 5 (Workbook, Part III—Laboratory Activity)

These exercises must be performed in a radiographic laboratory using a phantom or a student (without making exposure), an energized radiographic unit, illuminators for viewing radiographs, or monitors for viewing digital images. Arrange for a time when you can use your radiographic laboratory or a diagnostic radiographic room in a clinic setting.

This is one of the most important aspects of this learning series and should not be neglected or underemphasized. Students frequently have difficulty transferring the information they have learned about positioning to effective use in a clinical setting. Therefore you must carry out the laboratory activities as described in each chapter. Your instructors or lab assistants will assist you as needed in these exercises.

Each radiograph taken of the phantom or other radiographs provided by your instructor should be evaluated as described in your lab manual. Critique and evaluate each radiograph for errors of less-than-optimal positioning or exposure factors based on radiographic criteria provided in the textbook. Also, with the help of your instructor, learn how to discriminate between less-than-optimal, but passable radiographs, and those that need to be repeated. This generally requires additional experience and practice before you can make these judgments without assistance from a supervising technologist or radiologist.

SELF-TEST

Step 6

You should take the self-test only after you have completed all of the preceding steps. Treat the self-test like an actual exam. After completing the self-test, submit your test to your instructor. Unlike previous editions, the self-test answer keys are in the possession of the faculty. Instructors may elect to either provide students with the answer key or grade it themselves. If your score is less than 90% to 95%, you should go back and review the textbook again; pay special attention to the areas you missed before you take the final chapter evaluation exam provided by your instructor.

Note: Statistics prove that students who diligently complete all the exercises described in this section will invariably achieve higher grades in their positioning courses and will perform better in the clinical setting than those who do not. Avoid the temptation of taking shortcuts. If you bypass some of these exercises or just fill in the answers from the answer sheets, your instructors will know by your grade and by your clinical performance that you have taken these shortcuts. Most importantly, you will know that you are not doing your best and you will have difficulty competing with better-prepared technologists in the work place when you graduate.

Go to it and enjoy the feeling of satisfaction and success that only comes when you know you're doing your best!

Contents

1 Terminology, Positioning, and Imaging Principles

CHAPTER OBJECTIVES

After you have successfully completed the activities in this chapter, you will be able to:

A. General, Systemic, and Skeletal Anatomy and Arthrology

_____ 1. List the four basic types of tissues.

_____ 2. List the 10 systems of the body.

_____ 3. Match specific bodily functions to their correct anatomic system.

_____ 4. List the four general classifications of bone.

_____ 5. Identify specific characteristics and aspects of bone.

_____ 6. Classify specific joints by their structure and function.

_____ 7. Classify specific synovial joints by their movement.

B. Positioning Terminology

_____ 1. Define general radiographic and anatomic relational terminology.

_____ 2. Define the imaginary planes, sections, and surfaces of the body used to describe central ray angles or relationships among body parts.

_____ 3. Distinguish among a radiographic projection, position, and view.

_____ 4. Given various hypothetic situations, identify the correct radiographic projection.

_____ 5. Given various hypothetic situations, identify the correct radiographic position.

_____ 6. List the antonyms (terms with opposite meanings) of specific terms related to movement.

C. Positioning Principles

_____ 1. Given a hypothetic clinical situation, identify the response as required in the professional code of ethics.

_____ 2. Identify the correct sequence of steps taken to perform a routine radiographic procedure.

_____ 3. Given a set of circumstances, apply the three general rules of radiography concerning the minimal number of projections required for specific regions of the body.

_____ 4. Identify the correct way to view a conventional radiograph, computed tomography (CT) image, and magnetic resonance (MR) image.

D. Image Quality in Analog (Film-Screen) Imaging

_____ 1. Describe the major exposure factors that influence the diagnostic quality of the radiograph.

_____ 2. List the four image quality factors and their impact on a radiograph.

_____ 3. Define *radiographic density* and identify its controlling factors.

_____ 4. Given a hypothetic situation, select the correct factor to improve radiographic density.

_____ 5. Describe the correlation between radiographic density and the *anode heel effect*.

_____ 6. List three types of filters and which radiographic procedures are enhanced by their use.

_____ 7. Define *radiographic contrast* and identify its controlling factors.

_____ 8. Distinguish between long- and short-scale radiographic contrast.

_____ 9. Given a hypothetic situation, select the correct factor to improve radiographic contrast.

_____ 10. Given situations, identify the type of grid cutoff errors present and their effect on image quality.

_____ 11. Define *resolution* and identify its controlling factors.

_____ 12. List the three geometric factors that influence image sharpness.

_____ 13. Identify the best ways of controlling voluntary and involuntary motion.

_____ 14. Given a hypothetic situation, select the correct factor to improve radiographic detail.

_____ 15. Define *radiographic distortion* and identify its controlling factors.

_____ 16. Given a hypothetical situation, select the correct factor to minimize radiographic distortion.

E. Image Quality in Digital Radiography

_____ 1. List the six image quality factors specific to digital imaging.

_____ 2. Define *brightness* and identify its controlling factors in the digital image.

_____ 3. Define *contrast* and identify its controlling factors in the digital image.

_____ 4. List the two types of pixel sizes.

_____ 5. Define *spatial resolution* and identify its controlling factors in the digital image.

_____ 6. Define *distortion* and identify its controlling factors in the digital image.

_____ 7. Define *exposure indicator* and describe its relationship to the amount of radiation striking the image receptor (IR).

_____ 8. Explain the concept of the signal-to-noise ratio (SNR).

_____ 9. Define specific terms related to the post-processing of the digital image.

F. Applications of Digital Technology

_____ 1. List the major components of a storage phosphor-based digital systems (PSP) system.

_____ 2. Describe briefly how an image is recorded, processed, and viewed with a PSP system.

_____ 3. Explain the importance of correct centering, collimation, use of lead masking, and use of grids to the overall quality of the digital image.

_____ 4. Identify specific differences and similarities between PSP and digital radiography (FPD-TFT).

_____ 5. Define the terms PACS, RIS, HIS, HL7, and DICOM.

_____ 6. Compare and contrast different size image receptors between metric and English units of measurement.

_____ 7. Define specific imaging terms and acronyms.

G. Radiation Protection

_____ 1. List and define the traditional units and International System of Units (SI units) of radiation measurement and the conversion factors used to convert between systems.

_____ 2. List the specific annual dose-limiting recommendations of whole-body effective dose for the general population and occupationally exposed workers.

_____ 3. Define ALARA.

_____ 4. Apply the principles of ALARA to a given hypothetic situation.

_____ 5. Define and provide examples of effective dose (ED).

_____ 6. Identify specific methods to reduce exposure to the technologist during fluoroscopic and radiographic procedures.

_____ 7. Describe methods to reduce exposure to the patient during radiographic procedures.

_____ 8. Identify the major types of specific area shields and how they should be applied during radiographic procedures.

_____ 9. Define the 10-day rule and describe its limitations.

_____ 10. Define patient dose terminology for specific regions of the body.

_____ 11. Identify methods to ensure a dose to the patient is minimized when using digital imaging systems.

_____ 12. Explain the Image Wisely initiative and its purpose.

LEARNING EXERCISES

The following review exercises should be completed only after careful study of the associated pages in the textbook as indicated by each exercise. Because certain topics may be too advanced for the entry-level student, the review exercises for Chapter 1 are divided into sections A through C. You can complete specific sections of review exercises, as directed by your instructor, to best meet your learning needs.

After completing each of these individual exercises, check your answers with the answers provided at the end of the review exercises.

REVIEW EXERCISE A: General, Systemic, and Skeletal Anatomy and Arthrology (see textbook pp. 4-14)

1. The lowest level of the structural organization of the human body is the _____.

2. List the four basic types of tissues in the body.

   A. _____   C. _____

   B. _____   D. _____

3. List the 10 systems of the human body.

   A. _____   F. _____

   B. _____   G. _____

   C. _____   H. _____

   D. _____   I. _____

   E. _____   J. _____

4. Match the following functions to the correct body system.

   _____ 1. Eliminates solid waste from the body   A. Skeletal system

   _____ 2. Regulates fluid and electrolyte balance and volume   B. Circulatory system

   _____ 3. Maintains posture   C. Digestive system

   _____ 4. Regulates body activities with electrical impulses   D. Respiratory system

   _____ 5. Regulates bodily activities through various hormones   E. Urinary system

   _____ 6. Eliminates carbon dioxide from blood   F. Reproductive system

   _____ 7. Receives stimuli, such as temperature, pressure, and pain   G. Nervous system

   _____ 8. Reproduces the organism   H. Muscular system

   _____ 9. Helps regulate body temperature   I. Endocrine system

   _____ 10. Supports and protects many soft tissues of the body   J. Integumentary system

5. True/False: One of the six functions of the circulatory system is to protect against disease.

6. Which of the following body systems regulate body temperature?

   A. Endocrine

   B. Integumentary

   C. Digestive

   D. Circulatory

7. What is the largest organ system in the body?

   A. Digestive

   B. Nervous

   C. Integumentary

   D. Respiratory

8. List the two divisions of the human skeletal system.

   A. _____

   B. _____

9. True/False: The adult skeleton system contains 256 separate bones.

10. True/False: The scapula is part of the axial skeleton.

11. True/False: The skull is part of the axial skeleton.

12. True/False: The pelvis is part of the appendicular skeleton.

13. List the four classifications of bones.

   A. _____

   B. _____

   C. _____

   D. _____

14. The outer covering of a long bone, which is composed of a dense, fibrous membrane, is called what?

   A. Spongy or cancellous bone

   B. Compact bone

   C. Medullary aspect

   D. Periosteum

15. Which aspect of long bones is responsible for the production of red blood cells?

   A. Spongy or cancellous bone

   B. Compact bone

   C. Medullary aspect

   D. Periosteum

16. Which aspect of the long bone is essential for bone growth, repair, and nutrition?

   A. Medullary aspect

   B. Compact bone

   C. Periosteum

   D. Articular cartilage

17. Identify the primary and secondary growth centers for long bones.

   A. Primary growth center: _____

   B. Secondary growth center: _____

18. True/False: Epiphyseal fusion of the long bones is complete by the age of 16 years.

19. The _____ is the wider portion of a long bone in which bone growth in length occurs.

   A. Diaphysis

   B. Epiphysis

   C. Metaphysis

   D. Epiphyseal plate

20. List the three *functional* classifications of joints.

A. _____

B. _____

C. _____

21. List the three *structural* classifications of joints.

A. _____

B. _____

C. _____

22. Match the following joints to the correct structural classification.

_____ 1. First carpometacarpal of thumb   A. Fibrous joint

_____ 2. Roots around teeth   B. Cartilaginous joint

_____ 3. Proximal radioulnar joint   C. Synovial joint

_____ 4. Skull sutures

_____ 5. Epiphyses

_____ 6. Interphalangeal joints

_____ 7. Distal tibiofibular joint

_____ 8. Intervertebral disk space

_____ 9. Symphysis pubis

_____ 10. Hip joint

23. List the seven types of movement for synovial joints (give both of the preferred terms).

A. _____   E. _____

B. _____   F. _____

C. _____   G. _____

D. _____

24. Match the following synovial joints to the correct type of movement.

_____ 1. First carpometacarpal joint   A. Plane

_____ 2. Elbow joint   B. Ginglymus

_____ 3. Shoulder joint   C. Trochoidal

_____ 4. Intercarpal joint   D. Ellipsoidal

_____ 5. Wrist joint   E. Sellar

_____ 6. Temporomandibular joint   F. Spheroidal

_____ 7. First and second cervical vertebra joint   G. Bicondylar

_____ 8. Second interphalangeal joint

_____ 9. Distal radioulnar joint

_____ 10. Ankle joint

_____ 11. Knee joint

_____ 12. Third metacarpophalangeal joint

REVIEW EXERCISE B: Positioning Terminology (see textbook pp. 15-29)

1. A(n) _____ is an image of a patient's anatomic part(s) as produced by the actions of x-rays on an image receptor (radiograph).

2. The _____ is the aspect of an x-ray beam that has the least divergence (unless there is angulation).

3. An upright position with the arms abducted, palms forward, and head and feet directed straight ahead describes

    the _____ position.

4. The vertical plane that divides the body into equal right and left parts is the _____ plane.

5. The vertical plane that divides the body into equal anterior and posterior parts is the

    _____ plane.

6. A plane taken at right angles along any point of the longitudinal axis of the body is the

    _____ plane.

7. True/False: The *base plane of the skull* is a plane located between the infraorbital margin of the orbit and the superior margin of the external auditory meatus.

8. True/False: The *Frankfort horizontal plane* is also referred to as *the midcoronal plane*.

9. The direction or path of the central ray defines the following positioning term.

    A. Projection   C. Position

    B. View   D. Perspective

10. The positioning term that describes the general and specific body position is:

   A. Projection   C. Position
   B. View   D. Perspective

11. True/False: Oblique and lateral positions are described according to the side of the body closest to the image receptor.

12. True/False: Decubitus positions always use a horizontal x-ray beam.

13. What is the name of the position in which the body is turned 90° from a true anteroposterior (AP) or posteroanterior (PA) projection? _____

14. **Situation:** A patient is erect with the back to the image receptor. The left side of the body is turned 45° toward the image receptor. What is this position? _____

15. **Situation:** A patient is recumbent facing the image receptor. The right side of the body is turned 15° toward the image receptor. What is this position? _____

16. **Situation:** The patient is lying on his or her back. The x-ray beam is directed horizontally and enters the right side of the body and exits the left side of the body. An image receptor is placed against the left side of the patient.

   Which specific position has been used? _____

17. **Situation:** The patient is erect with the right side of the body against the image receptor. The x-ray beam enters the left side and exits the right side of the body. Which specific position has been performed?

   _____

18. **Situation:** A patient is lying on the left side on a cart. The x-ray beam is directed horizontally and enters the posterior surface and exits the anterior aspect of the body. The image receptor is against the anterior surface.

   Which specific position has been performed? _____

19. Match the following definitions to the correct term (using each term only once).

   _____ 1. Palm of the hand   A. Posterior

   _____ 2. Lying on the back facing upward   B. Anterior

   _____ 3. An upright position   C. Plantar

   _____ 4. Lying down in any position   D. Dorsum pedis

   _____ 5. Front half of the patient   E. Trendelenburg

   _____ 6. Top or anterior surface of the foot   F. Erect

   _____ 7. Position in which head is higher than the feet   G. Supine

   _____ 8. Posterior aspect of foot   H. Palmar

   _____ 9. Position in which head is lower than feet I. Recumbent

   _____ 10. Back half of the patient   J. Fowler's

20. What is the name of the projection in which the central ray enters the anterior surface and exits the posterior surface? _____

21. A projection using a CR angle of 10° or more directed parallel along the long axis of the body or body part is termed a/an _____ projection.

22. The specific position that demonstrates the apices of the lungs, without superimposition of the clavicles, is termed a/an _____ position.

23. True/False: Radiographic "view" is not a correct positioning term in the United States.

24. True/False: The term *varus* describes the bending of a part outward.

25. Match the following. (Indicate whether the following terms describe a **position** or **projection**.)

_____ 1. Anteroposterior	A. Position
_____ 2. Prone	B. Projection
_____ 3. Trendelenburg	
_____ 4. Left posterior oblique	
_____ 5. Left lateral chest	
_____ 6. Mediolateral ankle	
_____ 7. Tangential	
_____ 8. Lordotic	
_____ 9. Inferosuperior axial	
_____ 10. Left lateral decubitus	

26. For each of the following terms, list the word that has the **opposite** meaning.

A. Flexion: _____

B. Ulnar deviation: _____

C. Dorsiflexion: _____

D. Eversion: _____

E. Lateral (external) rotation: _____

F. Abduction: _____

G. Supination: _____

H. Retraction: _____

I. Depression: _____

27. Match the following relationship terms to the correct definition (using each term only once):

_____ 1. Near the source or beginning   A. Caudad or inferior

_____ 2. On the opposite side   B. Deep

_____ 3. Toward the center   C. Distal

_____ 4. Toward the head end of the body   D. Contralateral

_____ 5. Away from the source or beginning   E. Cephalad or superior

_____ 6. Outside or outward   F. Proximal

_____ 7. On the same side   G. Medial

_____ 8. Near the skin surface   H. Superficial

_____ 9. Away from the head end   I. Ipsilateral

_____ 10. Farther from the skin surface   J. Exterior

28. Moving or thrusting the jaw forward from the normal position is an example of

_____.

29. To turn or bend the wrist toward the radius side is called _____.

30. Which two types of information should be imprinted on **every** radiographic image?

A. _____

B. _____

REVIEW EXERCISE C: Positioning Principles (see textbook pp. 30-35)

1. True/False: A technologist has the right to refuse to perform an examination on a patient whom he or she finds offensive.

2. True/False: A technologist is responsible for the professional decisions he or she makes during care of a patient.

3. True/False: The technologist is responsible for communicating with the patient to obtain pertinent clinical information.

4. True/False: The technologist is expected to provide a preliminary interpretation of radiographic findings to the referring physician.

5. True/False: The technologist must reveal confidential information pertaining to a patient who is less than 18 years of age to the patient or guardian.

6. List the two rules or principles for determining positioning routines as they relate to the maximum number of projections required in a basic routine.

A. _____   B. _____

7. Indicate the minimum number of projections (1, 2, or 3) required for each of the following anatomic regions.

   A. Foot _____

   B. Chest _____

   C. Wrist _____

   D. Tibia/fibula _____

   E. Humerus _____

   F. Fifth toe _____

   G. Postreduction of wrist (image of wrist in cast) _____

   H. Left hip _____

   I. Knee _____

   J. Pelvis (non–hip injury) _____

8. **Situation:** A young child enters the emergency room with a fractured forearm. After one projection is completed that confirms a fracture, the child refuses to move the forearm for any additional projections.

   A. What is the minimum number of projections that should be taken for this forearm study?

      (a) One

      (b) Four

      (c) Three

      (d) Two

   B. If additional projections are required for a routine forearm series, what should the technologist do with the young patient described in this situation?

      (a) Because only one projection is required for a fractured forearm, the technologist is not required to take additional projections.

      (b) With the help of a parent or guardian, gently but firmly move the forearm for each additional projection required.

      (c) Rather than move the forearm for a second projection, place the image receptor (IR) and x-ray tube as needed for a second projection 90° from the first projection.

      (d) Ask the emergency room physician to move the forearm for a second projection. This eliminates any liability for the technologist in case the patient is injured further.

9. The physical localization of topographic landmarks on a patient is called _____.

10. Which two landmarks may not be palpated because of institutional policy?

    A. _____

    B. _____

11. True/False: Always place a radiograph for viewing as the image receptor "sees" the patient. (The patient's left is to the viewer's left on AP projections.)

12. True/False: Most CT and MRI images are viewed so that the patient's right is to the viewer's left.

REVIEW EXERCISE D: Image Quality in Analog (Film-Screen) Imaging (see textbook pp. 36-46)

1. The radiographic analog (film) image is composed of metallic _____ on a polyester base.

2. List the four image quality factors of a radiograph.

   A. _____

   B. _____

   C. _____

   D. _____

3. "The range of exposure over which a film produces an acceptable image" is the definition for:

   A. Density   C. Exposure latitude

   B. Contrast   D. Brightness

4. Which specific exposure factor controls the quality or penetrating ability of the x-ray beam?

   _____

5. Exposure time is usually expressed in units of _____.

6. The amount of blackness seen on a processed radiograph is called _____.

7. The primary controlling factor for the overall blackness on a radiograph is _____.

8. If the distance between the x-ray tube and image receptor is increased from 40 to 80 inches, what specific effect will it have on the radiographic density, if other factors are not changed?

   A. Increase density to 50%   C. No effect on density

   B. Decrease density to 25%   D. Decrease density to 50%

9. Which term is used to describe a radiograph that has too little density? _____

10. Doubling the mAs will result in _____ the density on the IR image.

11. True/False: kV must be altered to change radiographic density on the IR image.

12. When analog images, using manual technique settings, are underexposed or overexposed, a minimum change in

    mAs of _____ is required to make a visible difference in the radiographic density.

    A. 1% to 3%   C. 25% to 30%

    B. 10% to 15%   D. 50% to 100%

13. According to the anode heel effect, the x-ray beam is less intense at the _____ (cathode or anode) end of the x-ray tube.

14. To best use the anode heel effect, the thicker part of the anatomic structure should be placed under the

    _____ (cathode or anode) end of the x-ray tube.

15. What device or method (other than the anode heel effect) may be used to compensate for the anatomic part

    thickness difference and produce an acceptable density on the IR image? _____

16. List three common types of compensating filters.

    A. _____

    B. _____

    C. _____

17. Which type of compensating filter is used commonly for AP projections of the thoracic spine?

    _____ filter

18. Which type of compensating filter permits soft tissue and bony detail of the shoulder to be equally visualized?

    _____ filter

19. **Situation:** A radiograph of the foot is produced using conventional analog cassettes. The resulting radiograph demonstrates too little density and must be repeated. The original exposure was 5 mAs. What mAs is needed to correct the density on this radiograph? (Hint: Density needs to be doubled.)

    A. 5 mAs   C. 30 mAs

    B. 17.5 mAs   D. 10 mAs

20. The difference in density on adjacent areas of the radiograph defines _____.

21. What is the primary controlling factor for radiographic contrast? _____

22. List the two scales of radiographic contrast, and identify which is classified as high contrast and which is low contrast.

    A. _____   B. _____

23. Which scale of contrast is produced with a 110-kV technique? _____

24. True/False: A 50-kV technique produces a high-contrast image.

25. True/False: A low-contrast image demonstrates more shades of gray on the radiograph.

26. Which one of the following sets of exposure factors will result in the least patient exposure and produce long-scale contrast on a PA chest radiographic image?

    A. 50 kV, 800 mAs   C. 80 kV, 100 mAs

    B. 70 kV, 200 mAs   D. 110 kV, 10 mAs

27. **Situation:** A radiograph of the hand is underexposed and must be repeated. The original technique used was 55 kV with 2.5 mAs. The technologist decides to keep the mAs at the same level but change the kV to increase radiographic density. How much of an increase is needed in kilovoltage (kV) to double the density?

    A. 3- to 5-kV increase   C. 10- to 15-kV increase

    B. 8- to 10-kV increase   D. 15- to 20-kV increase

28. If an anatomic part measures greater than _____ cm, a grid must be used.

29. Identify the type of grid cutoff that is created by the following situations:

    A. The central ray (CR) and face of grid are not perpendicular.

        1. Off-center grid cutoff

        2. Off-level grid cutoff

        3. Off-focus grid cutoff

        4. Upside down grid cutoff

    B. The SID is set beyond the focal range of the grid.

        1. Off-center grid cutoff

        2. Off-level grid cutoff

        3. Off-focus grid cutoff

        4. Upside down grid cutoff

C. The back of the grid is facing the x-ray tube.

    1. Off-center grid cutoff

    2. Off-level grid cutoff

    3. Off-focus grid cutoff

    4. Upside down grid cutoff

30. The recorded sharpness of structures or objects on the radiograph defines _____.

31. The lack of visible sharpness is called _____.

32. List the three geometric factors that control or influence image resolution.

    A. _____

    B. _____

    C. _____

33. The term that describes the unsharp edges of the projected image is _____.

34. True/False: The use of a small focal spot will entirely eliminate the problem identified in the previous question.

35. The greatest contributor to image unsharpness as related to positioning is _____.

36. What is the best mechanism to control involuntary motion during an exposure?

    A. Use of a small focal spot

    B. Use of a grid

    C. Decrease object image receptor distance (OID)

    D. Shorten exposure time

37. Which one of the following changes will improve image resolution?

    A. Decrease OID

    B. Decrease source image receptor distance (SID)

    C. Use a large focal spot

    D. Use a higher kilovoltage

38. **Situation:** The technologist is performing an elbow series on a pediatric patient. Because of the nature of the injury, the technologist has been asked to produce radiographs that have the highest degree of recorded resolution possible. Which one of the following sets of factors will produce that level of detail?

    A. 0.3-mm focal spot and 30-inch SID

    B. 1.0-mm focal spot and 45-inch SID

    C. 0.5-mm focal spot and 40-inch SID

    D. 0.3-mm focal spot and 40-inch SID

39. The misrepresentation of an object size or shape projected onto a radiographic recording medium is called

_____.

40. True/False: Through careful selection and control of exposure and geometric factors, it is possible to eliminate all image distortion.

41. List the four primary controlling factors for distortion.

    A. _____   C. _____

    B. _____   D. _____

42. True/False: A decrease in SID reduces distortion.

43. True/False: An increase in OID reduces distortion.

44. True/False: Distortion is reduced when the central ray (CR) is kept perpendicular to the plane of the image receptor.

45. The SID for general radiographic procedures resulting in maximum recorded resolution is:

    A. 40 inches (102 cm)
    C. 44 inches (112 cm)
    B. 72 inches (183 cm)
    D. 48 inches (123 cm)

46. **Situation:** A chest x-ray on a patient with an enlarged heart has been requested. Which SID is recommended for this study?

    A. 40 inches (102 cm)
    C. 44 inches (112 cm)
    B. 72 inches (183 cm)
    D. 48 inches (123 cm)

47. True/False: Every radiographic image reflects some degree of penumbra or unsharpness, even if the smallest focal spot is used.

48. True/False: As the distance between the object and the image receptor is increased, magnification is reduced.

49. True/False: Image distortion increases as the angle of divergence increases from the center of the x-ray beam to the outer edges.

50. True/False: The greater the angle of inclination of the object or the IR, the greater the amount of distortion.

REVIEW EXERCISE E: Image Quality in Digital Radiography (see textbook pp. 47-51)

1. True/False: Digital imaging requires that images be chemically processed.

2. True/False: Digital images are a numeric representation of the x-ray intensities that are transmitted through the patient.

3. True/False: Digital imaging systems have a narrow dynamic range.

4. Digital processing involves the systematic application of highly complex mathematical formulas called:

    A. Matrices
    C. Analog-to-digital converters
    B. PACS
    D. Algorithms

5. The range or level of image contrast in the digital image is primarily controlled by:

    A. kV
    C. Digital processing
    B. mAs
    D. Matrix size

6. Exposure latitude with digital imaging is more _____ (narrow or wide) when compared with analog imaging.

7. List the six image quality factors to evaluate digital image.

    A. _____
    D. _____

    B. _____
    E. _____

    C. _____
    F. _____

8. In digital imaging, the term _____ replaces *density* as applied in analog (film)-based imaging.

   A. Brightness   C. Latitude

   B. Signal   D. Noise

9. True/False: Changes in mAs do not have a primary controlling effect on digital image brightness.

10. True/False: Brightness cannot be altered in the digital image once it has been processed.

11. A digital imaging system's ability to distinguish between similar tissues is termed:

    A. Brightness   C. Signal

    B. Image resolution   D. Contrast resolution

12. Radiographic contrast in the digital image is primarily affected by:

    A. kV   C. Application of processing algorithms

    B. Signal-to-noise ratio   D. Matrix size

13. The greater the bit depth of a digital imaging system, the greater the:

    A. Size of the matrix   C. Brightness

    B. Contrast resolution   D. Pixel size

14. List the terms describing the two pixel sizes used in digital imaging.

    A. _____

    B. _____

15. Which one of the two pixel sizes listed above is most critical in maintaining high-resolution digital images?

    _____

16. True/False: Focal spot size has no impact on the resolution of the digital image.

17. The current range of spatial resolution for digital radiographic imaging systems is between:

    A. 1.0 to 2.0 lp/mm   C. 0.5 to 1.0 lp/mm

    B. 10 to 50 lp/mm   D. 2.5 lp/mm to 5.0 lp/mm

18. In addition to acquisition pixel size, spatial resolution in the digital image is controlled by

    A. kV   C. SID

    B. Display matrix   D. Use of a grid

19. True/False: The factors that affect image distortion for the digital image are different from those that affect film-screen systems.

20. A numeric value that is representative of the exposure the digital image receptor receives is termed the

    _____.

21. List the four factors that affect the exposure indicator in the digital image.

    A. _____   C. _____

    B. _____   D. _____

22. If the recommended exposure indicator range for a well-exposed image is between 150 and 250, a value of

    350 would indicate _____ (overexposure or underexposure) of the image.

23. If the recommended exposure indicator range is between 2.0 and 2.4, then a value of 1.2 indicates

    _____ (overexposure or underexposure) of the image.

24. Verifying the exposure indicator for each exposure is essential in producing quality digital images with the

    _____.

25. A random disturbance that obscures or reduces clarity is the definition for _____.

26. SNR is the acronym for the _____.

27. When insufficient mAs is applied in the production of a digital image, it produces a

    _____ (high- or low-) SNR image.

28. Another term for image noise is:

    A. Variance   C. Mottle

    B. Static   D. Digital spam

29. Changing or enhancing the electronic image to improve its diagnostic quality is called

    _____.

30. Identify the type of post-processing described by listing the correct term for the following definitions.

    A. Adding text to images: _____

    B. Increasing brightness along the margins of structures to increase the visibility of the edges:

       _____

    C. Reversing the dark and light pixel values of an image: _____

    D. Enlarging all or part of an image: _____

    E. The application of specific image processing to reduce the display of noise in an image: _____

    F. Removing background anatomy to allow visualization of contrast media–filled structures: _____

REVIEW EXERCISE F: Applications of Digital Technology (see textbook pp. 52-57)

1. List the three components of a photostimulable storage phosphor plate (PSP-CR) system.

   A. _____

   B. _____

   C. _____

2. True/False: A PSP-based digital imaging system may be cassette based or cassette-less.

3. The term describing the image being transmitted to a digital archive for viewing and reading by the referring physician or radiologist is:

   A. Image archiving

   B. Image storage

   C. Image retrieval

   D. Image processing

4. When using a PSP image plate, patient data can be linked to the image by use of a(n):

   A. Bar code reader

   B. White light source

   C. Laser

   D. Ultraviolet light source

5. True/False: Once the PSP image plate has had an image recorded on it, it must be discarded.

6. True/False: The latent image on a PSP image plate is read by a laser within the CR reader.

7. True/False: The greater the exposure to the plate, the greater the intensity of the light emitted from the plate during the reading process.

8. Any residual latent image is erased on the PSP image plate by applying:

   A. Bright light

   B. Heat

   C. Low-level radiation

   D. Microwaves

9. The process of transferring the digital image to a storage device is termed _____.

10. Which one of the following technical factors does *not* apply to digital imaging (PSP radiography)?

   A. Close collimation

   B. Accurate centering of part and IR

   C. Use of lead masks

   D. A minimum of 72 inches (183 cm) is required for all projections.

11. True/False: Fifty percent of the IP must be exposed to produce a correct reading of the image.

12. True/False: The use of grids is optional with PSP because the IP is not as sensitive to scatter radiation as analog radiography.

13. Which of the following imaging components is *not* required with direct digital radiography (FPD-TFT)?

   A. IP

   B. Image reader

   C. Grid

   D. Both A and B

14. True/False: Patient dose may be lower with FPD-TFT as compared with analog radiography.

15. True/False: When using FPD-TFT for most nongrid procedures, one reason the grid is generally not removed is its fragile construction.

16. True/False: FPD-TFT and PSP-based systems does *not* provide the ability to view a previous image to evaluate for positioning errors and confirm the exposure indicator.

17. In addition to FPD-TFT and PSP-based systems, a third type of system is used to acquire radiographic images digitally which is:

   A. Electron capture systems

   B. PSB systems

   C. CCD-based systems

   D. Lens systems

18. Match the following metric measurements for image receptor sizes to the nearest equivalent traditional size.

   Metric   **Traditional (English)**

   _____ 1. 24 × 30 cm   A. 14 × 17 inches

   _____ 2. 18 × 24 cm   B. 7 × 17 inches

   _____ 3. 35 × 43 cm   C. 11 × 14 inches

   _____ 4. 30 × 35 cm   D. 10 × 12 inches

   _____ 5. 24 × 24 cm   E. 8 × 10 inches

   _____ 6. 18 × 43 cm   F. 9 × 9 inches

19. True/False: The size of the image receptor used is dependent primarily on the size of the body part being examined.

20. Define the acronym PACS.

   P: _____

   A: _____

   C: _____

   S: _____

21. True/False: A PACS automatically transports film-based images to the chemical processor after they have been exposed.

22. What do the following acronyms represent? (Write the complete term.)

   A. DICOM: _____

   B. RIS: _____

   C. HIS: _____

   D. HL7: _____

23. The electronic transmission of diagnostic imaging studies is termed _____.

24. The _____ receptor is made with amorphous selenium or amorphous silicon.

25. Provide the correct term for the following definitions.

_____ A. Series of "boxes" that gives form to the image

_____ B. Range of exposure intensities that produce an acceptable image

_____ C. The user adjusting the window level and window width

_____ D. Unsharp edges of the projected image

_____ E. Numeric value that is representative of the exposure the image receptor received in digital radiography

_____ F. Representative of the number of shades of gray that can be demonstrated by each pixel

_____ G. Misrepresentation of object size or shape as projected onto radiographic recording media

_____ H. Controls the energy (penetrating power) of the x-ray beam

_____ I. Random disturbance that obscures or reduces clarity

_____ J. The recorded sharpness of structures on the image

_____ K. Changing or enhancing the electronic image to view it from a different perspective or improve its diagnostic quality

26. List the complete term for the following acronyms.

A. RIS: _____

B. IR: _____

C. OID: _____

D. DR: _____

E. AEC: _____

F. HIS: _____

27. Match the following terms to the correct definition.

_____ A. Windowing   1. Term used by certain equipment manufacturers to imply exposure indicator

_____ B. Bit-depth   2. Range of exposure intensities that will produce an acceptable image

_____ C. Noise   3. Random disturbance that obscures or reduces clarity

_____ D. Exposure latitude 4. The point of least distortion of the projected image

_____ E. Exposure level   5. The user adjusting the window level and window width

_____ F. Central ray   6. Series of "boxes" that give form to the image

_____ G. Display matrix   7. Representative of the number of shades of gray that can be demonstrated by each pixel.

1. Which radiation unit is used to measure amount of ionizations created in air? (More than one answer is possible.)

   _____

2. Which unit of measurement is used to describe patient dose? _____

3. _____ dose allows comparisons of the relative risk from various imaging procedures.

4. What is the whole-body effective dose limit per year for a technologist? _____

5. What is the cumulative dose limit for a 35-year-old technologist? _____

6. For each of the following traditional units, list the equivalent SI unit of radiation measurement and its symbol.

   Traditional Unit   **SI Unit**

   A. Roentgen (R)   _____

   B. Radiation absorbed dose (rad)   _____

   C. Radiation equivalent man (rem)   _____

7. Convert the following doses, stated in traditional units, into the equivalent SI unit.

   A. 3 rad = _____ Gy   C. 38 rem = _____ Sv

   B. 448 mrad = _____ mGy   D. 15 rem = _____ mSv

8. What is the maximum dose limit for a pregnant technologist?

   A. Per month: _____

   B. For the entire gestational period: _____

9. The ED limit for minors under the age of 18 years is _____ per year.

10. Personnel monitoring devices must be worn if there is a possibility of acquiring

    _____% of the annual occupational effective dose limit.

    A. 1%   C. 15%

    B. 10%   D. 20%

11. Define the following dosimetry terms.

    A. TLD: _____

    B. OSL: _____

12. The acronym ALARA stands for _____.

13. **Situation:** A young child comes to the radiology department for a skull series. The child is combative and will not hold still for the procedure. Which one of the following individuals should be asked to restrain the patient (if mechanical restraints are not available)?

    A. A family member (if not pregnant)   C. The oldest technologist

    B. A student technologist   D. A nuclear medicine technologist

14. True/False: With accurate and close collimation, area shields do *not* need to be used.

15. True/False: Fluoroscopy procedures do not result in high exposures to the fetus of the pregnant technologist.

16. True/False: Exit dose is often a small percentage of the entrance dose.

17. True/False: ED describes gonadal dose levels only for each radiographic procedure.

18. What is one of the primary causes for repeat radiographs? (Select the *best* answer.)

    A. Excessive kilovoltage   C. Poor communication between technologist and patient

    B. Wrong IR selection   D. Distortion caused by incorrect SID

19. In addition to the primary causes identified in the previous question, what two other factors often lead to repeat exposures?

    A. _____   B. _____

20. List the two major forms of filtration found in x-ray tubes that affect the quality of the primary x-ray beam.

    A. _____

    B. _____

21. What are the most common metals used in filters for diagnostic radiology equipment?

    _____

22. List the two ways collimation will reduce patient exposure.

    A. _____

    B. _____

23. True/False: Safety standards require that collimators be accurate to within 10% of the selected SID.

24. True/False: Positive beam limitation (PBL) collimators restrict the size of the exposure field to the size of the cassette in a Bucky tray.

25. True/False: PBL collimators became optional on new equipment manufactured after May 1993 because of a change in Food and Drug Administration (FDA) regulations.

26. List the two general types of specific area shields.

    A. _____

    B. _____

27. The minimum thickness of a gonadal shield placed within the primary x-ray field should be:

    A. 0.1-mm lead equivalent   C. 1-mm lead equivalent

    B. 0.25-mm lead equivalent   D. 0.5-mm lead equivalent

28. If placed properly, gonadal shields absorb _____ of the primary beam in the 50- to 100-kV range.

    A. 95% to 99%   C. 70% to 80%

    B. 80% to 90%   D. 50% to 70%

29. An area shield should be used when radiation-sensitive tissues lie within _____

    inches (or _____ cm) of the primary beam.

30. Which type of area shield would be best suited for use during a sterile procedure?

    _____

31. True/False: The 10-day rule is considered by the International Commission on Radiological Protection (ICRP) and the American College of Radiology (ACR) to be obsolete.

32. **Situation:** A 20-year-old female enters the emergency room with a possible fracture of the pelvis and coccyx (tail bone). What should the technologist do in regard to gonadal shielding?

    A. Use it for all projections.   C. Ask the patient whether she is pregnant.

    B. Use it for the AP projections only.   D. Do not use shielding for initial pelvis projection.

33. What is the chief disadvantage of using faster-speed screens for all analog radiographic procedures?

    _____

34. True/False: Area shields must be used for all radiographic procedures with all patients.

35. What is the minimum lead equivalency recommended for a protective apron worn during fluoroscopy?

    _____

36. List the three cardinal principles for radiation protection.

    A. _____

    B. _____

    C. _____

37. True/False: kV ranges are typically 5 to 10 kV higher for digital systems as compared with analog kV ranges.

38. True/False: If the exposure indicator value is outside of the suggested range for that procedure, the projection(s) must be repeated.

39. What is the best method of reducing scatter to a worker's eyes and neck during fluoroscopy?

    _____

40. Which of the following is the best place for a technologist to stand during fluoroscopy to reduce occupational exposure?

    A. Head end of table   C. Behind the radiologist

    B. Foot end of table   D. Next to the radiologist

41. What is the federal set limit for exposure rates for intensified fluoroscopy units?

    A. 1 R/minute   C. 3 to 4 R/minutes

    B. 6 to 8 R/minutes   D. 10 R/minutes

42. In high-level fluoroscopy (HLF) mode, the exposure rate measured at tabletop *cannot* exceed

    _____.

43. With most modern fluoroscopy equipment, the average exposure rate is:

    A. 0.5 R/minute   C. 1 to 3 R/minutes

    B. 5 to 7 R/minutes   D. 10 R/minutes

44. Which of the following projections provides the greatest amount of dose to the ovaries? (Review the patient dose chart in the text.)

    A. PA chest   C. AP abdomen

    B. Lateral skull   D. AP thoracic spine

45. Which of the following projections provides the greatest amount of bone marrow dose? (review patient dose chart in text)

    A. AP lumbar spine   C. Retrograde pyelogram

    B. PA chest   D. Lateral skull

46. What are the two types of fluoroscopy readouts required by the FDA to monitor radiation output?

    A. _____

    B. _____

47. The minimum radiation dose that will produce temporary skin injury (epilation) is:

    A. 1 Gy (100 rad)   C. 5 Gy (500 rad)

    B. 3 Gy (300 rad)   D. 6 Gy (600 rad)

48. True/False: Pulsed fluoroscopy, when frames per minute are minimized, can produce a substantial dose reduction.

49. True/False: Radiation-attenuating surgical gloves offer minimal protection of the interventionist's hands, provide a false sense of protection, and therefore are not recommended.

50. True/False. The Image Wisely initiative is intended to minimize the radiation exposure to children.

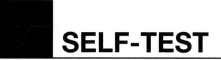 **SELF-TEST**

This series of self-tests should be taken only after completing all of the readings, review exercises, and laboratory activities for a particular section. This self-test is divided into seven sections. The purpose of this test is not only to provide a good learning exercise but also to serve as a strong indicator of what your final evaluation exam will cover. It is strongly suggested that if you do not get at least a 90% to 95% grade on each self-test, you should review those areas in which you missed questions before going to your instructor for the final evaluation exam.

SELF-TEST A: General, Systemic, and Skeletal Anatomy and Arthrology

1. Which of the following is (are) *not* one of the four basic types of tissue in the human body? (More than one answer is possible.)

   A. Integumentary   D. Osseous

   B. Connective   E. Muscular

   C. Nervous   F. Epithelial

2. How many separate bones are found in the adult human body?

   A. 180   C. 206

   B. 243   D. 257

3. Which one of the following systems distributes oxygen and nutrients to the cells of the body?

   A. Digestive   C. Skeletal

   B. Circulatory   D. Urinary

4. Which one of the following systems maintains the acid-base balance in the body?

   A. Digestive   C. Reproductive

   B. Urinary   D. Circulatory

5. Which one of the following systems is considered to be the largest organ system in the human body?

   A. Muscular   C. Skeletal

   B. Endocrine   D. Integumentary

6. The two divisions of the human skeleton are:

   A. Bony and cartilaginous   C. Vertebral and extremities

   B. Axial and appendicular   D. Integumentary and appendicular

7. Which portion of the long bones is responsible for the production of red blood cells?

   A. Spongy or cancellous   C. Hyaline

   B. Periosteum   D. Compact aspect

8. What type of tissue covers the ends of the long bones?

   A. Spongy or cancellous
   B. Periosteum
   C. Hyaline or articular cartilage
   D. Compact aspect

9. The narrow space between the inner and outer table of the flat bones in the cranium is called the:

   A. Calvarium
   B. Periosteum
   C. Medullary portion
   D. Diploe

10. What is the primary center for endochondral ossification in long bones?

    A. Diaphysis (shaft)
    B. Epiphyseal plate
    C. Epiphyses
    D. Medulla

11. What is the name of secondary growth centers of endochondral ossification found in long bones?

    A. Diaphysis (shaft)
    B. Epiphyseal plate
    C. Epiphyses
    D. Metaphysis

12. The aspect of long bones where bone growth in length occurs is termed:

    A. Diaphysis (shaft)
    B. Epiphyseal plate
    C. Epiphyses
    D. Metaphysis

13. A skull suture has the structural classification of a _____ joint.

    A. Fibrous
    B. Cartilaginous
    C. Synovial
    D. Diarthrosis

14. The symphysis pubis has the structural classification of a _____ joint.

    A. Fibrous
    B. Cartilaginous
    C. Synovial
    D. Synarthrosis

15. Which specific joint(s) is (are) the only true syndesmosis, amphiarthrodial, fibrous joint(s)?

    A. Joints between the roots of teeth and adjoining bone
    B. First carpometacarpal joint
    C. Distal tibiofibular joint
    D. Proximal and distal radioulnar joints

16. Match the following bones to their correct classification.

    _____ 1. Sternum   A. Long bone

    _____ 2. Femur   B. Short bone

    _____ 3. Tarsal bones   C. Flat bone

    _____ 4. Pelvic bones   D. Irregular bone

    _____ 5. Scapulae

    _____ 6. Humerus

    _____ 7. Vertebrae

    _____ 8. Calvarium

17. The three structural classifications of joints are synovial, cartilaginous, and:

   A. Amphiarthrodial   C. Diarthrodial

   B. Ellipsoidal   D. Fibrous

18. Classify the following synovial joints based on their type of movement.

   _____ 1. First carpometacarpal joint   A. Plane (gliding)

   _____ 2. Intercarpal joint   B. Ginglymus (hinge)

   _____ 3. Hip joint   C. Trochoidal (pivot)

   _____ 4. Proximal radioulnar joint   D. Ellipsoidal (condyloid)

   _____ 5. Interphalangeal joint   E. Sellar (saddle)

   _____ 6. Fourth metacarpophalangeal joint   F. Spheroidal (ball and socket)

   _____ 7. Knee joint   G. Bicondylar

   _____ 8. Wrist joint

   _____ 9. Joint between C1 and C2

   _____ 10. Ankle joint

SELF-TEST B: Positioning Terminology

1. Which plane divides the body into equal anterior and posterior parts?

   A. Midsagittal   B. Transverse   C. Midcoronal   D. Longitudinal

2. True/False: The terms *radiograph* and *image receptor* refer to the same thing.

3. A longitudinal plane that divides the body into right and left parts is the:

   A. Coronal plane   C. Sagittal plane

   B. Horizontal plane   D. Oblique plane

4. Match the following definitions to the correct term.

_____ 1. Near the source or beginning

_____ 2. Away from head end of the body

_____ 3. Inside of something

_____ 4. Increasing the angle of a joint

_____ 5. Outward stress of the foot

_____ 6. Movement of an extremity away from the midline

_____ 7. Turning palm downward

_____ 8. A backward movement

_____ 9. To move around in the form of a circle

_____ 10. Toward the center

_____ 11. Away from the source or beginning

_____ 12. On the opposite side of the body

A. Eversion

B. Circumduction

C. Pronation

D. Contralateral

E. Proximal

F. Medial

G. Interior

H. Retraction

I. Caudad

J. Extension

K. Abduction

L. Distal

5. Match the following definitions to the correct term.

_____ 1. Lying down in any position

_____ 2. Head lower than the feet position

_____ 3. Upright position, palms forward

_____ 4. Top of the foot

_____ 5. Frankfort horizontal plane

_____ 6. A plane at right angle to the longitudinal plane

_____ 7. Head higher than feet position

_____ 8. Palm of hand

_____ 9. Sole of foot

_____ 10. Front half of body

_____ 11. A plane that divides body into anterior and posterior halves

_____ 12. A recumbent position with knees and hips flexed with support for legs

A. Base plane of skull

B. Plantar

C. Palmar

D. Fowler's position

E. Lithotomy position

F. Anatomic position

G. Trendelenburg position

H. Horizontal plane

I. Midcoronal plane

J. Dorsum pedis

K. Anterior

L. Recumbent

6. The direction or path of the central ray of the x-ray beam defines the positioning term:

A. Position

B. View

C. Perspective

D. Projection

7. **Situation:** A patient is placed in a recumbent position facing downward. The left side of the body is turned 30° toward the image receptor. Which specific position has been performed?

   A. LAO

   B. Left lateral decubitus

   C. LPO

   D. RAO

8. **Situation:** A patient is placed into a recumbent position facing downward. The x-ray tube is directed horizontally and enters the left side and exits the right side of the body. An image receptor is placed against the right side of the patient. Which position has been performed?

   A. Dorsal decubitus

   B. Left lateral decubitus

   C. Ventral decubitus

   D. Right lateral decubitus

9. **Situation:** A patient is erect with her back to the image receptor. The central ray enters the anterior aspect and exits the posterior aspect of the body. Which projection has been performed?

   A. Posteroanterior

   B. Tangential

   C. Ventral decubitus

   D. Anteroposterior

10. **Situation:** A patient is lying down facing upward with the posterior surface of the body against the image receptor. The right side of the body is turned 45° toward the image receptor. The x-ray tube is directed vertically and enters the anterior surface of the body. Which position has been performed?

    A. LPO

    B. RAO

    C. RPO

    D. LAO

11. **Situation:** An elbow projection is taken with the posterior surface placed against the image receptor. The elbow is rotated 20° outwardly. Which specific projection has been performed?

    A. PA oblique with medial rotation

    B. PA oblique with lateral rotation

    C. AP oblique with medial rotation

    D. AP oblique with lateral rotation

12. **Situation:** A specific projection of the foot in which the central ray enters the anterior surface and exits the posterior surface is termed:

    A. Dorsoplantar

    B. Plantodorsal

    C. Axioplantar

    D. Posteroanterior

13. **Situation:** A patient is placed in a recumbent position with the body tilted so that the head is higher than the feet. The image receptor is under the patient and the x-ray tube is above the patient. Which is the general position of the patient?

    A. Trendelenburg

    B. Reid's

    C. Sims'

    D. Fowler's

14. **Situation:** The anterior surface of the right knee of the patient is facing the image receptor. The anterior aspect of the knee and lower leg is rotated 15° toward the midline. Which specific projection has been performed?

    A. AP oblique with medial rotation

    B. PA oblique with medial rotation

    C. PA oblique with lateral rotation

    D. AP oblique with lateral rotation

15. What is the name of the projection in which the central ray merely skims a body part?

    A. Tangential

    B. Decubitus

    C. Axial

    D. Trendelenburg

16. What is the name of the specific projection in which the central ray enters the left side of the chest and exits the opposite side?

   A. Parietoacanthial   C. Transthoracic

   B. Axial   D. Lordotic

17. What is the specific projection that enters the posterior aspect of the skull and exits the acanthion?

   A. Acanthioparietal   C. Axial

   B. Tangential   D. Parietoacanthial

18. Which one of the following is an example of an axial projection?

   A. Transthoracic lateral   C. AP chest with 20° cephalic angle

   B. Mediolateral ankle   D. AP abdomen with 30° rotation to left

19. Which one of the following positioning terms is no longer considered valid in the United States?

   A. Radiographic view   C. Radiographic projection

   B. Radiographic position   D. Semi-axial projection

20. Match each of the following positioning terms to the term that is its direct opposite.

   _____ 1. Proximal   A. Kyphosis

   _____ 2. Cephalad   B. Inferior

   _____ 3. Ipsilateral   C. External

   _____ 4. Medial   D. Distal

   _____ 5. Superficial   E. Plantodorsal

   _____ 6. Internal   F. Lateral

   _____ 7. Lordosis   G. PA

   _____ 8. AP   H. Caudad

   _____ 9. Superior   I. Contralateral

   _____ 10. Dorsoplantar   J. Deep

SELF-TEST C: Positioning Principles

1. True/False: If a patient is younger than 18 years of age, any confidential information obtained during the procedure must be shared with the parent or guardian.

2. True/False: The technologist must provide a preliminary interpretation of any radiographs if requested by the referring physician.

3. True/False: Personal patient information can be shared with another technologist even if he or she has no role in that patient's procedure.

4. True/False: The technologist can explain a radiographic procedure to the patient without permission from the referring physician or radiologist.

5. Indicate the minimum number of projections required for the following structures.

_____ 1. Knee   A. Two

_____ 2. Fourth finger   B. Three

_____ 3. Humerus

_____ 4. Sternum

_____ 5. Ankle

_____ 6. Tibia/fibula

_____ 7. Chest

_____ 8. Hand

_____ 9. Hip (proximal femur)

_____ 10. Forearm

6. Which of the following radiographic procedures requires only a single AP projection be taken?

A. Post-reduction forearm   C. Hand on a pediatric patient

B. Pelvis   D. Ribs

7. **Situation:** A patient enters the emergency room with a fractured forearm. The fracture is set, or reduced. The orthopedic physician orders a postreduction series. How many projections are required?

A. One   C. Two

B. Three   D. Four

8. **Situation:** A patient enters the emergency room with a dislocated elbow. The patient is in extreme pain. What is the minimum number of projections that must be performed?

A. One   C. Two

B. Three   D. Four

9. **Situation:** A patient comes to radiology for a rib study. What is the minimum number of projections that must be performed?

A. One   C. Two

B. Three   D. Four

10. **Situation:** A patient enters the emergency room with a possible fractured ankle. She can move it but is painful. What is the minimum number of projections that must be performed?

A. One   C. Two

B. Three   D. Four

11. **Situation:** A patient enters the emergency room with a small piece of wire embedded in the palm of the hand. What is the minimum number of projections required for this study?

A. One   C. Two

B. Three   D. Four

12. **Situation:** A patient has fallen on the ice and has a possible fractured hip (proximal femur). What is the minimum number of projections that should be taken for this patient?

A. One   C. Two

B. Three   D. Five

13. **Situation:** A patient enters the emergency room with a possible fractured little (fifth) toe. What is the minimum number of projections that must be taken?

A. One   C. Two

B. Three   D. Five

14. Which of the following positioning routines should be performed for a wrist study?

A. AP, PA, and lateral projections

B. AP and lateral projections

C. PA, oblique, and lateral projections

D. Oblique, axial, and lateral projections

15. Which of the following positioning routines should be performed for a chest study?

A. PA and lateral projections

B. PA, oblique, and lateral projections

C. AP, PA, and lateral projections

D. PA, RAO, and LAO projections

16. The technique for localizing bony and soft tissue of radiographic landmarks is termed:

A. Localization   C. Physical assessment

B. Tactile localization   D. Palpation

SELF-TEST D: Image Quality in Analog (Film-Screen) Imaging

1. Which one of the following is *not* one of the four primary image quality factors?

A. Density   D. Detail

B. Contrast   E. Distortion

C. Kilovoltage (kV)

2. The amount of blackness on a processed radiograph is called:

A. Density   C. Contrast

B. Milliampere seconds (mAs)   D. Penumbra

3. Which of the following exposure factors primarily controls radiographic density?

A. kV   C. Focal spot size

B. mAs   D. Source image receptor distance (SID)

4. True/False: For an underexposed radiograph, the mAs must be increased by a factor of four to produce a visible change in radiographic density.

5. **Situation:** A radiograph of the knee reveals that it is overexposed and must be repeated. The original technique used 10 mAs. Which one of the following changes will improve the image during the repeat exposure?

   A. Increase to 15 mAs

   B. Decrease to 5 mAs

   C. Increase to 20 mAs

   D. Decrease to 2 mAs

6. The primary controlling factor for radiographic contrast is:

   A. mAs

   B. kV

   C. Focal spot size

   D. SID

7. **Situation:** Chest radiography requires long-scale contrast. Which set of exposure factors will produce this?

   A. 50 kV, 20 mAs

   B. 65 kV, 15 mAs

   C. 110 kV, 2 mAs

   D. 80 kV, 5 mAs

8. Which one of the following sets of exposure factors will produce the highest (short-scale) radiographic contrast?

   A. 60 kV, 30 mAs

   B. 80 kV, 20 mAs

   C. 96 kV, 5 mAs

   D. 120 kV, 2 mAs

9. True/False: Kilovoltage is a secondary controlling factor for radiographic density.

10. True/False: A low-kilovoltage technique (50 kV) produces a long-scale contrast image.

11. **Situation:** A radiograph of the elbow reveals that it is overexposed. The technologist wants to adjust kV rather than mAs for the repeat exposure. This is contrary to common practice. The original analog exposure factors were 70 kV and 5 mAs. Which one of the following kV settings would reduce radiographic density by one-half?

    A. 80 kV and 5 mAs

    B. 66 kV and 5 mAs

    C. 60 kV and 5 mAs

    D. 56 kV and 5 mAs

12. Which one of the following techniques or devices will reduce the amount of scatter radiation striking the IR?

    A. Collimation

    B. Lower kV

    C. Grids

    D. All of the above

13. True/False: Recorded detail or spatial resolution is optimal with a long object image receptor distance (OID) and a short SID.

14. Which one of the following factors best controls involuntary cardiac motion artifact?

    A. Careful instructions given to the patient

    B. High kV technique

    C. Practicing with patient when to hold breath

    D. Shortening the exposure time

15. **Situation:** The technologist is asked to produce a high-quality image of the carpal (wrist) bones. The emergency room physician suspects that the patient has a very small fracture of one of the bones. Which one of following sets of technical factors will produce an image with the highest degree of radiographic resolution?

    A. 1.0-mm focal spot and 30-inch (77 cm) SID

    B. 2.0-mm focal spot and 36-inch (92 cm) SID

    C. 0.5-mm focal spot and 40-inch (102 cm) SID

    D. 0.3-mm focal spot and 40-inch (102 cm) SID

16. Rather than rely on the anode heel effect, what can be used to equalize density of specific anatomy?

   A. Inherent filtration   C. Added filtration

   B. Compensating filter   D. A diaphragm

17. Which type of compensating filter is recommended for an AP projection of the shoulder?

   A. Wedge   C. Trough

   B. Boomerang   D. Beveled

18. Which type of compensation filter is recommended for an axiolateral hip projection?

   A. Wedge   C. Trough

   B. Boomerang   D. Beveled

19. Which type of grid cutoff is created if the CR and the face of the grid are not perpendicular to each other?

   A. Off-level   C. Upside down grid

   B. Off-center   D. Off-focus

20. Which one of the following projections requires the use of a grid?

   A. PA hand   C. AP abdomen

   B. Axial calcaneus (heel)   D. AP elbow

21. The misrepresentation of an object's size or shape projected on a radiograph is called:

   A. Magnification   C. Unsharpness

   B. Blurring   D. Distortion

22. Which one of the following sets of factors *minimizes* radiographic distortion to the greatest degree?

   A. 40-inch (102-cm) SID and 8-inch (20-cm) OID

   B. 44-inch (113-cm) SID and 6-inch (15-cm) OID

   C. 72-inch (183-cm) SID and 3-inch (7.5-cm) OID

   D. 60-inch (154-cm) SID and 4-inch (10-cm) OID

23. True/False: To best use the anode heel effect, the thinner aspect of the anatomic part should be placed under the cathode aspect of the x-ray tube.

24. The best method to reduce distortion of the joints of the hand is to keep the fingers

   _____ to the IR.

   A. Perpendicular   C. At a 30° angle

   B. Parallel   D. Vertical

25. Which one of the following factors affects spatial resolution to the greatest degree?

   A. Use of a grid   C. Focal spot size

   B. kV   D. mAs

SELF-TEST E: Image Quality in Digital Radiography

1. Each digital image is formed by two-dimensional elements termed:
   - A. Pixels
   - B. Matrix
   - C. Voxels
   - D. Bytes

2. Highly complex mathematical formulas used in creating the digital image are termed:
   - A. Digital reconstructions
   - B. Bit processing matrices
   - C. Digital displays
   - D. Algorithms

3. True/False: Changes in kV have little impact on patient dose with digital imaging.

4. True/False: kV and mAs do not have the same direct effect on image quality with digital imaging as they do with IR-screen imaging.

5. True/False: A wide exposure latitude associated with digital imaging systems will reduce repeat exposures.

6. The intensity of light that represents the individual pixels in the image on the monitor is termed:
   - A. Latitude
   - B. Brightness
   - C. Contrast
   - D. Resolution

7. The primary controlling factor of contrast in the digital image is:
   - A. kV
   - B. mAs
   - C. Processing algorithms
   - D. Use of a grid

8. The greater the bit depth of a digital system, the greater the:
   - A. Contrast resolution
   - B. Brightness
   - C. Resolution
   - D. Noise

9. Which one of the following terms describes the minimum pixel size that can be displayed by a monitor?
   - A. Acquisition pixel size
   - B. Display pixel size
   - C. Monitor latent pixel size
   - D. Reconstructed pixel size

10. True/False: OID and SID have little impact on spatial resolution of the digital image.

11. True/False: The current range of spatial resolution for digital general radiographic imaging is between 2.5 to 5 line pairs per mm.

12. A numeric value that is representative of the exposure the image receptor received is termed:
    - A. Algorithm
    - B. Noise
    - C. Spatial resolution
    - D. Exposure indicator

13. Random disturbance that obscures or reduces clarity is the definition for:
    - A. Noise
    - B. Signal
    - C. Digital fluctuation
    - D. Signal variation

14. True/False: If an acceptable exposure indicator range is between 2.0 and 2.4, an exposure indicator of 4.0 would indicate overexposure of the image.

15. True/False: A high SNR results when insufficient mAs is used in creating a digital image.

16. Which one of the following factors will result in an increase in noise?

   A. Excessive mAs
   B. Scatter radiation
   C. High kV
   D. Decrease in pixel size

17. Changing or enhancing the electronic image to improve its diagnostic quality describes:

   A. Noise reduction
   B. Smoothing
   C. Post-processing
   D. Edge enhancement

18. _____ is the application of specific image processing that alters the pixel values across the image so as to present a more uniform image appearance.

   A. Smoothing
   B. Edge enhancement
   C. Brightness gain
   D. Equalization

19. Window width controls the _____ of the digital image.

   A. Edge enhancement
   B. Contrast
   C. Smoothing
   D. Brightness

20. True/False: Post-processing can correct for a low-SNR image.

SELF-TEST F: Applications of Digital Technology

1. Which one of the following statements is true in regard to PSP (computed radiography) imaging?

   A. PSP provides a wide exposure latitude.
   B. AEC cannot be used with PSP.
   C. Collimation should not be used.
   D. A longer SID must be used with PSP over film-screen systems.

2. Which one of the following processes is used to erase the PSP imaging plate following exposure?

   A. Ultraviolet light
   B. Low-level x-rays
   C. Bright light
   D. Laser

3. Patient information may be linked to the image on the CR imaging plate by:

   A. Light source
   B. Laser
   C. X-ray source
   D. Bar code reader

4. The PSP imaging plate is composed of:

   A. Calcium tungstate phosphor
   B. Zinc cadmium sulfate phosphor
   C. Silicon phosphor
   D. Photostimulable phosphor

5. The latent image recorded on the PSP image plate is read by a(n):

   A. Laser
   B. Bright light source
   C. Microwave source
   D. Ultraviolet light source

6. True/False: Close collimation must be avoided when acquiring an image on a PSP IP.

7. True /False: Grids cannot be used with a PSP system.

8. True/False: Grids are often used for extremity exams when using FPD-TFT (digital radiography).

9. True/False: FPD-TFT often requires less exposure than film-screen systems.

10. True/False: Close collimation should be avoided when using DR.

11. True/False: FPD-TFT can be either cassette-less or cassette-based systems.

12. True/False: RIS is a digital network that permits viewing and storage of both digital and film-screen produced images.

13. _____ controls the brightness of a digital image (within a certain range):

    A. Window width   C. Display pixel

    B. Window level   D. Bit depth

14. The acronym DICOM refers to:

    A. A set of standards to ensure communication among digital imaging systems

    C. A digital image transmission system

    D. A new-generation CR system

    B. A new direct digital "flat plate" receptor system

15. A digital transmission system for transferring radiographic images to remote locations is termed:

    A. PACS   C. HIS

    B. Direct DR   D. Teleradiography

16. CCD-based digital imaging systems have the advantage of _____ over other digital acquisition systems.

    A. using higher kV   C. rapid display of the image

    B. reducing mottle   D. enhanced noise reduction

17. A series of "boxes" that give form to the image is the definition for:

    A. Pixels   C. Display matrix

    B. Voxels   D. Acquisition matrices

18. A 30 × 35 cm IR is equivalent to a:

    A. 14 × 17 inches IR   C. 8 × 10 inches IR

    B. 11 × 14 inches IR   D. 10 × 12 inches IR

19. The application of specific image processing to reduce the display of noise in an image is the definition for:

    A. Windowing   C. Window width

    B. Edge enhancement   D. Smoothing

20. The recorded sharpness of structures on the image is the definition for:

    A. Spatial resolution   C. Equalization

    B. SNR   D. Bit depth

SELF-TEST G: Radiation Protection

1. What is the SI unit of radiation measurement for absorbed dose?

   A. Sievert

   B. Gray

   C. Coulombs per kilogram of air

   D. Roentgen

2. Which term is replacing "exposure" to describe skin dose?

   A. Sievert

   B. Gray

   C. Air kerma

   D. Rem

3. What is the annual whole-body effective dose (ED) for a technologist?

   A. 100 mSv or 10 rem

   B. 1 mSv or 0.1 rem

   C. 10 mSv or 1 rem

   D. 50 mSv or 5 rem

4. What is the cumulative lifetime ED for a 25-year-old technologist?

   A. 250 mSv

   B. 25 mSv

   C. 500 mSv

   D. 2500 mSv

5. What is the annual ED limit for an individual younger than 18 years of age?

   A. 50 mSv or 5 rem

   B. 1 mSv or 0.1 rem

   C. 1 mSv or 1 rem

   D. 100 mSv or 10 rem

6. The federal set maximum limit on exposure rates for intensified fluoroscopy units is:

   A. 3 to 4 R/minutes

   B. 0.5 R/minutes

   C. 1 R/minutes

   D. 10 R/minutes

7. For most modern equipment, the average fluoroscopy tabletop exposure rate is:

   A. 10 R/minutes

   B. 5 to 8 R/minutes

   C. 1 and 3 R/minutes

   D. 15 to 20 R/minutes

8. What is the primary purpose of x-ray tube filtration?

   A. Absorb lower (unusable) energy x-rays

   B. Reduce the x-ray intensity

   C. Increase quantity of the x-ray photons

   D. All of the above

9. Which of the following results in the highest ED for females (assuming no specific area shields are used)?

   A. Anteroposterior (AP) thoracic spine (7- × 17-inch collimation)

   B. AP thoracic spine (14- × 17-inch collimation)

   C. AP cervical spine (10- × 12-inch collimation)

   D. PA chest (14- × 17-inch collimation)

10. The use of a 1-mm lead equivalent gonadal shield reduces the gonadal dose by

    _____ if the gonads are within the primary x-ray field.

    A. 20% to 30%

    B. 40% to 50%

    C. 50% to 90%

    D. 100%

11. Which type of shield is ideal when the affected tissue is part of a sterile field?

   A. Contact shield
   B. Lead masking
   C. Shadow shield
   D. Gonadal-shaped shield

12. True/False: Low kV and high mAs techniques greatly reduce patient dose compared with high kV and low mAs techniques.

13. True/False: The total ED for females on an AP chest projection is more than double that for a PA chest.

14. True/False: The use of a positive beam limiting (PBL) collimator is no longer required by the FDA for new x-ray equipment manufactured after 1994.

15. True/False: Collimators must be accurate within 5% of the selected SID.

16. Which one of the following is not one of the cardinal principles of radiation protection?

   A. Distance
   B. Shielding
   C. Time
   D. Collimation

17. Which one of the following changes will best reduce patient dose?

   A. Decrease kV and increase mAs
   B. Using a grid
   C. Increase kV and lower mAs
   D. Increase mAs and lower kV

18. Where is the safest place for the technologist to stand during a fluoroscopic procedure?

   A. At the head end of the table
   B. At the foot end of the table
   C. On the floor behind the fluoroscopic tower
   D. Behind the radiologist

19. Which one of the following protection devices must be employed during a fluoroscopic procedure?

   A. Bucky slot shield
   B. Lead gloves
   C. Compensating filter
   D. Restraining devices

20. The ED for a pregnant technologist per month is:

   A. 1 mSv (0.1 rem)
   B. 0.5 mSv (0.05 rem)
   C. 5 mSv (500 mrem)
   D. 50 mSv (5 rem)

21. True/False: A fetal personnel dosimeter is worn at the level of the waist by a pregnant technologist during fluoroscopy.

22. True/False: All administrative staff in the radiology department must wear a personnel dosimeter even if not involved with patient care directly.

23. True/False: The ICRP and ACR have determined that the "10-day rule" is obsolete for procedures of the abdomen and pelvis.

24. Which one of the following statements is false in regard to digital imaging?

   A. The use of higher kV and lower mAs is recommended.

   B. A minimal 40-inch (102-cm) SID is encouraged with PSP and DR procedures.

   C. All radiographs should be within the exposure indicator.

   D. ALARA does not apply to digital imaging.

25. True/False: Using a different algorithm to process an overexposed CR image is an acceptable and ethical practice.

2 Chest

CHAPTER OBJECTIVES

After you have successfully completed the activities in this chapter, you will be able to:

_____ 1. List the parts of the bony thorax.

_____ 2. List specific topographic positioning landmarks of the chest.

_____ 3. Identify the parts and function of specific structures of the respiratory system.

_____ 4. List the four organs of the mediastinum.

_____ 5. Identify specific structures of the chest on line drawings.

_____ 6. Identify specific structures of the chest on posteroanterior (PA) and lateral radiographs.

_____ 7. Identify specific structures of the chest on a computed tomography (CT), transverse image.

_____ 8. Describe the methods to ensure proper degree of inspiration during chest radiography.

_____ 9. Describe the importance of using close collimation, gonadal shielding, and anatomic side markers during chest radiography.

_____ 10. Identify the common kVp ranges used during chest radiography.

_____ 11. Identify alterations in positioning routine and exposure factors specific to pediatric and geriatric patients.

_____ 12. List three reasons for taking chest radiographs with the patient in the erect position whenever possible.

_____ 13. Describe the three important positioning criteria that must be present on chest radiographs using erect PA and lateral positions.

_____ 14. Describe the advantages of the central ray placement method compared with the traditional method of centering for the PA and lateral chest projections.

_____ 15. Identify advantages and disadvantages in using CT, sonography, nuclear medicine, and magnetic resonance imaging (MRI) to demonstrate specific types of pathologic conditions in the chest.

_____ 16. Match various types of clinical indications to their correct definition.

_____ 17. For specific forms of chest pathology, indicate whether manual exposure factors need to be increased, decreased, or remain the same.

_____ 18. List the correct central ray placement, part position, and criteria for specific chest projections.

_____ 19. Given a hypothetic situation, identify the correct modifications of position, kV level, or both to improve the radiographic image.

_____ 20. Given a hypothetic situation, identify the correct position for a radiograph of specific pathologic conditions.

POSITIONING AND RADIOGRAPHIC CRITIQUE

_____ 1. Using a peer, position the patient for posteroanterior (PA), anteroposterior (AP), and lateral chest projections.

_____ 2. Using a chest phantom, use routine PA and lateral chest positions to produce satisfactory radiographs (if equipment is available).

_____ 3. Determine whether rotation is present on PA and lateral chest radiographs.

_____ 4. Critique and evaluate chest radiographs based on the five divisions of radiographic criteria: (1) anatomy demonstrated, (2) position, (3) collimation and central ray, (4) exposure, and (5) anatomic side markers.

_____ 5. Distinguish between acceptable and unacceptable chest radiographs based on exposure factors, motion, collimation, positioning, or other errors.

LEARNING EXERCISES

Complete the following review exercises after reading the associated pages in Chapter 2 of the textbook as indicated by each exercise. Answers to each review exercise are given at the end of the review exercises and laboratory activities.

PART I: RADIOGRAPHIC ANATOMY
REVIEW EXERCISE A: Radiographic Anatomy of the Chest (see textbook pp. 70-77)

1. The bony thorax consists of (A) the single _____ anteriorly, (B) two

   _____, (C) two _____, (D) twelve pairs of

   _____, and (E) twelve _____ posteriorly.

2. The two important bony landmarks of the thorax that are used for locating the central ray on a posteroanterior

   (PA) and anteroposterior (AP) chest projection are the (A) _____ and

   (B) _____, respectively.

3. The four divisions of the respiratory system are:

   A. _____   C. _____

   B. _____   D. _____

4. Identify correct anatomic terms for the following structures.

   A. Adam's apple _____   D. Shoulder blade _____

   B. Voice box _____   E. Collar bone _____

   C. Breastbone _____

5. List the three divisions of the structure located proximally to the larynx that serve as a common passageway for both food and air.

   A. _____   C. _____

   B. _____

6. What is the name of the structure that acts as a lid over the larynx to prevent foreign objects such as food particles

   from entering the respiratory system? _____

7. The trachea is located _____ (anteriorly or posteriorly) to the esophagus.

8. The _____ bone is seen in the anterior portion of the neck and is found just below
   the tongue or floor of the mouth.

9. If a person accidentally inhales a food particle, which bronchus is it most likely to enter, and why?

   A. The _____ bronchus

   B. Why? _____

10. A. What is the name of the prominence, or ridge, seen when looking down into the bronchus where it divides into

    the right and left bronchi? _____

    B. This prominence, or ridge, is approximately at the level of the _____ vertebra.

11. What is the term for the small air sacs located at the distal ends of the bronchioles, in which oxygen and carbon

    dioxide are exchanged in the blood? _____

12. A. The delicate, double-walled sac or membrane containing the lungs is called the

    _____.

    B. The outer layer of this membrane adhering to the inner surface of the chest wall and diaphragm is the

    _____.

    C. The inner layer adhering to the surface of the lungs is the _____, or

    _____.

    D. The potential space between these two layers (identified in B and C) is called the

    _____.

    E. Air or gas that enters the space identified in D results in a condition called

    _____.

13. Fill in the correct terms for the following portions of the lungs.

   A. Lower, concave portion: _____

   B. Central area in which bronchi and blood vessels enter the lungs: _____

   C. Upper, rounded portion above the level of the clavicles: _____

   D. Extreme, outermost lower corner of the lungs: _____

14. Explain why the right lung is smaller than the left lung and the right hemidiaphragm is positioned higher than

   the left hemidiaphragm. _____

15. List the four important structures located in the mediastinum.

   A. _____   C. _____

   B. _____   D. _____

16. Identify the following structures in Fig. 2-1

   A. _____ gland

   B. _____

   C. _____

   D. _____

   E. _____

   F. _____ gland

   G. _____

   H. _____

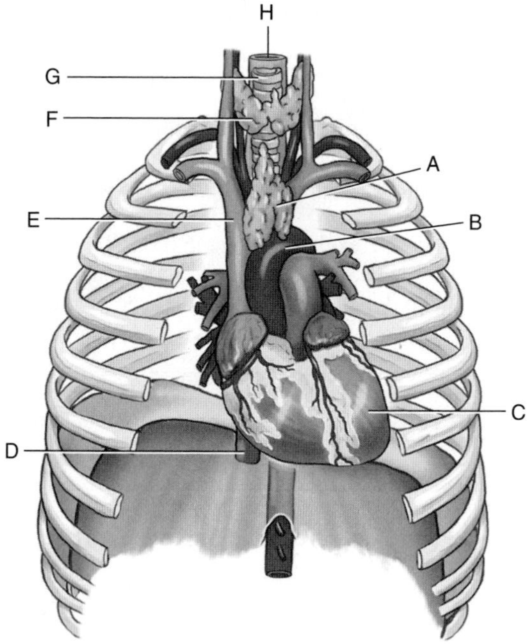

Fig. 2-1. Structures within the mediastinum.

17. The heart is enclosed in a double-walled membrane called the _____.

18. The three parts of the aorta are the _____ , _____ ,

   and _____.

19. Identify the following labeled structures as seen on PA and lateral chest radiographs in Figs. 2-2 and 2-3.

A. _____

B. _____

C. _____

D. _____

E. _____

F. _____

G. _____

H. _____

I. _____

J. _____

K. _____

L. _____

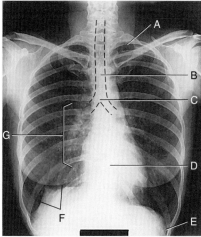

Fig. 2-2. Posteroanterior (PA) chest radiograph.

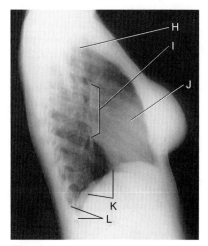

Fig. 2-3. Lateral chest radiograph.

20. Identify the labeled parts on this computed tomography (CT) image (Fig. 2-4) of a transverse section of the thorax at the level of T5, the fifth thoracic vertebra, which is also the level of the carina. (Hint: B, G, and H are major blood vessels.)

A. _____

B. _____

C. _____

D. _____

E. _____

F. _____

G. _____

H. _____

I. _____

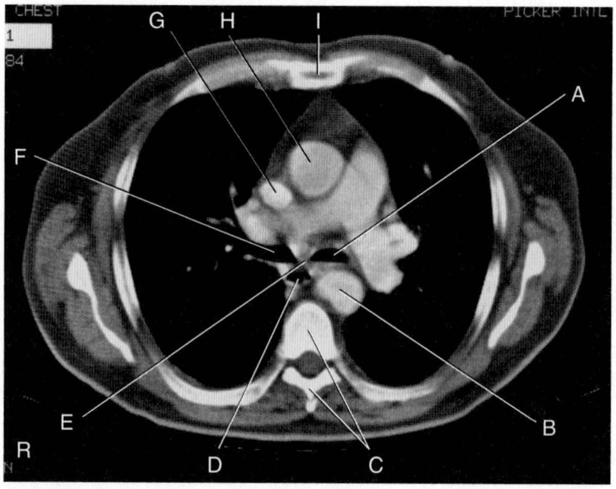

Fig. 2-4. Computed tomography (CT) transverse section of the thorax at the level of T5.

PART II: RADIOGRAPHIC POSITIONING
REVIEW EXERCISE B: Technical Considerations (see textbook pp. 78-88)

1. Which type of body habitus is associated with a broad and deep thorax?

   _____

2. Which one of the following types of body habitus may cause the costophrenic angles to be cut off if careful vertical collimation is not used?

   A. Hypersthenic

   B. Hyposthenic

   C. Sthenic

   D. Hyposthenic and asthenic

3. What is the minimum number of ribs that should be demonstrated above the diaphragm on a PA radiograph of an

   average adult chest with full inspiration? _____

4. Which of the following objects should be removed (or moved) before chest radiography? (Choose all that apply.)

   A. Necklace

   B. Bra

   C. Religious medallion around neck

   D. Dentures

   E. Pants

   F. Hair fasteners

   G. Oxygen lines

5. True/False: Chest radiography is the most commonly repeated radiographic procedure because of poor positioning or exposure factor selection errors.

6. Chest radiography for the adult patient usually employs a kilovoltage peak of _____

   to _____ kV.

7. True/False: Generally, you do not need to use radiographic grids for adult patients for PA or lateral chest radiographs.

8. Optimal technical factor selection ensures proper penetration of the:

   A. Heart   D. Hilar region

   B. Great vessels   E. All of the above

   C. Lung regions

9. Describe the way optimum density of the lungs and mediastinal structures can be determined on a PA chest

   radiograph _____.

10. True/False: Because the heart is always located in the left thorax, the use of anatomic side markers on a PA chest projection may not be necessary.

11. Which one of the following devices should be used for the erect PA and lateral chest projections for an infant?

    A. Upright chest device   C. Pigg-O-Stat

    B. Supine table Bucky   D. Plexiglas restraint board

12. Which one of the following sets of exposure factors is recommended for a chest examination of a young pediatric patient?

    A. 70 to 85 kV, short exposure time   C. 100 to 120 kV, short exposure time

    B. 90 to 100 kV, medium exposure time   D. 120 to 150 kV, long exposure time

13. True/False: Because they have shallower (superior-inferior dimension) lung fields, the central ray is often centered higher for geriatric patients.

14. To ensure better lung inspiration during chest radiography, exposure should be made during the

    _____ inspiration.

15. List four possible pathologic conditions that suggest the need for both inspiration and expiration PA chest radiographs.

    A. _____   C. _____

    B. _____   D. _____

16. List and explain briefly the three reasons chest radiographs should be taken with the patient in the erect position (when the patient's condition permits).

    A. _____   C. _____

    B. _____

17. Why do the lungs tend to expand more with the patient in an erect position than in a supine position?

    _____

18. Explain the primary purpose and benefit of performing chest radiography using a 72-inch (183-cm) source

    image receptor distance (SID). _____

19. What is a common radiographic sign seen on a chest radiograph for a patient with respiratory distress syndrome (RDS)?

    A. Enlargement of heart   C. Elevated diaphragms

    B. Fluid in apices   D. Air bronchogram

20. Which one of the following anatomic structures is examined to determine rotation on a PA chest radiograph?

A. Appearance of ribs   C. Symmetric appearance of sternoclavicular joints

B. Shape of heart   D. Symmetric appearance of costophrenic angles

21. Which positioning tip will help you prevent the patient's chin and neck from being superimposed over the upper airway and apices of the lungs for a PA chest radiograph?

_____

_____

22. For patients with the following clinical histories, which lateral projection would you perform—right or left?

A. Patient with severe pains in left side of chest _____

B. Patient with no chest pain but recent history of pneumonia in right lung _____

C. Patient with no chest pain or history of heart trouble _____

23. Why is it important to raise the patient's arms above the head for lateral chest projections?

_____

_____

24. The traditional central ray centering technique for the chest is to place the top of the image receptor (IR)

_____ inches (_____ cm) above the shoulders.

25. A recommended central ray centering technique for a PA chest projection requires the technologist to palpate the

_____ and measure down from that bony landmark _____ inches (_____ cm) for

a male and _____ inches (_____ cm) for a female patient.

26. A. Should the 14- × 17-inch (35- × 43-cm) image receptor be aligned lengthwise or crosswise for a PA chest

projection of a hypersthenic patient? _____

B. For a hyposthenic patient? _____

27. Which one of the following bony landmarks is palpated for centering of the AP chest projection?

A. Vertebra prominens   C. Thyroid cartilage

B. Jugular notch   D. Sternal angle

28. True/False: With most digital chest units, the question of IR placement into either vertical or crosswise positions is eliminated because of the larger IR.

29. True/False: In general, for an average patient more collimation should be visible on the lower margin of the chest image than on the top for a PA or lateral chest projection.

30. True/False: For most patients, the central ray level for a PA chest projection is near the inferior angle of the scapula.

31. True/False: The height, or vertical dimension, of the average-to-large person's chest is greater than the width, or horizontal dimension.

32. True/False: Single-photon emission computed tomography (SPECT) is frequently used to diagnose myocardial infarction.

33. True/False: Ultrasound is not an effective modality to detect pleural effusion.

34. True/False: Echocardiography and electrocardiography are basically the same procedure.

35. Match each of the following descriptions of clinical indicators to its correct term.

_____ 1. One of the most common inherited diseases	A. Atelectasis
_____ 2. Condition most frequently associated with congestive heart failure	B. Bronchiectasis
	C. Bronchitis
_____ 3. Dyspnea	D. Chronic obstructive pulmonary disease (COPD)
_____ 4. Accumulation of air in pleural cavity	
_____ 5. Accumulation of pus in pleural cavity	E. Shortness of breath
_____ 6. A form of occupational lung disease	F. Cystic fibrosis
_____ 7. A contagious disease caused by an airborne bacterium	G. Empyema
	H. Pleurisy
_____ 8. Irreversible dilation of bronchioles	I. Pneumothorax
_____ 9. Most common form is emphysema	J. Pulmonary edema
_____ 10. Acute or chronic irritation of bronchi	K. Tuberculosis
_____ 11. Collapse of all or portion of lung	L. Silicosis
_____ 12. Inflammation of pleura	

36. For the following types of pathologic conditions, indicate whether manual exposure factors would be increased (+), decreased (−), or generally remain the same (0) compared with standard chest exposure factors.

_____ Left lung atelectasis

_____ Lung neoplasm

_____ Severe pulmonary edema

_____ Respiratory distress syndrome (RDS) or adult respiratory distress syndrome (ARDS), known as hyaline membrane disease (HMD) in infants

_____ Secondary tuberculosis

_____ Advanced emphysema

_____ Large pneumothorax

_____ Pulmonary emboli

_____ Primary tuberculosis

_____ Advanced asbestosis

37. Which one of the following is not a form of occupational lung disease?

A. Anthracosis   C. Silicosis

B. Emphysema   D. Asbestosis

38. Which one of the following chest projections/positions is recommended to detect calcifications or cavitations within the upper lung region near the clavicles?

A. Left lateral decubitus   C. RPO and LPO

B. PA   D. AP lordotic

REVIEW EXERCISE C: Positioning of the Chest (see textbook pp. 90-101)

1. Why is a PA chest preferred to an AP projection? _____

2. The CR is placed at the level of the _____ vertebra for a PA chest projection.

3. The shoulders need to be rolled forward for the PA projection to allow the _____ to move laterally and be clear of the lung fields.

4. Why should a left lateral be performed unless departmental protocol indicates otherwise?

5. How much separation of the posterior ribs on a lateral chest projection indicates excessive rotation from a true

   lateral position? _____ (Note: Less separation than this is caused by the divergent x-rays.)

6. To prevent the clavicles from obscuring the apices on an AP projection of the chest, the central ray should

   be angled (A) _____ (caudad or cephalad) so that it is perpendicular to the

   (B) _____.

7. What is the name of the condition characterized by fluid entering the pleural cavity?

   _____

8. Which specific position would be used if a patient were unable to stand but the physician suspected the patient

   had fluid in the left lung? _____

9. What is the name of the condition characterized by free air entering the pleural cavity?

   _____

10. Which specific position would be used if the patient were unable to stand but the physician suspected the patient

    had free air in the left pleural cavity? _____

11. What circumstances or clinical indications suggest that an AP lordotic projection should be ordered?

    _____

12. What position/projection would be used for a patient who is too ill or weak to stand for an AP lordotic projection?

    _____

13. A. Which anterior oblique projection would best demonstrate the left lung—right anterior oblique (RAO) or left

    anterior oblique (LAO)? _____

    B. Which posterior oblique projection would best demonstrate the left lung—RPO or LPO?

    _____

14. For certain studies of the heart, the _____ (right or left) anterior oblique requires a

    rotation of _____ °.

15. True/False: A grid is not recommended for a LPO projection of the adult chest.

16. Where is the central ray placed for a lateral projection of the upper airway? _____

17. Careful collimation during a chest radiograph will improve image quality by decreasing

    _____ radiation to the IR.

18. What are the recommended patient instructions when performing an erect PA chest on a female patient with large

    pendulous breasts? _____

19. True/False: No lead shielding is necessary for male patients or women greater than age 65 during radiographic
    imaging of the chest.

20. An erect chest PA radiograph aids the patient to achieve full inspiration and helps to prevent

    _____ and _____ of the pulmonary vessels.

REVIEW EXERCISE D: Problem Solving for Technical and Positioning Errors

The following radiographic problems involve technical and positioning errors that lead to substandard images. Other
questions involve situations pertaining to various conditions and pathologic findings. As you analyze these problems and
situations, use your textbook to help you find solutions to these questions.

1. A radiograph of a PA view of the chest reveals the sternoclavicular (SC) joints are not the same distance from
   the spine. The right SC joint is closer to the midline than is the left SC joint. What is the positioning error?

   _____

2. A radiograph of a PA projection of the chest shows only seven posterior ribs above the diaphragm. What caused
   this problem, and how could it be prevented on the repeat exposures?

   _____

   _____

3. A radiograph of a PA and left lateral projection of the chest reveals the mediastinum of the chest is underpenetrated. The
   technologist used the following factors for the radiograph: a 72-inch (183-cm) SID, an upright Bucky, a full-inspiration
   exposure, 75-kV and 600-mA, and a ¹⁄₆₀-second exposure time.

   A. Which one of these factors is the most likely cause of the problem? Briefly explain.

      _____

   B. How can the technologist improve the image when making the repeat exposure?

      _____

4. A radiograph of a PA projection of the chest reveals the top of the apices are cut off and a wide collimation border
   can be seen below the diaphragm. In what way can this be corrected during the repeat radiograph?

   _____

5. **Situation:** A patient with a clinical history of advanced emphysema comes to the radiology department for a chest x-ray. AEC will not be used. How should the technologist alter the manual exposure settings for this patient?

   A. Do not alter them. Use the standard exposure factors.

   B. Decrease the kV moderately ($--$).

   C. Increase the kV slightly ($+$).

   D. Increase the kV moderately ($++$).

6. **Situation:** A patient with severe pleural effusion comes to the radiology department for a chest x-ray. Automatic exposure control (AEC) will not be used. How should the technologist alter the manual exposure settings for this patient?

   A. Do not alter them. Use the standard exposure factors.

   B. Decrease the kV moderately ($--$).

   C. Increase the kV slightly ($+$).

   D. Increase the kV moderately ($++$).

7. **Situation:** A patient comes to the radiology department for a presurgical chest examination. The clinical history indicates a possible situs inversus of the thorax (transposition of structures within the thorax). Which positioning step or action must be taken to perform a successful chest examination?

   _____

8. A radiograph of a lateral projection of the chest reveals the posterior ribs and costophrenic angles are separated more than ½ inch, or 1 cm, indicating excessive rotation. Describe a possible method of determining the direction

   of rotation. _____

9. **Situation:** A patient enters the emergency room with a possible hemothorax in the right lung caused by a motor vehicle accident (MVA). The patient is unable to stand or sit erect. Which specific projection would

   best demonstrate this condition, and why? _____

10. **Situation:** A young child enters the emergency room with a possible foreign body in one of the bronchi of the lung. The foreign body, a peanut, cannot be seen on the PA and lateral projections of the chest projection. Which additional projection(s) could the technologist perform to locate the foreign body?

    _____

11. **Situation:** A routine chest series indicates a possible mass beneath a patient's right clavicle. The PA and lateral projections are inconclusive. What additional projection(s) could be taken to rule out this condition?

    _____

12. **Situation:** A patient has a possible small pneumothorax. Routine chest projections (PA and lateral) fail to reveal the pneumothorax conclusively. Which additional projections could be taken to rule out this condition?

    _____

13. **Situation:** A patient with a history of pleurisy comes to the radiology department. Which one of the following radiographic series should be performed?

    A. Soft tissue lateral of the upper airway   C. Erect PA and lateral

    B. Right and left lateral decubitus   D. CT scan of the chest

14. **Situation:** A patient with a possible neoplasm in the right lung apex comes to the radiology department for a chest examination. The PA and lateral projections do not clearly demonstrate the neoplasm because of superimposition of the clavicle over the apex. The patient is unable to stand or sit erect. Which additional projection can be taken to clearly demonstrate the neoplasm and eliminate the superimposition of the clavicle and the left lung apex?

_____

15. **Situation:** PA and left lateral projections demonstrate a suspicious region in the left lung. The radiologist orders an oblique projection that will best demonstrate or "elongate" the left lung. Which specific oblique projections will best elongate the left lung? (More than one oblique projection will accomplish this goal.)

_____

PART III: LABORATORY ACTIVITIES

You must gain experience in chest positioning before performing the following exams on actual patients. You may gain experience with positioning and radiographic evaluation of these projections by performing exercises using radiographic phantoms and practicing on other students (although not taking actual exposures).

The following suggested activities assume your teaching institution has an energized lab and radiographic phantoms. If not, perform only Laboratory Exercise B, the physical positioning activities. (Check off each step and projection as you complete it.)

Laboratory Exercise A: Energized Laboratory

1. Using the chest radiographic phantom, produce radiographs using:

_____ PA and AP projections   _____ Lateral projection

2. Evaluate the radiographs you produced above, additional radiographs provided by your instructor, or both for the following criteria.

_____ Rotation   _____ Anatomic side markers

_____ Collimation   _____ Proper exposure factors

_____ Part and central ray centering   _____ Motion

Laboratory Exercise B: Physical Positioning

1. On another person, simulate taking all of the following routine and special projections of the chest. Follow the suggested positioning steps and sequence as listed below and as described in Chapter 2 of your textbook:

_____ PA chest   _____ AP supine or semisupine

_____ Anterior and posterior obliques   _____ Lateral decubitus

_____ Lateral chest   _____ AP lordotic

_____ AP and lateral upper airway

Step 1. General Patient Positioning

_____ Select the size and number of image receptors needed.

_____ Prepare the radiographic room. Check that the x-ray tube is centered to the center of the IR holder (or the centerline of the table for Bucky exams).

_____ Correctly identify the patient and bring the patient into the room.

_____ Explain to the patient what you will be doing.

_____ Assist the patient to the proper place and position for the first radiograph.

Step 2. Measuring Part Thickness

_____ Measure the body part being radiographed and set correct exposure factors (manual technique). (If using an AEC system, select the correct chamber cells on the control panel.)

Step 3. Part Positioning

_____ Align and center the body part to the central ray or vice versa for chest positioning with the chest board. (For Bucky exams on a table, move the patient and tabletop together as needed [with floating-type tabletop]).

Step 4. Image Receptor (IR) Centering

_____ After the part has been centered to the central ray, the IR is also centered to the central ray. (*Note:* This step can be omitted on most chest units where the x-ray tube and IR unit are attached and move together.)

Additional Steps or Actions

_____ 1. Collimate accurately to include only the area of interest.

_____ 2. Place the correct side marker within the exposure field (so that you do not superimpose pertinent anatomic structures).

_____ 3. Restrain or provide support for the body part to prevent motion.

_____ 4. Use contact lead shielding as needed (e.g., gonadal, breast, thyroid).

_____ 5. Give clear breathing instructions and make the exposure while watching patient through the console window.

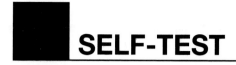

SELF-TEST

This self-test should be taken only after completing all of the readings, review exercises, and laboratory activities for a particular section. The purpose of this test is not only to provide a learning exercise but also to serve as a strong indicator of what your final unit evaluation exam will cover. It is strongly suggested that if you do not receive at least a 90% to 95% grade on each self-test, you should review those areas in which you missed questions before going to your instructor for the final unit evaluation exam.

1. Match each of the following structures with its correct anatomic term.

   _____ 1. Breastbone   A. Clavicle

   _____ 2. Adam's apple   B. Larynx

   _____ 3. Shoulder blade   C. Thyroid cartilage

   _____ 4. Voice box   D. Scapula

   _____ 5. Collar bone   E. Sternum

2. The correct term for the seventh cervical vertebrae is:

   A. Xiphoid process   C. Axis

   B. Jugular notch   D. Vertebra prominens

3. A notch, or depression, located on the superior portion of the sternum is called the:

   A. Sternal notch   C. Jugular notch

   B. Xiphoid notch   D. Sternal angle

4. The trachea bifurcates and forms the:

   A. Right and left bronchi C. Costophrenic angles

   B. Right and left hilum   D. Pulmonary arteries

5. A specific prominence, or ridge, found at the point where the internal distal trachea divides into the right and left bronchi is called the:

   A. Hilum   C. Epiglottis

   B. Carina   D. Alveoli

6. The area of each lung where the bronchi and blood vessels enter and leave is called the:

   A. Carina   C. Base

   B. Apex   D. Hilum

7. The structures within the lung where oxygen and carbon dioxide gas exchange occurs are called:

   A. Carina   C. Hilum

   B. Alveoli   D. Bronchi

8. Which of the following is *not* an aspect of the pleura?

   A. Parietal pleura   C. Pleural cavity

   B. Hilar pleura   D. Pulmonary pleura

9. The condition in which blood fills the potential space between the layers of pleura is called:

   A. Pneumothorax   C. Atelectasis

   B. Hemothorax   D. Empyema

10. The extreme, outermost lower corner of each lung is called the:

    A. Costophrenic angle   C. Base

    B. Apex   D. Hilar region

11. Which one of the following structures is *not* found in the mediastinum?

    A. Thymus gland   C. Epiglottis

    B. Heart and great vessels   D. Trachea

12. A narrow thorax that is shallow from the front to back but very long in the vertical dimension is characteristic of

    a(n) _____ body habitus.

    A. Hypersthenic   C. Hyposthenic

    B. Sthenic   D. Asthenic

13. Identify the best kV level for adult chest radiography from the following choices.

    A. 85 kV, 40-inch (102-cm) SID

    B. 110 kV, 40-inch (102-cm) SID

    C. 120 kV, 60-inch (153-cm) SID

    D. 125 kV, 72-inch (183-cm) SID

14. Match the correct answers for the structures labeled on this midsagittal section of the pharynx and upper airway (Fig. 2-5).

_____ A.

_____ B.

_____ C.

_____ D.

_____ E.

_____ F.

_____ G.

_____ H.

_____ I.

_____ J.

_____ K.

_____ L.

_____ M.

1. Laryngopharynx

2. Uvula

3. Epiglottis

4. Esophagus

5. Spinal cord

6. Oral cavity

7. Hyoid bone

8. Nasopharynx

9. Thyroid gland

10. Oropharynx

11. Larynx

12. Hard palate

13. Thyroid cartilage

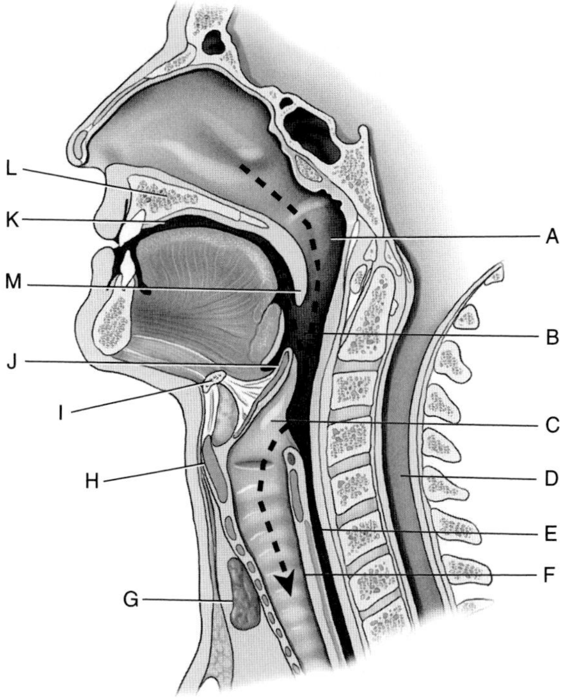

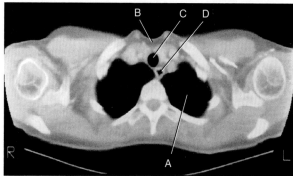

Fig. 2-5. Midsagittal section of the pharynx and upper airway.

15. Identify the structures labeled on this computed tomography (CT) axial section of the thorax at the level of T3 (the third thoracic vertebra) (Fig. 2-6).

A. _____

B. _____

C. _____

D. _____

Fig. 2-6. Computed tomography (CT) axial section of the thorax at the level of T3.

16. Identify the structures on this CT axial section of the thorax at the approximate level of T4-T5, 1 cm proximal to carina (Hint: B, E, and F are major blood vessels) (Fig. 2-7).

A. _____

B. _____

C. _____

D. _____

E. _____

F. _____

G. _____

H. _____

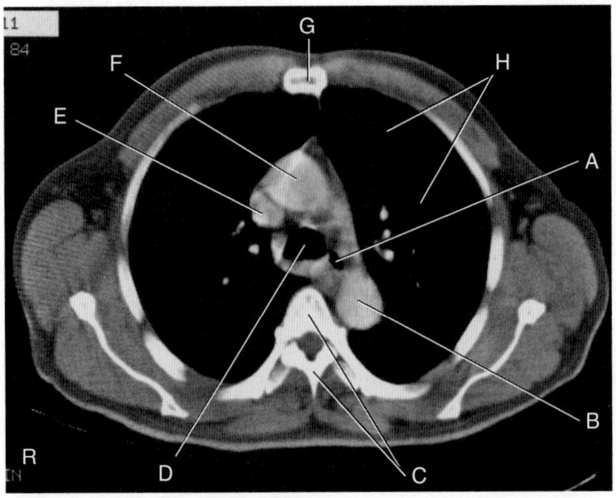

Fig. 2-7. Computed tomography (CT) axial section of the thorax at the approximate level of T4-T5.

17. What is the name of the special immobilization device used for pediatric chest studies?

   A. Pigg-O-Stat   C. Chest immobilizer

   B. Restraining chair   D. Franklin unit

18. Which one of the following exposure factors is recommended for a chest study of a young pediatric patient?

   A. 110-125 kV, short exposure time   C. 70-85 kV, short exposure time

   B. 90-105 kV, medium exposure time   D. 60-75 kV, long exposure time

19. Which of the following is *not* a valid reason to perform chest projections with the patient in the erect position?

   A. To reduce patient dose

   B. To demonstrate air and fluid levels

   C. To allow the diaphragm to move down farther

   D. To prevent hyperemia of pulmonary vessels

20. Why are the shoulders pressed downward and toward the IR for a posteroanterior (PA) projection of the chest?

   A. To remove scapulae from lung fields

   B. To prevent hyperemia of pulmonary vessels

   C. To allow the diaphragm to move down farther

   D. To reduce chest rotation

21. Why are the shoulders rolled forward for a PA projection of the chest?

   A. To remove scapulae from lung fields

   B. To prevent hyperemia of pulmonary vessels

   C. To allow the diaphragm to move down farther

   D. To reduce chest rotation

22. Where is the central ray placed for an anteroposterior (AP) supine projection of the chest?

    A. 7 to 8 inches (18 to 20 cm) below vertebra prominens

    B. 1 to 2 inches (2.5 to 5 cm) below jugular notch

    C. 3 to 4 inches (8 to 10 cm) below jugular notch

    D. 3 to 4 inches (8 to 10 cm) below thyroid cartilage

23. Which one of the following terms is defined as a "shortness of breath"?

    A. Dyspnea   C. Pleurisy

    B. Bronchiectasis   D. Atelectasis

24. A condition in which all or a portion of the lung is collapsed is:

    A. Atelectasis   C. Pneumothorax

    B. Pleural effusion   D. Pneumoconiosis

25. A condition in which excess fluid builds in the lungs as a result of obstruction of the pulmonary circulation is termed:

    A. Pulmonary emboli   C. Pulmonary edema

    B. Pneumothorax   D. Bronchopneumonia

26. A sudden blockage of an artery in the lung is called:

    A. Pleurisy   C. Adult respiratory distress syndrome (ARDS)

    B. Pulmonary emboli   D. Chronic obstructive pulmonary disease (COPD)

27. Which one of the following is *not* a form of occupational lung disease?

    A. Asbestosis   C. Anthracosis

    B. Silicosis   D. Tuberculosis

28. Manual exposure factors for a patient with a large pneumothorax should:

    A. Be reduced   C. Be increased

    B. Remain the same   D. Change from automatic exposure control (AEC) to manual technique

29. A PA chest radiograph reveals that the left sternoclavicular joint is superimposed over the spine (in comparison with the right joint). What specific positioning error is involved?

    A. Poor inspiration

    B. Rotation into a right anterior oblique (RAO) position

    C. Rotation into a left anterior oblique (LAO) position

    D. Tilting of the chest toward the left

30. A PA chest radiograph demonstrates 10 posterior ribs above the diaphragm.

    Is this an acceptable degree of inspiration? _____ Yes _____ No

31. A PA and lateral chest radiographic study has been completed. The PA projection reveals the right costophrenic angle was collimated off, but both angles are included on the lateral projection.

    Would you repeat the PA projection? _____ Yes _____ No

32. A lateral chest radiograph demonstrates the soft tissue of the upper limbs is superimposed over the apices of the lungs. How can this situation be prevented?

   A. Deeper inspiration   C. Slight rotation to the patient's left

   B. Extend chin   D. Raise upper limbs higher

33. A lateral chest radiograph reveals that the posterior ribs and costophrenic angles are separated by approximately

   ½ inch (slightly less than 1 cm). Should the technologist repeat this projection? _____ Yes _____ No

34. **Situation:** A radiograph of an AP lordotic projection reveals the clavicles are projected within the apices. The clinical instructor informs the student technologist that the study is unacceptable, but during the repeat exposure the patient complains of being too unsteady to lean backward for another projection. What other options are available if the student wants to complete the study?

   A. Perform the PA lordotic projection   C. Perform both lateral decubitus projections

   B. Perform an AP semiaxial projection   D. Perform inspiration and expiration PA projections

35. **Situation:** An ambulatory patient with a clinical history of advanced emphysema enters the emergency room. The patient is having difficulty breathing and is receiving oxygen. The physician has ordered a PA and lateral chest study. Should the technologist alter the typical exposure factors for this patient?

   A. No. Use the standard exposure factors.

   B. Yes. Increase the exposure factors.

   C. Yes. Decrease the exposure factors.

   D. No. Increase the SID instead of changing the exposure factors.

36. **Situation:** A patient enters the ER with an injury to the chest. The ER physician suspects a pneumothorax may be present in the right lung. The patient is unable to stand or sit erect. Which specific position or projection can be performed to confirm the presence of the pneumothorax?

   A. Left lateral decubitus   C. Right lateral decubitus

   B. Inspiration and expiration PA   D. AP lordotic

37. **Situation:** A PA and lateral chest study reveals a suspicious mass located near the heart in the right lung. The radiologist would like a radiograph of the patient in an anterior oblique position to delineate the mass from the heart. Which position or projection should the technologist use to accomplish this objective?

   A. 45° LAO   C. 60° LAO

   B. 45° RAO   D. AP lordotic

38. **Situation:** A patient with a history of pulmonary edema comes to the radiology department and is unable to stand. The physician suspects fluid in the left lung. Which specific projection should be used to confirm this diagnosis?

   A. Right lateral decubitus   C. AP lordotic

   B. AP semiaxial   D. Left lateral decubitus

39. For the following image evaluation questions, refer to textbook p. 102 (Fig. C2-92) (PA chest).

    A. Which positioning error(s) is (are) visible on this radiograph? (More than one answer may be selected.)

       (a) All essential anatomic structures are not demonstrated.

       (b) Central ray is incorrectly centered.

       (c) Collimation is not evident.

       (d) Exposure factors are incorrect.

       (e) No anatomic side marker is visible.

       (f) Rotation into the RAO position is evident. (The spine is shifted to the right.)

       (g) Rotation into the LAO position is evident. (The spine is shifted to the left.)

       (h) The chin is not elevated.

    B. Which error(s) on this radiograph is (are) considered "repeatable"?

    C. Which of the following modifications must be made during the repeat exposure? (More than one answer may be selected.)

       (a) Increase closer collimation.

       (b) Center CR correctly to T7.

       (c) Decrease exposure factors.

       (d) Increase exposure factors.

       (e) Place anatomic side marker on IR before exposure.

       (f) Correct for rotation of shoulders and hips.

       (g) Place image receptor crosswise.

       (h) Elevate chin higher.

40. For the following image evaluation questions, refer to textbook p. 102 (Fig. C2-94) (Lateral chest).

    A. What positioning error(s) is (are) seen on this radiograph? (More than one answer may be selected.)

       (a) All essential anatomy is not demonstrated on the radiograph.

       (b) CR centering is incorrect.

       (c) Collimation is not evident.

       (d) Exposure factors are incorrect.

       (e) No anatomic side marker is seen on radiograph.

       (f) Excessive rotation of the chest is demonstrated.

    B. Which error(s) on this radiograph is (are) considered "repeatable"?

    C. Which of the following modifications must be made during the repeat exposure? (More than one answer may be selected.)

       (a) Center the central ray correctly—to T7.

       (b) Decrease the exposure factors.

       (c) Increase the exposure factors.

       (d) Place an anatomic marker correctly on the IR before exposure.

       (e) Ensure that the shoulders and hips are superimposed to eliminate rotation.

       (f) Raise the upper limbs higher.

3 Abdomen

_____ 20. Given various hypothetic situations, identify the correct modification of position, exposure factors, or both to improve the radiographic image.

_____ 21. Given various hypothetic situations, identify the correct position for a specific pathologic feature or condition.

POSITIONING AND RADIOGRAPHIC CRITIQUE

_____ 1. Use another student as a model to practice putting a patient in supine, erect, and lateral decubitus abdominal positions.

_____ 2. Using an abdomen phantom, produce an AP projection of the abdomen that results in a satisfactory radiograph (if equipment is available).

_____ 3. Determine whether rotation, tilt, or both are present on a radiograph of an AP projection of the abdomen.

_____ 4. Critique and evaluate abdominal radiographs based on the five divisions of radiographic criteria: (1) anatomy demonstrated, (2) position, (3) collimation and central ray, (4) exposure, and (5) anatomic side markers.

_____ 5. Distinguish between acceptable and unacceptable abdominal radiographs based on exposure factors, motion, collimation, positioning, or other errors.

_____ 6. Identify specific bony and soft tissue structures seen radiographically.

_____ 7. Discriminate among radiographs taken in supine, erect, or lateral decubitus positions.

LEARNING EXERCISES

Complete the following review exercises after reading the associated pages in Chapter 3 of the textbook as indicated by each exercise. Answers to each review exercise are given at the end of the review exercises.

PART I: RADIOGRAPHIC ANATOMY
REVIEW EXERCISE A: Abdominopelvic Anatomy (see textbook pp. 104-111)

1. The two large muscles found in the posterior abdomen adjacent to the lumbar vertebra and usually visible on

   an anteroposterior (AP) radiograph are called the _____

2. The medical prefix for stomach is _____.

3. List the three parts of the small intestine.

   A. _____   B. _____   C. _____

4. Which portion of the small intestine is considered to be the longest? _____.

5. The large intestine begins in the _____ quadrant with a saclike area called the

   _____

6. The sigmoid colon is located between the _____ and

   _____ of the large intestine.

7. Which one of the following organs is considered to be part of the lymphatic system?
   A. Liver   C. Pancreas
   B. Spleen   D. Gallbladder

8. List the three accessory digestive organs.

A. _____   B. _____   C. _____

9. Circle the correct term. The pancreas is located **anteriorly** or **posteriorly** to the stomach.

10. Which one of the following organs is *not* directly associated with the digestive system?

A. Gallbladder   C. Jejunum

B. Spleen   D. Pancreas

11. Why is the right kidney found in a more inferior position than the left kidney? _____

12. Which endocrine glands are superomedial to each kidney? _____

13. True/False: The correct term for the radiographic study of the urinary system is intravenous pyelogram (IVP).

14. The double-walled membrane lining the abdominopelvic cavity is called the _____.

15. The organs located posteriorly to, or behind, the serous membrane lining of the abdominopelvic cavity are referred

to as _____.

16. Which one of the following structures helps stabilize and support the small intestine?

A. Omentum   C. Viscera

B. Peritoneum   D. Mesentery

17. Which one of the following structures is a double fold of peritoneum that connects the transverse colon to the greater curvature of the stomach?

A. Mesocolon   C. Greater omentum

B. Lesser omentum   D. Mesentery

18. Match the following structures to the correct location of the peritoneum.

_____ 1. Liver   A. Intraperitoneum

_____ 2. Urinary bladder   B. Retroperitoneum

_____ 3. Kidneys   C. Infraperitoneum

_____ 4. Spleen

_____ 5. Ovaries

_____ 6. Duodenum

_____ 7. Transverse colon

_____ 8. Testes

_____ 9. Adrenal glands

_____ 10. Stomach

_____ 11. Pancreas

_____ 12. Ascending and descending colon

19. For each of the following organs, identify the correct abdominal quadrant in which the organ is found—left upper quadrant (LUQ), left lower quadrant (LLQ), right lower quadrant (RLQ), or right upper quadrant (RUQ).

A. Liver _____

B. Spleen _____

C. Sigmoid colon _____

D. Left colic flexure _____

E. Stomach _____

F. Appendix _____

G. Two-thirds of jejunum _____

20. What is the correct name for the abdominal region found directly in the middle of the abdomen?

A. Epigastric   C. Umbilical

B. Inguinal   D. Pubic

21. Which one of the following abdominal regions contains the rectum?

A. Pubic   D. Epigastric

B. Inguinal   E. Hypochondriac

C. Umbilical   F. Lumbar

22. Identify the bony landmarks in Fig. 3-1.

A. _____

B. _____

C. _____

D. _____

E. _____

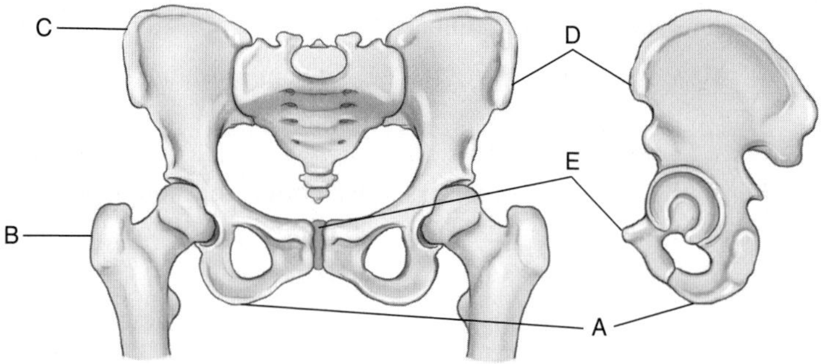

Fig. 3-1. Landmarks of the pelvis.

23. The prominence of the greater trochanter is about the same level of the _____

symphysis pubis, and the lower margins of the ischial tuberosities is about _____ inches (_____ cm) _____

(proximal or distal) to the symphysis pubis.

24. Which topographic landmark corresponds to the inferior margin of the abdomen and is formed by the anterior

junction of the two pelvic bones? _____

25. Which topographic landmark is found at the level of L2-L3? _____

26. The iliac crest is at the level of the _____ vertebra.

27. Identify the labeled parts of the digestive system (Fig. 3-2).

A. _____

B. _____

C. _____

D. _____ valve

E. _____

F. _____

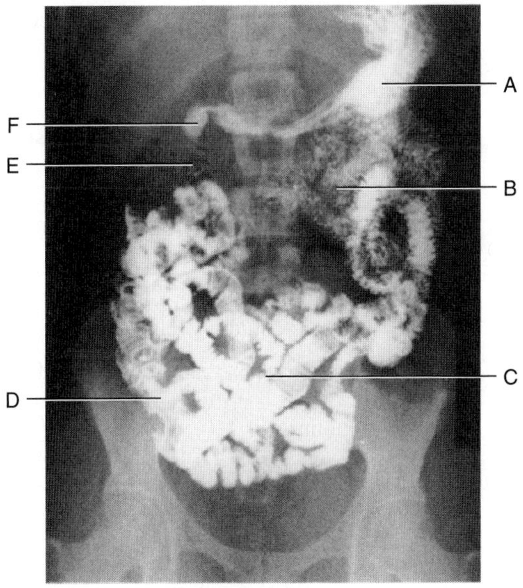

Fig. 3-2. Radiograph of the digestive tract.

28. Identify the labeled structures present on the computed tomography (CT) image (Fig. 3-3).

A. _____

B. _____

C. _____

D. _____

E. _____

F. _____

G. _____

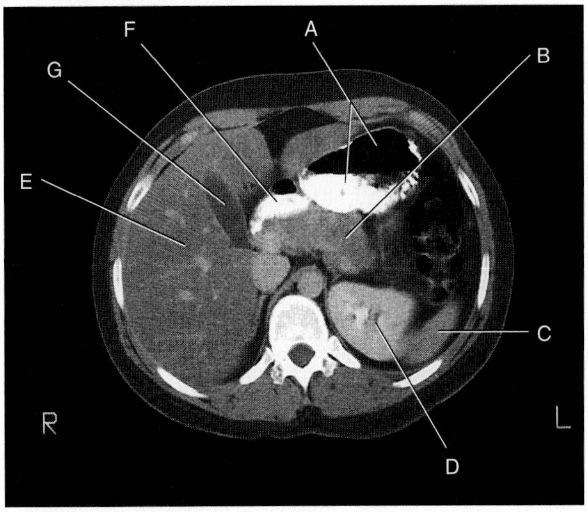

Fig. 3-3. Computed tomography (CT) cross-sectional image of abdomen at the level of L1 or L2.

PART II: RADIOGRAPHIC POSITIONING AND OTHER PATIENT CONSIDERATIONS
REVIEW EXERCISE B: Shielding, Exposure Factors, and Positioning (see textbook pp. 112-114)

1. What are the two causes of voluntary motion?

A. _____   B. _____

2. Voluntary motion can best be prevented by _____ to the patient.

3. What is the primary cause for involuntary motion in the abdomen?

_____

4. What is the best mechanism to control involuntary motion?

_____

5. True/False: Because the liver margin is visible in the right upper quadrant of the abdomen, it is not necessary to place a right or left anatomic side marker on the cassette before exposure.

6. True/False: For an adult abdomen, a collimation margin must be visible on all four sides of the radiograph.

7. Gonadal shielding should *not* be used during abdomen radiography if:

   A. It obscures essential anatomy

   B. The patient requests that it not be used

   C. The technologist does not elect to use it

   D. The patient is 40 years or older

8. Gonadal shielding for _____ may be impossible for studies of the lower abdominopelvic region.

   A. Males

   B. Females

   C. Both males and females

   D. Small children

9. Gonadal shielding for females involves placing the top of the shield at or slightly above the level of the

   _____, with the bottom at the _____.

10. Which one of the following exposure considerations would be most ideal for an AP abdomen of an average-size adult?

    A. 110-120 kV, grid, 40-inch (102-cm) SID

    B. 85-95 kV, grid, 40-inch (102-cm) SID

    C. 70-80 kV, grid, 40-inch (102-cm) SID

    D. 60-70 kV, grid, 40-inch (102-cm) SID

11. Which of the following technical considerations is essential when performing abdomen studies on a young pediatric patient?

    A. Short exposure times

    B. High-speed image receptor

    C. Reduced kV and mAs

    D. All of the above

12. True/False: A radiolucent pad should be placed underneath geriatric patients for added comfort.

13. With the use of iodinated contrast media, _____ is able to distinguish between a simple cyst or tumor of the liver.

    A. Ultrasound

    B. Nuclear medicine

    C. CT

    D. MRI

14. The preferred imaging modality for examining the gallbladder quickly is:

    A. Ultrasound

    B. Nuclear medicine

    C. Barium enema study

    D. MRI

15. _____ is being used to evaluate patients with acute appendicitis.

    A. Ultrasound

    B. Nuclear medicine

    C. CT

    D. MRI

16. Match the following definitions to the correct clinical indication.

_____ 1. Free air or gas in the peritoneal cavity

_____ 2. Inflammatory condition of the colon

_____ 3. Telescoping of a section of bowel into another loop of bowel

_____ 4. Abnormal accumulation of fluid in the peritoneal cavity

_____ 5. Bowel obstruction caused by a lack of intestinal peristalsis

_____ 6. A twisting of a loop of bowel creating an obstruction

_____ 7. Chronic inflammation of the intestinal wall that may result in bowel obstruction

A. Volvulus

B. Adynamic ileus

C. Ascites

D. Ulcerative colitis

E. Pneumoperitoneum

F. Intussusception

G. Crohn's disease

17. Match each of the following radiographic appearances of the abdomen to its corresponding type of pathologic condition.

_____ 1. Distended loops of air-filled small intestine

_____ 2. Air-filled "coiled spring" appearance

_____ 3. General abdominal haziness

_____ 4. Thin crest-shaped radiolucency underneath diaphragm

_____ 5. Deep air-filled mucosal protrusions of colon wall

_____ 6. Large amount of air trapped in sigmoid colon with a tapered narrowing at the site of obstruction

A. Ascites

B. Volvulus

C. Pneumoperitoneum

D. Ulcerative colitis

E. Intussusception

F. Crohn's disease

18. The central ray is centered to the level of the _____ for a supine AP projection of the abdomen.

19. Exposure for an AP projection of the abdomen should be taken on _____ (inspiration or expiration).

20. Rotation can be determined on a KUB radiograph by the loss of symmetric appearance of:

A. _____   C. _____

B. _____   D. _____

21. Which type of body habitus may require two crosswise images to be taken if the entire abdomen is to be included?

_____

22. True/False: A tall asthenic patient may require two 35- × 43-cm (14- × 17-inch) image receptors placed lengthwise if the entire abdomen is to be included.

23. True/False: It is always acceptable during KUB imaging practice to indicate the side of the body with a digital marker.

24. Why is it recommended to take abdominal radiographs at the end of patient expiration?

_____

25. Which one of the following abdominal structures is not visible on a properly exposed KUB?

    A. Kidneys   C. Pancreas

    B. Margin of liver processes   D. Lumbar transverse processes

26. Why may the PA projection of a KUB generally be less desirable than the AP projection?

_____

27. Which decubitus position of the abdomen best demonstrates intraperitoneal air in the abdomen?

_____

28. Why should a patient be placed in the decubitus position for a minimum of 5 minutes before exposure?

_____

29. Which decubitus position best demonstrates possible aneurysms, calcifications of the aorta, or umbilical hernias?

_____

30. Which projection best demonstrates a possible aortic aneurysm in the prevertebral region of the abdomen?

_____

31. List the projections commonly performed for an acute abdominal series or three-way abdomen series.

    A. _____   B. _____   C. _____

32. Which projection of the three-way acute abdominal series best demonstrates free air under the diaphragm?

_____

33. Which positioning routine should be used for an acute abdominal series if the patient is too ill to stand?

_____

34. Which one of the following projections requires a kV setting of 110 to 125?

    A. Erect abdomen for ascites

    B. Supine abdomen for intraabdominal mass

    C. PA, erect chest for free air under diaphragm

    D. Dorsal decubitus abdomen for calcified aorta

35. To ensure the diaphragm is included on an erect abdomen projection, the central ray should be at the level of

_____, which places the top of the 35- × 43-cm (14- × 17-inch) IR at the level of

the _____.

36. What is the recommended overlap when using two crosswise images for an AP projection of a supine abdomen of

a broad hypersthenic-type patient? _____

37. What scale of contrast is recommended for visualization of the abdominal structures on an abdominal x-ray?

    A. Short scale

    B. Long scale

REVIEW EXERCISE C: Problem Solving for Technical and Positioning Errors

The following radiographic problems involve technical and positioning errors that may lead to substandard images. As you analyze these problems, review your textbook to find solutions to these questions.

Other questions involve situations pertaining to various patient conditions and pathologic findings. If you need more information about a particular pathologic condition, review your textbook or a medical dictionary to learn more about it.

1. A KUB radiograph reveals that the symphysis pubis was cut off along the bottom of the image. Is this an acceptable radiograph? If it is not, how can this problem be prevented during the repeat exposure?

2. A radiograph of an AP projection of an average-size adult abdomen was produced using the following exposure factors: 90 kV, 400 mA, $\frac{1}{10}$ second, grid, and 40-inch (102-cm) SID using film/screen (analog) imaging system. The overall density of the radiograph was acceptable, but the soft tissue structures, such as the psoas muscles and kidneys, were not visible. Which adjustment to the technical considerations will enhance the visibility of these structures on the repeat exposure?

3. A radiographic image of an AP projection of the abdomen demonstrates motion. The following exposure factors were selected: 78 kV, 200 mA, $\frac{2}{10}$ second, grid, and 40-inch (102-cm) SID. The technologist is sure that the patient did not breathe or move during the exposure. What may have caused this blurriness? What can be done to correct this problem on the repeat exposure?

4. A radiograph of an AP abdomen reveals the left iliac wing is more narrowed than the right. What specific positioning error caused this?

5. **Situation:** A patient with a possible dynamic ileus enters the emergency room. The patient is able to stand. The physician has ordered an acute abdominal series. What specific positioning routine should be used?

6. **Situation:** A patient with a possible perforated duodenal ulcer enters the emergency room. The ER physician is concerned about the presence of free air in the abdomen. The patient is in severe pain and *cannot* stand. What positioning routine should be used to diagnose this condition?

7. **Situation:** The ER physician suspects a patient has a kidney stone. The patient is sent to the radiology department to confirm the diagnosis. What specific positioning routine would be used to rule out the presence of a kidney stone?

_____

_____

8. **Situation:** A patient in intensive care may have developed intra-abdominal bleeding. The patient is in critical condition and cannot go to the radiology department. The physician has ordered a portable study of the abdomen. Which specific position or projection can be used to determine the extent of the bleeding?

_____

_____

9. **Situation:** A patient with a history of ascites comes to the radiology department. Which one of the following positions best demonstrates this condition?

   A. Erect AP abdomen   C. Supine KUB

   B. Erect PA chest   D. Prone KUB

10. **Situation:** A KUB radiograph reveals that the gonadal shielding is superior to the upper margin of the symphysis pubis. The female patient has a history of kidney stones. What is the next step the technologist should take?

   A. Accept the radiograph because the kidneys were not obscured by the shielding.

   B. Repeat the exposure without using gonadal shielding.

   C. Repeat the exposure only if the patient complains of pain in the lower abdomen.

   D. Repeat the exposure with gonadal shielding, but position it below the symphysis pubis.

11. **Situation:** A hypersthenic patient comes to the radiology department for a KUB. The radiograph reveals that the symphysis pubis is included on the image, but the upper abdomen, including the kidneys, is cut off. What is the next step the technologist should take?

   A. Accept the radiograph.

   B. Repeat the exposure, but expose it during inspiration to force the kidneys lower into the abdomen.

   C. Ask the radiologist whether the upper abdomen really needs to be seen. Repeat only if requested.

   D. Repeat the exposure. Use two 35- × 43-cm (14- × 17-inch) image receptors crosswise to include the entire abdomen.

12. **Situation:** A patient comes from the ER with a large distended abdomen caused by an ileus. The physician suspects that the distention is caused by a large amount of bowel gas that is trapped in the small intestine. The standard analog technique for a KUB on an adult is 76 kV, 30 mAs. Should the technologist change any of these exposure factors for this patient? (AEC is not being used.)

   A. No. Use the standard exposure settings.

   B. Yes. Decrease the milliamperage seconds (mAs).

   C. Yes. Increase the milliamperage seconds (mAs).

   D. Yes. Increase the kilovoltage (kV).

13. **Situation:** A child goes to radiology for an abdomen study. It is possible that he swallowed a coin. The ER physician believes it may be in the upper GI tract. Which of the following routines would best identify the location of the coin?

   A. KUB and left lateral decubitus

   B. Acute abdominal series

   C. KUB and lateral abdomen

   D. Supine and erect KUB

PART III: LABORATORY EXERCISES

You must gain experience in chest positioning before performing the following exams on actual patients. You may gain experience in positioning and radiographic evaluation of these projections by performing exercises using radiographic phantoms and practicing on other students (although you will not be taking actual exposures).

The following suggested activities assume your teaching institution has an energized lab and radiographic phantoms. If not, perform only Laboratory Exercise B, the physical positioning activities. (Check off each step and projection as you complete it.)

Laboratory Exercise A: Energized Laboratory

1. Using the abdominal radiographic phantom, produce a radiograph of:

   _____ KUB

2. Evaluate the KUB radiograph, additional radiographs provided by your instructor, or both for the following criteria:

   _____ Rotation   _____ Part and central ray centering

   _____ Proper exposure factors   _____ Motion

   _____ Collimation   _____ Anatomic side markers

Laboratory Exercise B: Physical Positioning

1. On another person, simulate taking all of the following basic and special projections of the chest. Follow the suggested positioning steps and sequence as listed below and as described in Chapter 3 of your textbook.

   _____ KUB of the abdomen   _____ Dorsal decubitus

   _____ Left lateral decubitus   _____ Acute abdominal series to include: AP supine, AP erect, PA chest

Step 1. General Patient Positioning

_____ Select the size and number of IR needed.

_____ Prepare the radiographic room. Check that the x-ray tube is centered to the center of the IR holder (or the centerline of the table for Bucky exams).

_____ Correctly identify the patient and bring the patient into the room.

_____ Explain to the patient what you will be doing.

_____ Assist the patient to the proper place and position for the first radiograph.

Step 2. Measuring Part Thickness

_____ Measure the body part being radiographed and set the correct exposure factors (technique). (If using an AEC system, select the correct chamber cells on the control panel.)

Step 3. Part Positioning

_____ Align and center the body part to the central ray or vice versa. For Bucky exams on a table, move the patient and tabletop together as needed (with floating type of tabletop). (*Note:* In cases in which the correct central ray position is of primary importance, the central ray icon is included in the textbook on the appropriate positioning page.)

Step 4. IR Centering

_____ After the part has been centered to the central ray, the IR is also centered to the central ray.

Additional Steps or Actions

_____ 1. Collimate accurately to include only the area of interest.

_____ 2. Place the correct marker within the exposure field (so that you do not superimpose pertinent anatomic structures).

_____ 3. Restrain or provide support for the body part to prevent motion.

_____ 4. Use contact lead shielding as needed.

_____ 5. Give clear breathing instructions and make the exposure while watching the patient through the console window.

This self-test should be taken only after completing all of the readings, review exercises, and laboratory activities for a particular section. The self-test is divided into six sections. The purpose of this test is not only to provide a good learning exercise but also to serve as a strong indicator of what your final unit evaluation exam will cover. It is strongly suggested that if you do not receive at least a 90% to 95% grade on each self-test, you should review those areas in which you missed questions before going to your instructor for the final unit evaluation exam.

1. The double-walled membrane lining the abdominal cavity is called the:

    A. Greater omentum   C. Lesser omentum

    B. Mesentery   D. Peritoneum

2. Which of the following soft tissue structures are seen on a properly exposed KUB?

    A. Spleen   C. Psoas muscles

    B. Pancreas   D. Stomach

3. The first portion of the small intestine is called the:

    A. Duodenum   C. Jejunum

    B. Ileum   D. Pylorus

4. At the junction of the small and large intestine is the:

    A. Sigmoid colon   C. Ileocecal valve

    B. Rectum   D. Ascending colon

5. Match the correct answers to the structures labeled on Fig. 3-4.

    _____ 1.   A. Sigmoid colon

    _____ 2.   B. Liver

    _____ 3.   C. Jejunum

    _____ 4.   D. Oral cavity

    _____ 5.   E. Spleen

    _____ 6.   F. Stomach

    _____ 7.   G. Esophagus

    _____ 8.   H. Oropharynx

    _____ 9.   I. Pancreas

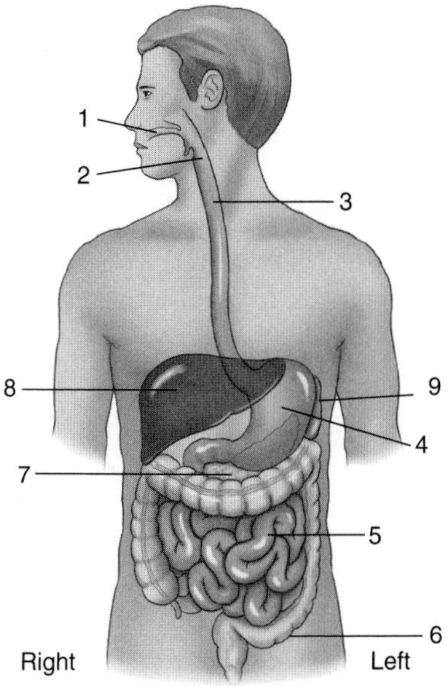

Fig. 3-4. Digestive tract and surrounding structures.

6. Which one of the following is not an accessory organ of digestion?

   A. Liver   C. Pancreas

   B. Gallbladder   D. Kidney

7. The kidneys are connected to the bladder by way of the:

   A. Urethra   C. Ureter

   B. Renal artery   D. Renal vein

8. Which structure stores and releases bile?

   A. Liver   C. Pancreas

   B. Spleen   D. Gallbladder

9. Which one of the following structures connects the small intestine to the posterior abdominal wall?

   A. Greater omentum   C. Lesser omentum

   B. Peritoneum   D. Mesentery

10. For each of the following organs, identify the correct abdominal quadrant(s) in which the organ would be found on an average sthenic patient—left upper quadrant (LUQ), left lower quadrant (LLQ), right lower quadrant (RLQ), or right upper quadrant (RUQ) (*Note:* Some organs may be found in more than one quadrant.)

    A. Cecum _____

    B. Liver _____

    C. Spleen _____

    D. Stomach _____

    E. Right colic flexure _____

    F. Sigmoid colon _____

    G. Appendix _____

    H. Pancreas _____

    I. Gallbladder _____

11. Which region of the abdomen contains the spleen?

    A. Epigastric   C. Left hypochondriac

    B. Umbilical   D. Left inguinal

12. Match the following structures to the correct compartment of the peritoneum.

    _____ 1. Cecum   A. Intraperitoneum

    _____ 2. Jejunum   B. Retroperitoneum

    _____ 3. Ascending colon   C. Infraperitoneum

    _____ 4. Liver

    _____ 5. Adrenal glands

    _____ 6. Gallbladder

    _____ 7. Ovaries

    _____ 8. Duodenum

    _____ 9. Urinary bladder

    _____ 10. Pancreas

13. The xiphoid process corresponds with which vertebral level?

A. T9-T10   C. L2-L3

B. L4-L5   D. T4-T5

14. Identify the topographic positioning landmarks as labeled on Figs. 3-5 and 3-6.

    _____ 1. Iliac crest

    _____ 2. Ischial tuberosity

    _____ 3. Xiphoid process

    _____ 4. Pubic symphysis

    _____ 5. Greater trochanter

    _____ 6. Lower costal margin

    _____ 7. Anterior superior iliac spine (ASIS)

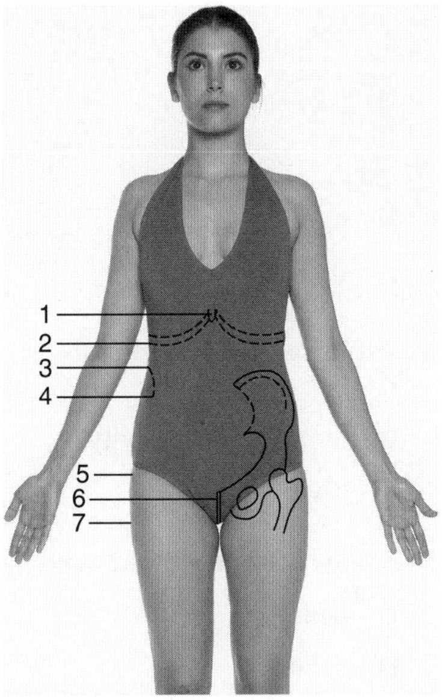

Fig. 3-5. Anterior surface landmarks. 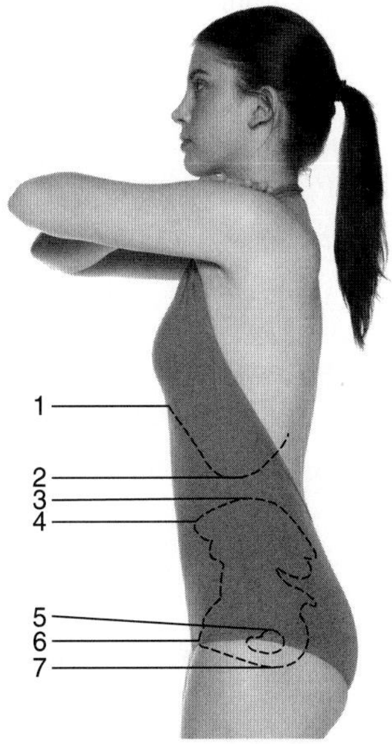   **Fig. 3-6.** Lateral surface landmarks.

15. To identify the inferior margin of the abdomen, the technologist can palpate the symphysis pubis or:

A. Iliac crest   C. ASIS

B. Greater trochanter   D. Ischial tuberosity

16. An important anatomic landmark that is commonly used to locate the center of the abdomen is the:

    A. Iliac crest   C. ASIS

    B. Greater trochanter   D. Ischial tuberosity

17. Which one of the following factors best controls the involuntary motion of a young, pediatric patient during abdominal radiography?

    A. Short exposure time

    B. High kV (100-125)

    C. Clear, concise breathing instructions

    D. Use of compression band across the abdomen

18. An abnormal accumulation of fluid in the abdominal cavity is called:

    A. Ileus   C. Volvulus

    B. Ulcerative colitis   D. Ascites

19. Another term describing a nonmechanical bowel obstruction is:

    A. Pneumoperitoneum   C. Ascites

    B. Paralytic ileus   D. Intussusception

20. The telescoping of a section of bowel into another loop is called:

    A. Intussusception   C. Volvulus

    B. Ascites   D. Ulcerative colitis

21. A chronic disease involving inflammation of the large intestine is:

    A. Ascites   C. Crohn's disease

    B. Volvulus   D. Ulcerative colitis

22. Free air or gas in the peritoneal cavity is:

    A. Pneumothorax   C. Pneumoperitoneum

    B. Ileus   D. Volvulus

23. Free air in the intraabdominal cavity rises to the level of the _____ in a patient who is in the erect position.

    A. Greater omentum   C. Intraperitoneal cavity

    B. Diaphragm   D. Liver

24. Which one of the following conditions is demonstrated radiographically as general abdominal haziness?

    A. Pneumoperitoneum   C. Ileus

    B. Ascites   D. olvulus

25. Which one of the following conditions is demonstrated radiographically as distended, air-filled loops of the small bowel?

    A. Ascites   C. Pneumoperitoneum

    B. Ulcerative colitis   D. Ileus

26. Identify the structures labeled on this AP KUB radiograph (Fig. 3-7).

A. _____

B. _____

C. _____

D. _____

E. _____

F. _____

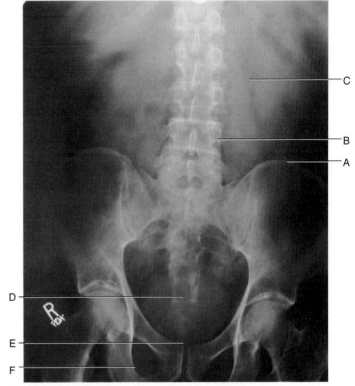

Fig. 3-7. Anteroposterior (AP) KUB radiograph.

27. Identify the organs or structures labeled on this computed tomography (CT) image (Fig. 3-8) at the level of L1-L2.

A. _____

B. _____

C. _____

D. _____

E. _____

F. _____

G. _____

H. _____

I. _____

J. _____

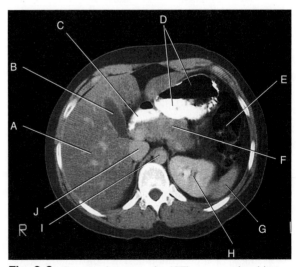

Fig. 3-8. Computed tomography (CT) cross-sectional image at the level of L1-L2.

28. Which one of the following sets of exposure factors would be the best for abdominal radiography (for an average-size adult)?

    A. 110 kV, grid, 40-inch (102-cm) SID

    B. 78 kV, grid, 40-inch (102-cm) SID

    C. 78 kV, grid, 72-inch (183-cm) SID

    D. 65 kV, grid, 40-inch (102-cm) SID

29. A radiograph of an AP projection of the abdomen reveals that the right iliac wing is wider than the left. What type of positioning error was involved?

    A. Rotation toward the left   C. Rotation toward the right

    B. Tilt to the left   D. Tilt to the right

30. Most abdominal projections are taken:

    A. Upon expiration   C. Upon inspiration

    B. During shallow breathing   D. During deep breathing

31. A KUB radiograph on a large hypersthenic patient reveals that the entire abdomen is not included on the 35- × 43-cm (14- × 17-inch) IR. What can be done to correct this on the repeat radiograph?

    A. Use two cassettes placed lengthwise.   C. Expose during deep inspiration.

    B. Use two cassettes placed crosswise.   D. Perform KUB with patient in the erect position.

32. What is the minimum amount of time a patient should be upright before taking a projection to demonstrate intra-abdominal free air?

    A. 20 minutes   C. 2 minutes

    B. 30 minutes   D. 5 minutes

33. If the posteroanterior (PA) chest projection is *not* performed for the acute abdomen series, centering for the erect abdomen projection *must* include the:

    A. Inferior liver margin   C. Entire kidneys

    B. Diaphragm   D. Bladder

34. Which specific decubitus position of the abdomen should be used in an acute abdomen series if the patient cannot stand?

    A. Left lateral decubitus   C. Right lateral decubitus

    B. Dorsal decubitus   D. Ventral decubitus

35. **Situation:** A patient with a possible ileus enters the emergency room. The physician orders an acute abdominal series. The patient can stand. Which specific position best demonstrates air/fluid levels in the abdomen?

    A. AP supine abdomen   C. Dorsal decubitus

    B. Right lateral decubitus   D. AP erect abdomen

36. **Situation:** A patient with a possible perforated bowel caused by trauma enters the ER. The patient is unable to stand. Which projection best demonstrates any possible free air within the abdomen?

    A. Dorsal decubitus   C. AP supine abdomen

    B. Left lateral decubitus   D. Right lateral decubitus

37. **Situation:** A patient with a clinical history of a possible umbilical hernia comes to the radiology department. The KUB is inconclusive. Which additional projection can be taken to help confirm the diagnosis?

    A. AP erect abdomen   C. Dorsal decubitus

    B. Left lateral decubitus   D. Ventral decubitus

38. **Situation:** A patient comes to the radiology department with a clinical history of pneumoperitoneum. The patient is able to stand. Which one of the following projections best demonstrates this condition?

    A. AP supine abdomen   C. Dorsal decubitus

    B. AP erect abdomen   D. Left lateral decubitus

39. **Situation:** A patient comes to the radiology department with a clinical history of ascites. The patient is unable to stand or sit erect. Which one of the following projections best demonstrates this condition?

    A. AP supine abdomen   C. Dorsal decubitus

    B. Left lateral decubitus   D. AP supine chest

40. **Situation:** A patient comes in the ER with possible gallstones. The patient is in severe pain. Which of the following imaging modalities or projections provides the quickest method for confirming the presence of gallstones?

    A. Sonography   C. MRI

    B. Acute abdomen series   D. KUB

41. **Situation:** A patient comes into the ER with the history of Crohn's disease. An acute abdomen series is ordered on this patient. Which of the following is the reason for this order?

    A. Verify diagnosis   C. Identify location of gallstones

    B. Identify current inflammation   D. Verify current infection

42. Which one of the following alternative imaging modalities is most effectively used to evaluate GI motility and reflux?

    A. CT   C. Sonography

    B. MRI   D. Nuclear medicine

43. Which one of the following technical factors is essential when using computed radiography (CR) to ensure a high-quality image is produced?

    A. Low kV   C. Large focal spot

    B. 72-inch (183-cm) SID   D. Close collimation

44. For the following critique questions, refer to the textbook, p. 123 (Fig. C3-49) (AP supine KUB).

    A. Which positioning error(s) is (are) visible on this radiograph? (More than one answer may be selected.)

        (a) All essential anatomic structures are not demonstrated.

        (b) CR-to-IR centering is incorrect.

        (c) CR-to-anatomy centering is incorrect.

        (d) Collimation is not evident.

        (e) Exposure factors are incorrect.

        (f) No marker is seen on the radiograph.

        (g) Rotation is toward the right.

        (h) Rotation is toward the left.

B. Which error(s) on this radiograph is (are) considered "repeatable"?

_____

C. Which of the following modifications must be made during the repeat exposure? (More than one answer may be selected.)

    (a) Open up collimation.

    (b) Center CR-to-IR correctly.

    (c) Center CR-to-anatomy correctly.

    (d) Decrease exposure factors.

    (e) Increase exposure factors.

    (f) Place marker on IR before exposure.

    (g) Ensure that ASISs are equal distance from tabletop to eliminate rotation.

45. For the following critique questions, refer to Fig. C3-51 (AP erect abdomen) on p. 123 in your textbook.

    A. Which positioning error(s) is (are) visible on this radiograph? (More than one answer may be selected.)

        (a) All essential anatomic structures are not demonstrated.

        (b) CR-to-IR centering is incorrect.

        (c) Collimation is not evident.

        (d) Exposure factors are incorrect.

        (e) No marker is seen on the radiograph.

        (f) Rotation is toward the right.

        (g) Rotation is toward the left.

    B. Which error(s) on this radiograph is (are) considered "repeatable"?

_____

    C. Which of the following modifications must be made during the repeat exposure? More than one answer may be selected.

        (a) Open up collimation.

        (b) Center CR-to-IR correctly.

        (c) Decrease exposure factors.

        (d) Increase exposure factors.

        (e) Place marker on IR before exposure.

        (f) Ensure that ASISs are equal distance from tabletop to eliminate rotation.

4 Upper Limb

CHAPTER OBJECTIVES

After you have successfully completed the activities in this chapter, you will be able to:

_____ 1. List the total number of bones of the hand and wrist.

_____ 2. Identify specific aspects of the phalanges, metacarpals, and carpal bones.

_____ 3. On drawings and radiographs, identify specific anatomic structures of the hand and wrist.

_____ 4. List and describe the location, size, and shape of each carpal bone of the wrist.

_____ 5. Match specific joints of the hand and wrist according to classification and movement type.

_____ 6. List four specific ligaments of the wrist.

_____ 7. On drawings and radiographs, identify specific fat pads and stripes of the upper limb.

_____ 8. Distinguish between ulnar and radial deviation wrist movements.

_____ 9. Identify specific parts of the forearm, elbow, and distal humerus.

_____ 10. On drawings and radiographs, identify specific anatomic structures of the forearm, elbow, and distal humerus.

_____ 11. List the technical factors commonly used for upper limb radiography.

_____ 12. Match specific clinical indications of the upper limb to their correct definition.

_____ 13. Match specific clinical indications of the upper limb to their correct radiographic appearance.

_____ 14. For select pathologic conditions of the upper limb, indicate whether manual exposure factors should be increased or decreased or remain the same.

_____ 15. Identify the correct central ray placement, part position, and radiographic criteria for specific positions of the fingers, thumb, hand, wrist, forearm, and elbow.

_____ 16. Identify which structures are best seen with each routine and special projection of the upper limb.

_____ 17. Based on clinical situations, describe the preferred positioning routine to assist the physician with the diagnosis of a specific condition or disease process.

_____ 18. Identify and apply the exposure conversion chart for various sizes of plaster and fiberglass casts.

_____ 19. List the three radiographic criteria for a true lateral elbow position.

_____ 20. Given various hypothetic situations, identify the correct modification of a position, exposure factors, or both to improve the radiographic image.

_____ 21. Given various hypothetic situations, identify the correct position for a specific clinical indication or pathologic feature.

_____ 22. Given radiographs of specific upper limb positions, identify specific positioning and exposure factor errors.

POSITIONING AND RADIOGRAPHIC CRITIQUE

_____ 1. Using another student as a model, practice routine and special projections of the upper limb.

_____ 2. Using a hand and elbow radiographic phantom, produce satisfactory radiographs of the hand, thumb, wrist, and elbow (if equipment is available).

_____ 3. Critique and evaluate upper limb radiographs based on the five divisions of radiographic criteria: (1) anatomy demonstrated, (2) position, (3) collimation and central ray, (4) exposure, and (5) anatomic side markers.

_____ 4. Distinguish between acceptable and unacceptable upper limb radiographs based on exposure factors, motion, collimation, positioning, or other errors.

LEARNING EXERCISES

Complete the following review exercises after reading the associated pages in the textbook as indicated by each exercise. Answers to each review exercise are given at the end of the review exercises.

PART I: RADIOGRAPHIC ANATOMY
REVIEW EXERCISE A: Anatomy of the Hand and Wrist (see textbook pp. 126-129)

1. Identify the number of bones for each of the following.

   A. Phalanges (fingers and thumb) _____   C. Carpals (wrist) _____

   B. Metacarpals (palm) _____   D. Total _____

2. The two portions of the thumb (first digit) are the:

   A. _____

   B. _____

3. The three portions of each finger (second through fifth digits) are the:

   A. _____

   B. _____

   C. _____

4. The three parts of each phalanx, starting distally, are the:

   A. _____   B. _____   C. _____

5. List the three parts of each metacarpal, starting proximally:

   A. _____   B. _____   C. _____

6. The name of the joint between the proximal and distal phalanges of the first digit is the

   _____.

7. The joints between metacarpals and phalanges are the _____.

8. Fill in the names and parts of the following bones and joints of the right hand as labeled on Fig. 4-1. Include abbreviations for joints if applicable.

A. _____

B. _____

C. _____

D. _____

E. _____

F. _____

G. _____

H. _____

I. _____

J. _____

K. _____

L. _____

M. _____

N. _____

O. _____

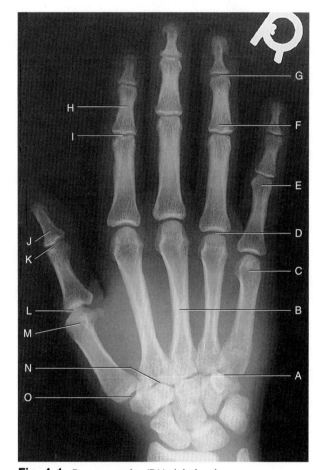

Fig. 4-1. Posteroanterior (PA) right hand.

9. Match each of the carpal bones labeled in Figs. 4-2 and 4-3 with its correct name.

_____ A.   1. Lunate

_____ B.   2. Hamate

_____ C.   3. Trapezium

_____ D.   4. Pisiform

_____ E.   5. Triquetrum

_____ F.   6. Trapezoid

_____ G.   7. Capitate

_____ H.   8. Scaphoid

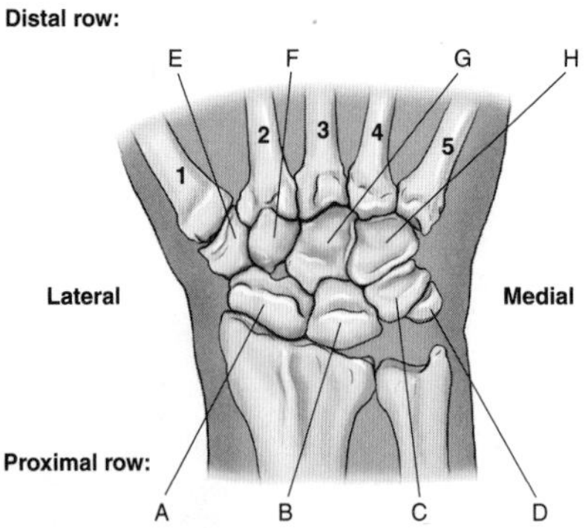

Fig. 4-2. Posterior view of wrist.

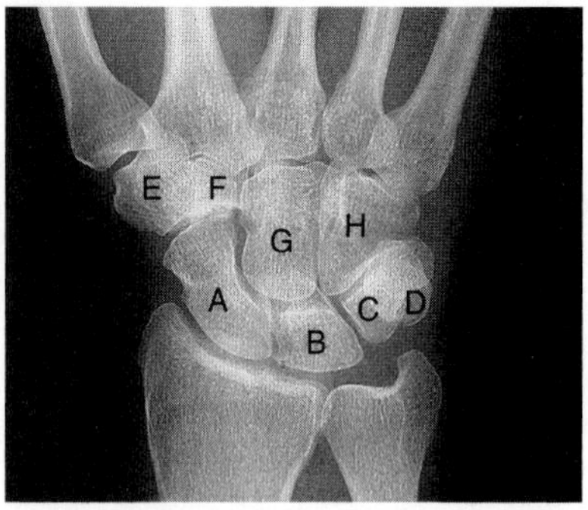

Fig. 4-3. Posteroanterior (PA) wrist.

10. Which is the largest of the carpal bones? _____

11. What is the name of the hooklike process extending anteriorly from the hamate? _____

12. Which is the most commonly fractured carpal bone? _____

13. List one of the mnemonics given in the textbook that uses the first letter of each of the preferred terms of the eight

    carpal bones. _____

14. Match each of the structures labeled on Figs. 4-4 and 4-5 with the correct term.

_____ A.   1. Capitate

_____ B.   2. Scaphoid

_____ C.   3. Base of first metacarpal

_____ D.   4. Pisiform

_____ E.   5. Trapezoid

_____ F.   6. Hamulus (hamular process)

_____ G.   7. Triquetrum

_____ H.   8. Hamate

_____ I.   9. Trapezium

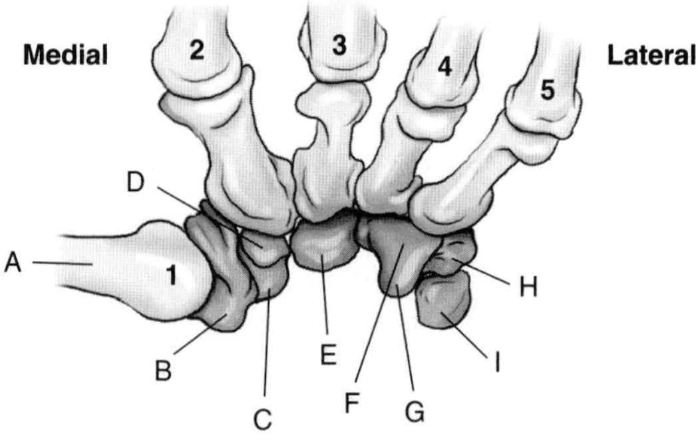

Fig. 4-4. Carpal canal, inferosuperior projection.

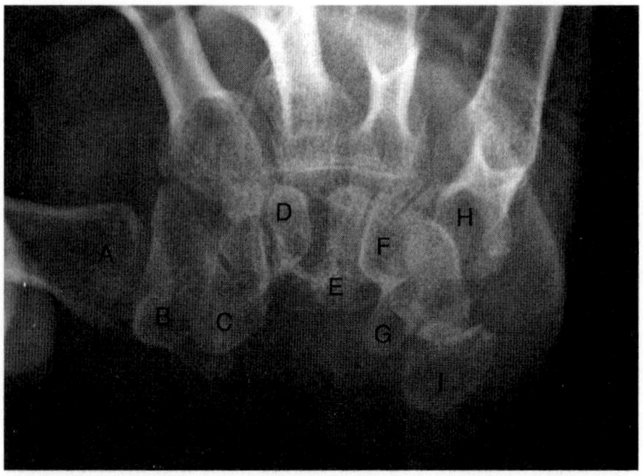

Fig. 4-5. Carpal canal, inferosuperior projection.

15. Identify the carpals and other structures labeled on Fig. 4-6.

A. _____

B. _____

C. _____

D. _____

E. _____

F. _____

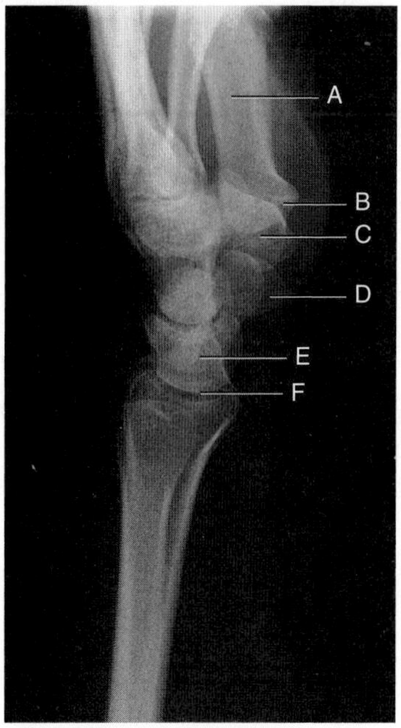

Fig. 4-6. Lateral wrist.

REVIEW EXERCISE B: Anatomy of the Forearm, Elbow, and Distal Humerus (see textbook pp. 130-132)

1. A. In the anatomic position, which of the bones of the forearm is located on the lateral (thumb) side?

   _____

   B. Which is on the medial side? _____

2. Indicate whether the following structures are part of the radius (R), ulna (U), or distal humerus (H) by listing the appropriate letter next to the structure.

   _____ A. Trochlear notch   _____ E. Coronoid tubercle

   _____ B. Radial notch   _____ F. Coronoid process

   _____ C. Olecranon fossa   _____ G. Olecranon process

   _____ D. Trochlea   _____ H. Coronoid fossa

3. Which joint permits the forearm to rotate during pronation? _____

4. A. The articular portion of the medial aspect of the distal humerus is called the

   _____.

   B. The similar structure found on the lateral aspect of the distal humerus is called the

   _____.

5. The deep depression located on the posterior aspect of the distal humerus is the

   _____.

6. The criteria for evaluating a true lateral position of the elbow are the appearance of three concentric arcs (Fig. 4-7). These arcs include:

A. The first and smallest of the arcs:

   _____

B. The intermediate double arc, consisting of the outer ridges of:

   (a) The smaller arc: _____

   (b) The larger arc: _____

C. The third arc, which is part of the ulna:

   _____

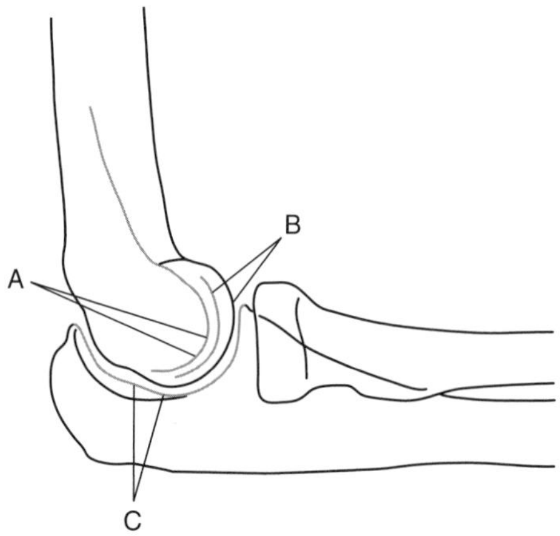

Fig. 4-7. The lateral elbow. Three concentric circles.

7. Match the following articulations with the correct joint movement types.

   _____ A. Interphalangeal   1. Ginglymus

   _____ B. Carpometacarpal of first digit   2. Ellipsoidal

   _____ C. Elbow joint (humeroulnar and humeroradial)   3. Trochoidal

   _____ D. Metacarpophalangeal of second to fifth digits   4. Plane

   _____ E. Radiocarpal   5. Sellar

   _____ F. Intercarpal

   _____ G. Elbow joint

   _____ H. Proximal radioulnar joint

8. Ellipsoidal joints are classified as freely movable, or _____, and allow movement

   in _____ directions.

9. True/False: In addition to the ulnar and radial collateral ligaments, the following five additional ligaments are also important in stability of the wrist joint.

   A. Dorsal radiocarpal   D. Scapulolunate

   B. Palmar radiocarpal   E. Lunotriquetral

   C. Triangular fibrocartilage complex (TFCC)

10. Which ligament of the wrist extends from the styloid process of the radius to the lateral aspect of the scaphoid and

    trapezium bones? _____

11. What is the name of the two special turning or bending positions of the hand and wrist that demonstrate medial and lateral aspects of the carpal region?

     A. _____   B. _____

12. Of the two positions listed in the previous question, which one is most commonly performed to detect a fracture

     of the scaphoid bone? _____

13. How does the forearm appear radiographically if pronated for a posteroanterior (PA) projection?

     _____

14. The two important fat stripes or bands around the wrist joint are the:

     A. _____   B. _____

15. The fat pads around the elbow joint are valuable diagnostic indicators if the following three technical/positioning requirements are met with the lateral position.

     A. _____

     B. _____

     C. _____

16. True/False: If the posterior fat pad of the elbow is not visible radiographically, it suggests that a nonobvious radial head or neck fracture is present.

17. True/False: Excessive kV (analog imaging) may obscure the visibility of a fat pad.

18. True/False: Trauma or infection makes the anterior fat pad more difficult to see on a lateral elbow radiograph.

19. Which routine projections best demonstrate the scaphoid fat pad?

     _____

20. Which routine projection best demonstrates the pronator fat stripe?

     _____

21. Identify the parts labeled on Figs. 4-8 and 4-9.

A. _____

B. _____

C. _____

D. _____

E. _____

F. _____

G. _____

H. _____

I. _____

J. _____

K. _____

L. _____

M. _____

N.* _____

O.* _____

P.* _____

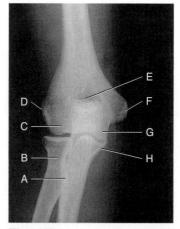

Fig. 4-8. Anteroposterior (AP) elbow.

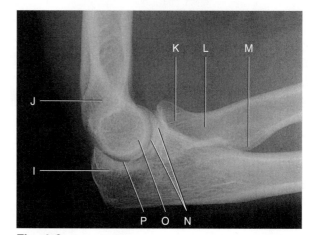

Fig. 4-9. Lateral elbow.

_____

*Hint: These are concentric arcs as evidence of a true lateral position.

22. Identify the parts labeled on Figs. 4-10 and 4-11.

A. _____

B. _____

C. _____

D. _____

E. _____

F. _____

G. _____

H. _____

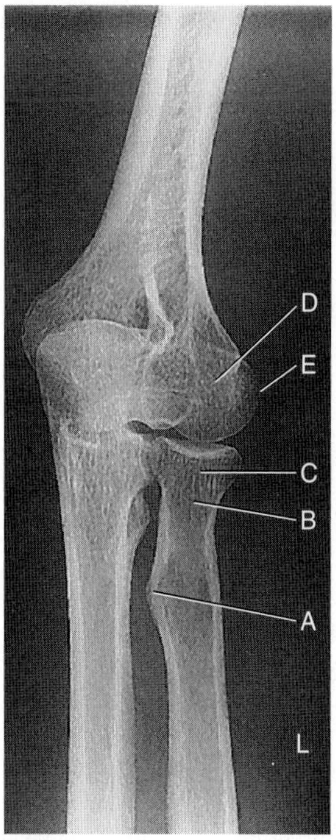

Fig. 4-10. Lateral (external) rotation of the elbow.

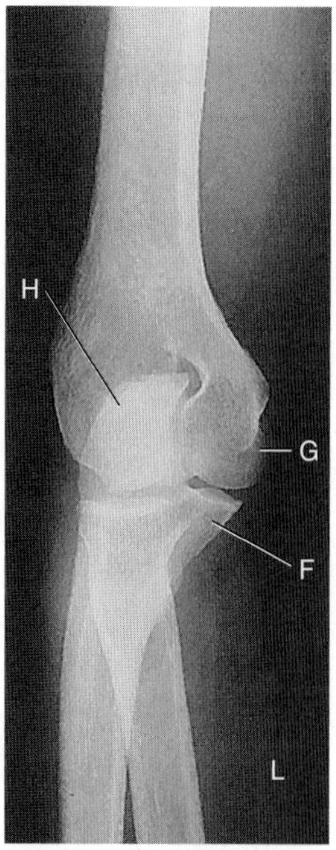

Fig. 4-11. Medial (internal) rotation of the elbow.

PART II: RADIOGRAPHIC POSITIONING
REVIEW EXERCISE C: Positioning of the Fingers, Thumb, Hand, and Wrist (see textbook pp. 141-161)

1. Identify the following technical factors most commonly used for upper limb radiography.

A. kV range (analog and digital): _____

B. Long or short exposure time: _____

C. Large or small focal spot: _____

D. Most common minimum source image receptor distance (SID): _____

E. Grids are used if the body part measures greater than _____ cm.

F. Type of intensification screens most commonly used for analog imaging: _____

G. Small to medium dry plaster casts: Increase _____ kV.

H. Large plaster casts: Increase _____ kV.

I. Fiberglass casts: Increase _____ kV.

J. Correctly exposed radiographs: Visualize _____ margins and

_____ markings of all bones.

2. The general rule for collimation for upper limb radiography states: _____.

3. Circle all pertinent factors that help reduce image distortion during upper limb radiography.

   A. kV

   B. 40 to 44 inches (102 to 113 cm) SID

   C. Milliamperage seconds (mAs)

   D. Minimal object image receptor distance (OID)

   E. Correct central ray placement and angulation

   F. Use of small focal spot

4. True/False: Lead (protective) shielding is only required for upper limb studies performed on patients who are child-bearing age or younger.

5. True/False: Guardians of young pediatric patients who are having upper limb studies can be asked to hold their child during the radiographic study.

6. _____ is a radiographic procedure that uses contrast media injected into the joint capsule to visualize soft tissue pathology of the wrist, elbow, and shoulder joints.

7. What is the routine positioning routine for the second through fifth digits of the hand?

   _____

   _____

8. How much of the metacarpals should be included for PA projection of the digits?

   _____

   _____

9. List the two radiographic criteria used to determine whether rotation is present on the PA projection of the digits.

   A. _____

   B. _____

10. Identify which positioning modification(s) should be used for a study of the second digit to reduce distortion for each of the following:

    A. PA oblique projection: _____

    B. Lateral position: _____

11. Where is the central ray centered for a PA oblique projection of the second digit?

    _____

12. Why is it important to keep the affected digit parallel to the image receptor (IR) for the PA oblique and lateral projections?

    A. To prevent distortion of the phalanx   C. To demonstrate small, nondisplaced fractures near the joint

    B. To prevent distortion of the joints   D. All of the above

13. Why is the anteroposterior (AP) projection of the thumb recommended instead of the PA?

    _____

14. Which projection of the thumb is achieved naturally by placing the palmar surface of the hand in contact with the

    cassette? _____

15. Which IR size should be used for a thumb projection? _____

16. A sesamoid bone is frequently found adjacent to the _____ joint of the thumb.

17. True/False: The entire metacarpal and trapezium must be demonstrated on all projections of the thumb.

18. Where is the central ray centered for an AP projection of the thumb?

    A. First interphalangeal (IP) joint   C. First metacarpophalangeal (MCP) joint

    B. Midaspect of proximal phalanx   D. First proximal interphalangeal (PIP) joint

19. A Bennett's fracture involves:

    A. Base of first metacarpal   C. Scaphoid bone

    B. Trapezium bone   D. Fracture extending through first IP joint

20. A. Which special positioning method can be performed to demonstrate a Bennett's fracture?

    _____

    B. What degree of central ray angulation is required for this projection? _____

21. Where is the central ray centered for a PA projection of the hand?

    A. Third MCP joint   C. Second MCP joint

    B. Midaspect of third metacarpal   D. Third PIP joint

22. A minimum of _____ inch(es) (_____ cm) of the forearm should be included radiographically for a PA projection of the hand.

23. True/False: Slight superimposition of the distal third, fourth, and fifth metacarpals may occur with a well-positioned PA oblique projection of the hand.

24. Which preferred lateral position of the hand best demonstrates the phalanges without excessive superimposition?

    _____

25. Which lateral projection of the hand best demonstrates a possible foreign body in the palm of the hand?

    _____

26. What is the proper name for the position referred to as the "ball-catcher's position"?

    _____

27. The "ball-catcher's position" is commonly used to evaluate for early signs of:

    A. Osteoporosis   C. Osteopetrosis

    B. Osteomyelitis   D. Rheumatoid arthritis

28. The elbow generally should be flexed _____° for the routine positions of the wrist.

29. How much rotation is required for an oblique projection of the wrist?

_____

30. Which alternative projection to the routine PA wrist best demonstrates the intercarpal joint spaces and wrist joint?

_____

31. Which positioning error is involved if a majority of the carpal bones are superimposed in a PA oblique wrist

    projection? _____

32. Which one of the following fractures is not demonstrated in a wrist routine?

    A. Barton's   C. Smith's

    B. Pott's   D. Colles'

33. During the PA axial scaphoid projection with central ray angle and ulnar flexion, the central ray must be angled

    _____° _____ (**distally** or **proximally**).

34. How much are the hand and wrist elevated from the IR for the modified Stecher method?

    A. None   C. 20°

    B. 10°   D. 15°

35. How much central ray angulation to the long axis of the hand is required for the carpal canal (tunnel) projection?

_____

36. Which special projection of the wrist best demonstrates the interspaces on the ulnar side of the wrist between the

    lunate, triquetrum, pisiform, and hamate bones? _____

37. Which special projection of the wrist helps rule out abnormal calcifications in the carpal sulcus?

_____

38. How much central ray angulation from the long axis of the forearm is required for the carpal bridge (tangential)

    projection? _____

39. The hand and wrist form a _____° angle to the forearm with the carpal bridge (tangential) projection.

REVIEW EXERCISE D: Clinical Features of the Fingers, Thumb, Hand, and Wrist (see textbook pp. 138-139)

1. List the correct pathology term for each of the following definitions.

   A. _____ Fracture and dislocation of the posterior lip of the distal radius

   B. _____ Most common type of primary malignant tumor occurring in bone

   C. _____ Reduction in the quantity of bone or atrophy of skeletal tissue

   D. _____ Sprain or tear of the ulnar collateral ligament

   E. _____ An abnormality of the cartilage affecting long bones

   F. _____ Transverse fracture extending through the distal aspect of the metacarpal neck, most often the fifth metacarpal

   G. _____ Hereditary condition marked by abnormally dense bone

   H. _____ Transverse fracture of the distal radius with posterior displacement of the distal fragment

2. Match the clinical indication or disease to its radiographic appearance.

   _____ A. Narrowing of joint space with periosteal growths on the joint margins   1. Osteomyelitis

   _____ B. Fluid-filled joint space with possible calcification   2. Bursitis

   _____ C. Possible calcification in the carpal sulcus   3. Carpal tunnel syndrome

   _____ D. Soft tissue swelling and loss of fat-pad detail visibility   4. Osteoarthritis

   _____ E. Mixed areas of sclerotic and cortical thickening along with radiolucent lesions   5. Osteopetrosis

3. For the following types of pathologic conditions, indicate whether the manual exposure factors should be increased (+), decreased (−), or remain the same (0) as compared with the manual exposure factors.

   _____ Advanced Paget's disease   _____ Osteoporosis

   _____ Joint effusion   _____ Osteopetrosis

   _____ Advanced rheumatoid arthritis   _____ Bursitis

REVIEW EXERCISE E: Positioning of the Forearm, Elbow, and Humerus (see textbook pp. 162-171)

1. Which routine projections are required for a study of the forearm? _____

2. True/False: For a forearm study, the technologist needs to include only the joint closest to the site of the injury.

3. To properly position the patient for an AP projection of the elbow, the epicondyles must be

   _____ to the IR.

4. If the patient cannot fully extend the elbow for the AP projection, what alternative projection(s) should be

   performed? _____

5. Which routine projection of the elbow best demonstrates the radial head, neck, and tuberosity with slight (if any)

   superimposition of the ulna? _____

6. True/False: Lead (gonadal) shielding is not required for upper limb radiographs if the patient can sit upright for these exams.

7. Which projection of the elbow best demonstrates the coronoid process in profile?

   _____

8. The best position to evaluate the posterior fat pads of the elbow joint is

   _____.

9. Which special projection(s) of the elbow should be performed instead of the routine AP if the patient's elbow is tightly flexed and cannot be extended at all?

   _____

10. How much is the upper limb rotated for a lateral (rotation) oblique projection of the elbow?

    _____

11. How much and in which direction should the central ray be angled for the trauma axial lateral projection (Coyle method) involving the radial head?

    _____

12. How much and in which direction should the central ray be angled for the trauma axial lateral projection (Coyle method) involving the coronoid process?

    _____

13. What is the amount of elbow flexion required for the trauma lateral projection (Coyle method) to demonstrate the

    coronoid process? _____

14. What is the only difference among the four radial head lateral projections of the elbow?

    _____

REVIEW EXERCISE F: Problem Solving for Technical and Positioning Errors

The following radiographic problems involve technical and positioning errors that may lead to substandard images. As you analyze these problems, review your textbook to find solutions to these questions.

Other questions involve situations pertaining to various patient conditions and clinical indications. If you need more information about a particular pathologic condition, review your textbook or a medical dictionary to learn more about it.

1. A three-projection study of the hand was taken using the following analog exposure factors: 64 kV, 1000 mA, $\frac{1}{100}$ second, large focal spot, 36-inch (92-cm) SID, and high-speed screens. Which of these factors should be changed on future hand studies to produce more optimal images?

   _____

2. A radiograph of a PA projection of the second digit reveals that the phalanges are not symmetric on both sides of the bony shafts. Which specific positioning error is involved?

   _____

3. A radiograph of a PA oblique projection of the hand reveals that the fourth and fifth metacarpals are superimposed. Which specific positioning error is involved?

_____

4. In a radiographic study of the forearm, the proximal radius crossed over the ulna in the frontal projection. Which specific positioning error led to this radiographic outcome?

_____

5. A PA axial scaphoid projection of the wrist using a 15° distal central ray angle and ulnar flexion was performed. The resultant radiograph reveals that the scaphoid bone is foreshortened. How must this projection be modified to produce a more diagnostic image of the scaphoid?

_____

6. A radiograph of an AP elbow projection reveals considerable superimposition between the proximal radius and ulna. Which specific positioning error is involved?

_____

7. A routine radiograph of an AP oblique elbow with lateral rotation reveals that the radial tuberosity is superimposed on the ulna. In what way must this position be modified during the repeat exposure?

_____

8. A radiograph of a lateral projection of the elbow reveals that the humeral epicondyles are not superimposed and the trochlear notch is not clearly demonstrated. Which specific type of positioning error is involved?

_____

9. **Situation:** A patient with a possible fracture of the radial head enters the emergency room. When the technologist attempts to place the arm in the AP oblique-lateral rotation position, the patient is unable to extend or rotate the elbow laterally. Which other positions can be used to demonstrate the radial head and neck without superimposition on the proximal ulna?

_____

10. **Situation:** A patient with a metallic foreign body in the palm of the hand enters the emergency room. Which specific positions should be used to locate the foreign body?

_____

11. **Situation:** A patient with a trauma injury enters the ER with an evident Colles' fracture. Which positioning routine should be used to determine the extent of the injury?

_____

12. **Situation:** A patient with a dislocated elbow enters the ER. The patient has the elbow tightly flexed and is careful not to move it. Which specific positioning routine can be used to determine the extent of the injury?

_____

13. **Situation:** A patient with a possible fracture of the trapezium enters the ER. The routine projections do not clearly demonstrate a possible fracture. Which other special projection can be taken?

_____

14. **Situation:** A patient with a history of carpal tunnel syndrome comes to the radiology department. The orthopedic physician suspects that bony changes in the carpal sulcus may be causing compression of the median nerve. Which special projection best demonstrates this region of the wrist?

_____

15. **Situation:** A patient comes to the radiology department for a hand series to evaluate early evidence of rheumatoid arthritis. Which special position can be used in addition to the routine hand projections to evaluate this patient?

_____

16. **Situation:** A patient is referred to radiology with a possible injury to the ulnar collateral ligament. The patient complains of pain near the first MCP joint. Initial radiographs of the hand do not indicate any fracture or dislocation. Which special projection can be performed to rule out an injury to the ulnar collateral ligament?

_____

17. **Situation:** A patient enters the ER with a possible foreign body in the dorsal aspect of the wrist. Initial wrist radiographs are inconclusive in demonstrating the location of the foreign body. What additional projection can be performed to demonstrate this region of the wrist?

_____

18. **Situation:** A patient has a routine elbow series performed. The AP projection indicates a possible deformity or fracture of the coronoid process. However, the patient is unable to pronate the upper limb for the AP oblique-medial rotation projection because of an arthritic condition. What other projection could be performed to demonstrate the coronoid process?

_____

REVIEW EXERCISE G: Critique Radiographs of the Upper Limb (see textbook p. 172)

The following questions relate to the radiographs found at the end of Chapter 4 in the textbook. Evaluate these radiographs for the radiographic criteria categories (A through F) that follow. Describe the corrections needed to improve the overall image. The major, or "repeatable," errors are specific errors that indicate the need for a repeat exposure, regardless of the nature of the other errors.

A. PA hand (Fig. C4-159)

Description of possible error:

1. Anatomy demonstrated: _____

2. Part positioning: _____

3. Collimation and central ray: _____

4. Exposure: _____

5. Anatomic side markers: _____

Repeatable error(s): _____

B. Lateral wrist (Fig. C4-160)

Description of possible error:

    1. Anatomy demonstrated: _____

    2. Part positioning: _____

    3. Collimation and central ray: _____

    4. Exposure: _____

    5. Anatomic side markers: _____

Repeatable error(s): _____

C. AP elbow (Fig. C4-161)

Description of possible error:

    1. Anatomy demonstrated: _____

    2. Part positioning: _____

    3. Collimation and central ray: _____

    4. Exposure: _____

    5. Anatomic side markers: _____

Repeatable error(s): _____

D. PA wrist (Fig. C4-162)

Which special wrist projection is demonstrated on this radiograph?

Description of possible error:

    1. Anatomy demonstrated: _____

    2. Part positioning: _____

    3. Collimation and central ray: _____

    4. Exposure: _____

    5. Anatomic side markers: _____

Repeatable error(s): _____

E. PA forearm (Fig. C4-163)

Description of possible error:

   1. Anatomy demonstrated: _____

   2. Part positioning: _____

   3. Collimation and central ray: _____

   4. Exposure: _____

   5. Anatomic side markers: _____

Repeatable error(s): _____

F. Lateral elbow (Fig. C4-164)

Description of possible error:

   1. Anatomy demonstrated: _____

   2. Part positioning: _____

   3. Collimation and central ray: _____

   4. Exposure: _____

   5. Anatomic side markers: _____

Repeatable error(s): _____

PART III: LABORATORY EXERCISES

You must gain experience in upper limb positioning before performing the following exams on actual patients. You can get experience in positioning and radiographic evaluation of these projections by performing exercises using radiographic phantoms and practicing on other students (although you will not be taking actual exposures).

   The following suggested activities assume that your teaching institution has an energized lab and radiographic phantoms. If not, perform Laboratory Exercises B and C, the radiographic evaluation and the physical positioning exercises. (Check off each step and projection as you complete it.)

Laboratory Exercise A: Energized Laboratory

   1. Using the hand radiographic phantom, produce radiographs of the following positioning routines:

      _____ Hand (PA, oblique, lateral)   _____ Thumb (AP, oblique, lateral)

      _____ Wrist (PA, oblique, lateral)

   2. Using the elbow radiographic phantom, produce radiographs of the following positioning routines:

      _____ AP   _____ AP oblique, medial rotation

      _____ Lateral elbow   _____ AP oblique, lateral rotation

Laboratory Exercise B: Radiographic Evaluation

1. Evaluate and critique the radiographs produced above, additional radiographs provided by your instructor, or both. Evaluate each radiograph for the following points:

   _____ Evaluate the completeness of the study. (Are all of the pertinent anatomic structures included on the radiograph?)

   _____ Evaluate for positioning or centering errors (e.g., rotation, off centering).

   _____ Evaluate for correct exposure factors and possible motion. (Are the density [brightness] and contrast of the images acceptable?)

   _____ Determine whether anatomic side markers and an acceptable degree of collimation and/or area shielding are seen on the images.

Laboratory Exercise C: Physical Positioning

1. On another person, simulate performing all of the following routine and special projections of the upper limb. Include the six steps listed below and described in the textbook. (Check off each step when completed satisfactorily.)

   Step 1. Appropriate size and type of IR with correct side markers

   Step 2. Correct central ray placement and centering of part to central ray and/or IR

   Step 3. Accurate collimation

   Step 4. Area shielding of patient where advisable

   Step 5. Use of proper immobilizing devices when needed

   Step 6. Approximate correct exposure factors, breathing instructions where applicable, and initiating exposure

Projections	*Step 1*	*Step 2*	*Step 3*	*Step 4*	*Step 5*	*Step 6*
● Second to fifth digit routines (PA, oblique, lateral)	_____	_____	_____	_____	_____	_____
● Thumb routine (AP, oblique, lateral)	_____	_____	_____	_____	_____	_____
● Hand (PA, oblique, lateral)	_____	_____	_____	_____	_____	_____
● Wrist routine (PA, oblique, lateral)	_____	_____	_____	_____	_____	_____
● Scaphoid, carpal canal, and carpal bridge projections	_____	_____	_____	_____	_____	_____
● Elbow routine (AP, oblique, lateral)	_____	_____	_____	_____	_____	_____
● Partial flexion AP	_____	_____	_____	_____	_____	_____
● Acute flexion AP	_____	_____	_____	_____	_____	_____
● Trauma axial lateral (Coyle)	_____	_____	_____	_____	_____	_____
● Radial head projections	_____	_____	_____	_____	_____	_____
● Forearm routine (AP, lateral)	_____	_____	_____	_____	_____	_____

This self-test should be taken only after completing all of the readings, review exercises, and laboratory activities for a particular section. The purpose of this test is not only to provide a good learning exercise but also to serve as a strong indicator of what your final unit evaluation exam will cover. It is strongly suggested that if you do not get at least a 90% to 95% grade on each self-test, you should review those areas in which you missed questions before going to your instructor for the final unit evaluation exam.

1. A. How many bones make up the phalanges of the hand?

    A. 14   C. 5

    B. 8   D. 16

  B. How many bones make up the carpal region?

    A. 14   C. 5

    B. 8   D. 7

  C. What is the total number of bones that make up the hand and wrist?

    A. 21   C. 26

    B. 27   D. 32

2. Match the following joint locations with the correct term.

    _____ A. Between the two phalanges of the first digit (thumb)   1. Radiocarpal

    _____ B. Between the first metacarpal and the proximal phalanx of the thumb   2. Fourth DIP

    _____ C. Between the middle and distal phalanges of the fourth digit   3. Fourth PIP

    _____ D. Between the carpals and the first metacarpal   4. First MCP

    _____ E. Between the forearm and the carpals   5. First CMC

    _____ F. Between the distal radius and ulna   6. Distal radioulnar

                                                               7. IP

3. Match each of the structures labeled on Fig. 4-12 to its correct term.

_____ A.   1. Distal phalanx of fourth digit

_____ B.   2. Head of fifth metacarpal

_____ C.   3. Base of fourth metacarpal

_____ D.   4. Scaphoid

_____ E.   5. Base of first metacarpal

_____ F.   6. Pisiform

_____ G.   7. Trapezoid

_____ H.   8. Body of proximal phalanx of fifth digit

_____ I.   9. Fifth carpometacarpal joint

_____ J.   10. Triquetrum

_____ K.   11. Radius

_____ L.   12. Proximal phalanx of first digit

_____ M.   13. Radiocarpal joint

_____ N.   14. Hamate

_____ O.   15. Capitate

_____ P.   16. Distal interphalangeal joint of fifth digit

_____ Q.   17. Trapezium

_____ R.   18. First metacarpophalangeal joint

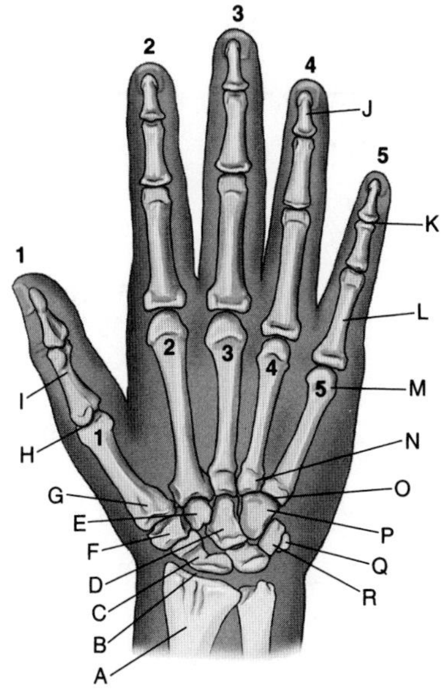

Fig. 4-12. Osteology of the hand and wrist.

4. Which carpal contains a "hooklike" process?

   A. Scaphoid   C. Hamate
   B. Trapezium   D. Pisiform

5. Which carpal articulates with the base of thumb?

   A. Scaphoid   C. Trapezoid
   B. Lunate   D. Trapezium

6. Which carpal is most commonly fractured?

   A. Scaphoid   C. Trapezium
   B. Capitate   D. Triquetrum

7. Which two carpal bones are located most anteriorly as seen on a lateral wrist radiograph? (HINT: They are on the radial side of the wrist.)

   A. Hamate and pisiform   C. Capitate and lunate
   B. Trapezium and trapezoid   D. Scaphoid and trapezium

8. Match each of the structures of the wrist labeled on Figs. 4-13, 4-14, and 4-15 to its correct term.

_____ A.   1. Pisiform

_____ B.   2. Trapezoid

_____ C.   3. Scaphoid

_____ D.   4. Triquetrum

_____ E.   5. Base of first metacarpal

_____ F.   6. Radius

_____ G.   7. Lunate

_____ H.   8. Trapezium

_____ I.   9. Hamate

_____ J.   10. Ulna

_____ K.   11. Capitate

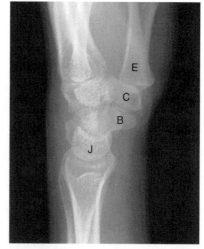

Fig. 4-13. Lateral wrist.

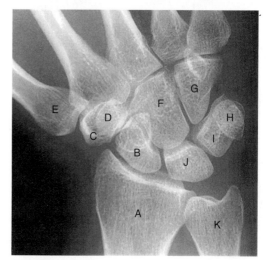

Fig. 4-14. Wrist.

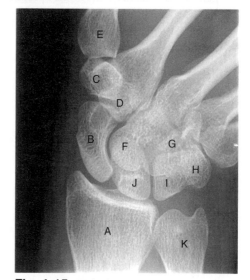

Fig. 4-15. Wrist.

9. Which wrist projection does Fig. 4-14 represent?

    A. PA wrist

    B. PA—ulnar deviation

    C. PA—radial deviation

    D. Carpal canal

10. Which one of the following carpals is *not* well seen in the projection in Fig. 4-14?

    A. Pisiform

    B. Lunate

    C. Scaphoid

    D. Triquetrum

11. Which projection does Fig. 4-15 represent?

    A. PA—ulnar deviation

    B. Carpal canal

    C. PA—radial deviation

    D. Modified Stecher method

12. Which one of the following carpal bones is best demonstrated in the projection in Fig. 4-15?

    A. Trapezium

    B. Scaphoid

    C. Trapezoid

    D. Hamate

13. Which bone of the upper limb contains the coronoid process?

    A. Humerus

    B. First metacarpal

    C. Radius

    D. Ulna

14. Where are the coronoid and radial fossae located?

    A. Anterior aspect of distal humerus

    B. Posterior aspect of distal humerus

    C. Proximal radius and ulna

    D. Distal end of radius

15. Which two bony landmarks are palpated to assist with positioning of the upper limb?

    A. Coronoid and olecranon processes

    B. Pisiform and hamate

    C. Lateral and medial epicondyles

    D. Radial and ulnar styloid processes

16. Where is the coronoid tubercle located?

    A. Medial aspect of coronoid process

    B. Anterior aspect of distal humerus

    C. Lateral aspect of proximal radius

    D. Posterior aspect of distal humerus

17. In an erect anatomic position, which one of the following structures is considered to be most inferior or distal?

    A. Head of ulna

    B. Olecranon process

    C. Radial tuberosity

    D. Head of radius

18. Match the following articulations to the correct joint movement type (each joint movement type may be used more than once).

    _____ A. Intercarpal joints

    _____ B. Radiocarpal joint

    _____ C. Elbow joint

    _____ D. First carpometacarpal joint

    _____ E. Third carpometacarpal joint

    1. Sellar

    2. Ginglymus

    3. Ellipsoidal

    4. Plane

19. The following four radiographs represent the most common routine projections for the elbow. Match each of these projections to the correct figure number.

_____ A. Fig. 4-16   1. AP projection

_____ B. Fig. 4-17   2. Lateral position

_____ C. Fig. 4-18   3. AP oblique—lateral rotation

_____ D. Fig. 4-19   4. AP oblique—medial rotation

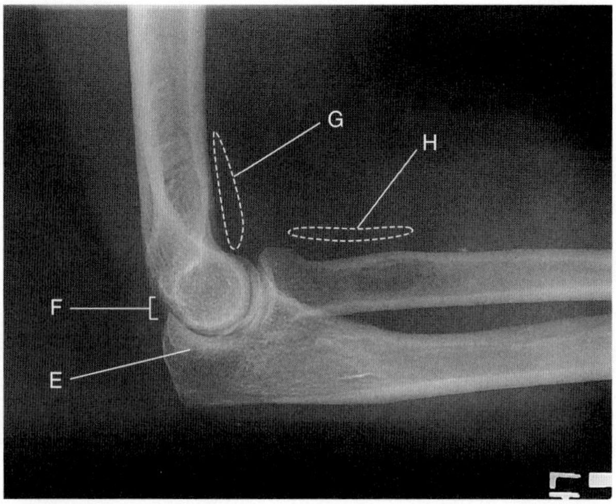

Fig. 4-16.

Identify the soft tissue and bony structures labeled on Figs. 4-16, 4-17, 4-18, and 4-19. (Terms may be used more than once.)

_____ E.   1. Trochlea

_____ F.   2. Olecranon process

_____ G.   3. Coronoid process

_____ H.   4. Medial epicondyle

_____ I.   5. Supinator fat pad

_____ J.   6. Capitulum

_____ K.   7. Anterior fat pad

_____ L.   8. Radial head and neck

_____ M.   9. Region of posterior fat pad

_____ N.   10. Coronoid tubercle

_____ O.

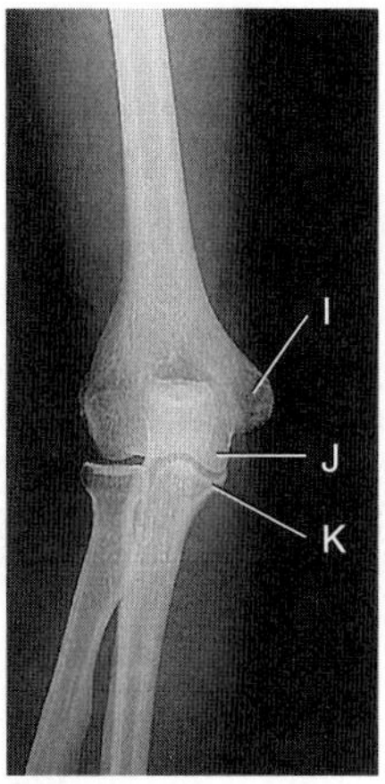

Fig. 4-17. 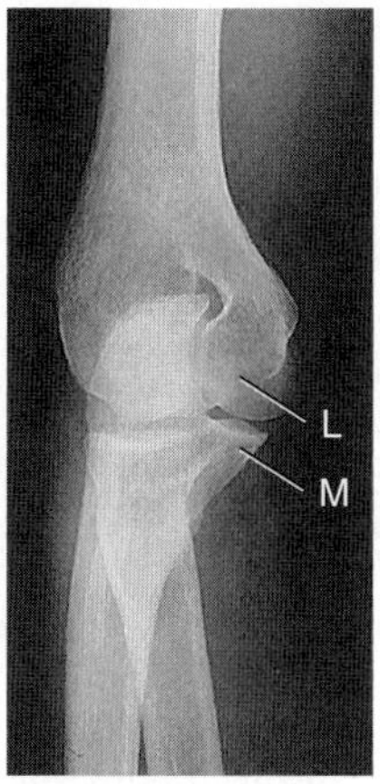   **Fig. 4-18.** 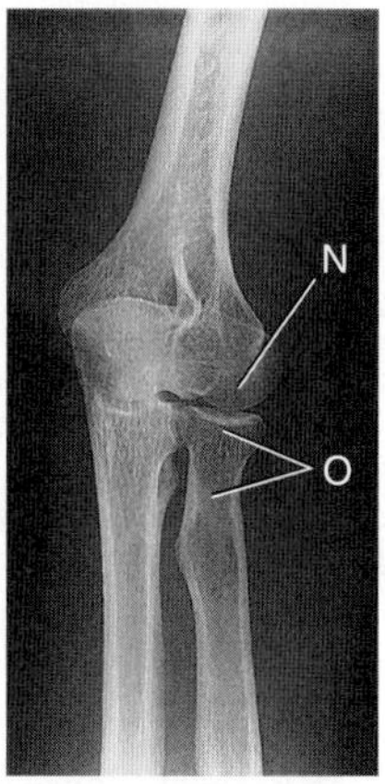   **Fig. 4-19.**

20. Identify each of the structures labeled on Figs. 4-20 and 4-21 with its correct term.

_____ A.

_____ B.

_____ C.

_____ D.

_____ E.*

_____ F.*

_____ G.

_____ H.

_____ I.

_____ J.

_____ K.

1. Coronoid fossa

2. Medial epicondyle

3. Head of radius

4. Trochlea

5. Radial tuberosity

6. Coronoid process

7. Lateral epicondyle

8. Capitulum

9. Trochlear sulcus

10. Coronoid tubercle

11. Radial fossa

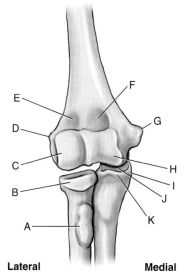

Lateral   Medial

Fig. 4-20. Anterior view of the elbow.

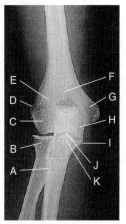

Fig. 4-21. Elbow. Anteroposterior (AP) extended.

21. True/False: To visualize fat pads surrounding the elbow, exposure factors must be adjusted to see both bony and soft tissue structures.

22. True/False: Anterior and posterior fat pads of the elbow are best seen on correctly positioned and correctly exposed anteroposterior (AP) elbow projections.

23. Why should a forearm never be taken as a PA projection?

A. Too painful for the patient

B. Causes the proximal radius to cross over the ulna

C. Causes the distal radius to cross over the ulna

D. Increases the object image receptor distance (OID) of the distal radius

---

*Not visible on radiograph.

24. In what position should the hand be for an AP elbow projection?

    A. Supinated   C. Rotated 20° from supinated position

    B. Pronated   D. True lateral position

25. In what position should the hand be for an AP medial rotation oblique elbow position?

    A. Supinated   C. Rotated 20° from supinated position

    B. Pronated   D. True lateral position

26. Match the projection of the elbow that best demonstrates each of the following structures:

    _____ A. Coronoid process in profile   1. Lateral elbow

    _____ B. Radial head and tuberosity without superimposition   2. AP elbow

    _____ C. Olecranon process in profile   3. AP, medial rotation oblique

    _____ D. Coronoid tubercle   4. AP, lateral rotation oblique

    _____ E. Trochlear notch in profile

    _____ F. Capitulum and lateral epicondyle in profile

    _____ G. Olecranon process seated in olecranon fossa

27. True/False: Placing multiple images on the same digital IP is recommended as long as close collimation is applied for each projection.

28. The long axis of the anatomic part being imaged should be placed:

    A. Perpendicular to the long axis of the IR

    B. Parallel to the long axis of the IR

    C. 30° angle to the long axis of the IR

    D. Any way that will accommodate multiple images being placed on a single IR

29. *Arthrography* is a radiographic study of:

    A. Fat pads and stripes

    B. Epiphyses of long bones

    C. Medullary aspect of long bones

    D. Soft tissues structures within certain synovial joints

30. Match each of the following pathologic terms to its correct definition.

_____ 1. Accumulated fluid within the joint cavity

_____ 2. A reduction in the quantity of bone or atrophy of skeletal tissue

_____ 3. Local or generalized infection of bone or bone marrow

_____ 4. Reverse of a Colles' fracture

_____ 5. Inflammation of the fluid-filled sacs enclosing the joints

_____ 6. Fracture of the base of the first metacarpal

_____ 7. Sprain or tear of the ulnar collateral ligament

_____ 8. Painful disorder of hand and wrist from compression of the median resulting nerve

A. Skier's thumb

B. Bursitis

C. Carpal tunnel syndrome

D. Bennett's fracture

E. Smith fracture

F. Joint effusion

G. Osteomyelitis

H. Osteoporosis

31. Which one of the following clinical indications requires a decrease in manual exposure factors?

A. Paget's disease
B. Advanced osteopetrosis
C. Advanced osteoporosis
D. Joint effusion

32. Where is the central ray centered for a PA projection of the second digit?

A. Affected PIP joint
B. Affected middle phalanx
C. Affected MCP joint
D. Affected CMC joint

33. Why is it important to keep the long axis of the digit parallel to the IR?

A. To reduce distortion of the phalanges
B. To properly visualize joints
C. To demonstrate small fractures
D. All of the above

34. Where is the central ray placed for a PA projection of the hand?

A. Second MCP joint
B. Third MCP joint
C. Middle phalanx of third digit
D. Third PIP joint

35. What is the major disadvantage of performing a PA projection of the thumb rather than an AP?

A. Increased OID
B. Increase in patient dose
C. More painful for patient
D. Awkward position for patient

36. What type of fracture is best demonstrated with a modified Robert's method?

A. Barton fracture
B. Colles' fracture
C. Bennett's fracture
D. Smith fracture

37. True/False: Both hands are examined with one single exposure when using the Norgaard method.

38. True/False: The hand(s) is (are) placed in a true PA position when using the Norgaard method.

39. Choose the *best* set of exposure factors for upper limb radiography using an analog (film-based) system.

   A. 75 kV, 200 mA, ¹⁄₂₀ second, small focal spot, 40-inch (102-cm) SID, high-speed screens

   B. 75 kV, 600 mA, ¹⁄₆₀ second, large focal spot, 40-inch (102-cm) SID, detail-speed screens

   C. 64 kV, 100 mA, ¹⁄₁₀ second, small focal spot, 40-inch (102-cm) SID, high-speed screens

   D. 64 kV, 200 mA, ¹⁄₂₀ second, small focal spot, 40-inch (102-cm) SID, detail-speed screens

40. A radiograph of a PA oblique of the hand reveals that the third, fourth, and fifth metacarpals are superimposed. What must be done to correct this positioning problem on the repeat exposure?

   A. Increase obliquity of the hand   C. Decrease obliquity of the hand

   B. Spread fingers out further   D. Form a tight fist with the fingers

41. A radiograph of an AP elbow projection demonstrates total separation between the proximal radius and ulna. What must be done to correct this positioning error on the repeat exposure?

   A. Rotate upper limb medially   C. Angle central ray 5° to 10° caudad

   B. Rotate upper limb laterally   D. Fully extend elbow

42. A radiograph of the carpal canal (inferosuperior) projection reveals that the pisiform and hamulus are superimposed. What can be done to correct this problem on the repeat exposure?

   A. Flex wrist slightly   C. Rotate wrist laterally 5° to 10°

   B. Extend wrist slightly   D. Rotate wrist medially 5° to 10°

43. A radiograph of an AP oblique-medial rotation reveals that the coronoid process is not in profile and the radial head is not superimposed over the ulna. What specific positioning error was involved?

   A. Insufficient medial rotation   C. Excessive extension of elbow

   B. Excessive medial rotation   D. Excessive flexion of elbow

44. A radiograph of a lateral projection of the elbow reveals that the epicondyles are not superimposed and the trochlear notch is not clearly seen. What must be done to correct this positioning error during the repeat exposure?

   A. Angle central ray 45° toward shoulder   C. Angle central ray 45° away from shoulder

   B. Place humerus/forearm in same horizontal plane   D. Extend elbow to form an 80° horizontal plane angle

45. **Situation:** A patient with a possible Barton fracture enters the emergency room. Which positioning routine should be performed to confirm the diagnosis?

   A. Elbow   C. Hand

   B. Wrist   D. Thumb

46. **Situation:** A patient with a possible Smith fracture enters the emergency room. Which positioning routine should be performed to confirm this diagnosis?

   A. Hand   C. Wrist/forearm

   B. Thumb   D. Elbow

47. **Situation:** A patient has a Colles' fracture reduced, and a large plaster cast is placed on the upper limb. The orthopedic surgeon orders a postreduction study. The original technique, used before the cast placement, involved 60 kV and 5 mAs (analog system). How should the exposure factors be altered with a large plaster cast?

   A. Same exposure factors   C. 65 kV

   B. 75 to 78 kV   D. 68 to 70 kV

48. **Situation:** A pediatric patient with a possible radial head fracture is brought into the emergency room. It is too painful for the patient to extend the elbow beyond 90° or rotate the hand. What type of special (i.e., optional) projection could be performed on this patient to confirm the diagnosis without causing further discomfort?

    A. Coyle method   C. Norgaard method

    B. Modified Robert's method   D. Modified Stecher method

49. For the following critique questions, refer to the AP elbow projection radiograph shown in Fig. C4-161 in your textbook.

    A. Which positioning error(s) is (are) visible on this radiograph? (More than one answer may be selected.)

        (a) All essential anatomic structures are not demonstrated.

        (b) Central ray is centered incorrectly.

        (c) Collimation is not evident.

        (d) Exposure factors are incorrect.

        (e) No anatomic side marker is visible.

        (f) Excessive rotation in the lateral direction is evident.

        (g) Insufficient rotation in the lateral direction is evident.

        (h) Excessive flexion of the joint is evident.

    B. Which criteria error(s) identified in the preceding is (are) considered "repeatable"?

        _____.

    C. Which of the following modifications must be made during the repeat exposure? (More than one answer may be selected.)

        (a) Increase collimation.

        (b) Center central ray correctly.

        (c) Decrease exposure factors.

        (d) Increase exposure factors.

        (e) Place anatomic side marker on IR before exposure.

        (f) Rotate elbow slightly more in the medial direction.

        (g) Rotate elbow slightly more in the lateral direction.

        (h) Extend elbow completely.

50. For the following critique questions, refer to the PA wrist projection (shown in Fig. C4-162 in the textbook).

  A. Which special wrist projection does this represent?

   (a) Ulnar deviation

   (b) Radial deviation

  B. Which positioning error(s) is (are) visible on this radiograph? (More than one answer may be selected.)

   (a) All essential anatomic structures are not demonstrated.

   (b) Central ray is centered incorrectly.

   (c) Exposure factors are incorrect.

   (d) No anatomic marker is visible.

   (e) Excessive rotation in the lateral direction is evident.

   (f) Excessive rotation in the medial direction is evident.

   (g) Excessive deviation of the joint is evident.

  C. Which criteria error(s) identified in the preceding is (are) considered "repeatable"?

   _____

  D. Which of the following modifications must be made during the repeat exposure? (More than one answer may be selected.)

   (a) Open up collimation to include all soft tissue and bony structures.

   (b) Center central ray correctly to midcarpal region.

   (c) Decrease exposure factors.

   (d) Increase exposure factors.

   (e) Place marker on IR before exposure.

   (f) Pronate hand toward IR.

   (g) Supinate hand away from IR.

   (h) Extend wrist.

   (i) Increase deviation movement.

   (j) Decrease deviation movement.

5 Humerus and Shoulder Girdle

CHAPTER OBJECTIVES

After you have successfully completed the activities in this chapter, you will be able to:

_____ 1. Identify the bones and specific features of the humerus and shoulder girdle.

_____ 2. On drawings and radiographs, identify specific anatomic structures of the humerus and shoulder girdle.

_____ 3. Match specific joints of the shoulder girdle to their structural classification and movement type.

_____ 4. Describe anatomic relationships of prominent structures of the humerus and shoulder girdle.

_____ 5. On radiographic images, identify rotational positions of the humerus.

_____ 6. List the technical and shielding considerations commonly used for humerus and shoulder girdle radiography.

_____ 7. Match specific clinical indications of the shoulder girdle to the correct definition.

_____ 8. Match specific clinical indications of the shoulder girdle to the correct radiographic appearance.

_____ 9. For select forms of pathologic conditions of the shoulder girdle, indicate whether manual exposure factors should be increased or decreased or remain the same.

_____ 10. List routine and special projections of the humerus and shoulder, including the type and size of IR holder, the central ray location with correct angles, and the structures best demonstrated.

_____ 11. Given various hypothetic situations, identify the correct modification of a position and/or exposure factors to improve the radiographic image.

_____ 12. Given various hypothetic situations, identify the correct position for a specific pathologic feature or condition.

_____ 13. Given radiographs of specific humerus and shoulder girdle projections, identify specific positioning and exposure factor errors.

POSITIONING AND RADIOGRAPHIC CRITIQUE

_____ 1. Using a peer, position the patient for routine and special projections of the humerus and shoulder girdle.

_____ 2. Using a shoulder radiographic phantom, produce satisfactory radiographs of the shoulder girdle (if equipment is available).

_____ 3. Critique and evaluate shoulder girdle radiographs based on the five divisions of radiographic criteria: (1) anatomy demonstrated, (2) position, (3) collimation and central ray, (4) exposure, and (5) anatomic side markers.

_____ 4. Distinguish between acceptable and unacceptable shoulder girdle radiographs based on exposure factors, motion, collimation, positioning, or other errors.

Complete the following review exercises after reading the associated pages in the textbook as indicated by each exercise. Answers to each review exercise are given at the end of the review exercises.

PART I: RADIOGRAPHIC ANATOMY
REVIEW EXERCISE A: Radiographic Anatomy of the Humerus and Shoulder Girdle (see textbook pp. 174-178)

1. The shoulder girdle consists of (A) _____ , (B) _____ ,

   and (C) _____ .

2. Identify the labeled parts on Figs. 5-1 and 5-2. Include secondary terms in parentheses where indicated.

   A. _____ (_____)

   B. _____ (_____)

   C. _____

   D. _____

   E. _____ (_____)

   F. _____

   G. Which projection (internal, external, or neutral rotation) of the proximal humerus is represented by this drawing and radiograph?

   _____

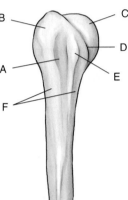

Fig. 5-1. Frontal view, proximal humerus.

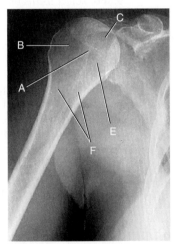

Fig. 5-2. Radiograph, proximal humerus.

3. The three aspects of the clavicle are the (A) _____, (B) _____,

   and (C) _____.

4. The _____ (male or female) clavicle tends to be thicker and more curved in shape.

5. The three angles of the scapula include the (A) _____, (B) _____,

   and (C) _____.

6. The anterior surface of the scapula is referred to as the _____ surface.

7. What is the anatomic name for the armpit? _____

8. What are the names of the two fossae located on the posterior scapula?

   A. _____   B. _____

9. All of the joints of the shoulder girdle are classified as being _____.

10. List the movement types for the following joints:

    A. Scapulohumeral: _____

    B. Sternoclavicular: _____

    C. Acromioclavicular: _____

11. Match each of the following anatomic structures with its correct location.

    _____   1. Greater tubercle   A. Scapula

    _____   2. Coracoid process   B. Clavicle

    _____   3. Crest of spine   C. Proximal humerus

    _____   4. Coronoid process   D. Not part of the shoulder girdle

    _____   5. Acromial extremity

    _____   6. Intertubercular groove

    _____   7. Condylar process

    _____   8. Surgical neck

12. Identify the following structures labeled on Figs. 5-3 and 5-4. Include secondary terms in parentheses where indicated.

A. _____

B. _____

   (_____)

C. _____

D. _____

E. _____

F. _____

G. _____

   (_____) border

H. _____

   (_____) border

I. _____

   (_____) surface

J. _____

   (_____) surface

K. _____

L. _____

M. _____

N. _____

   (_____)

O. _____

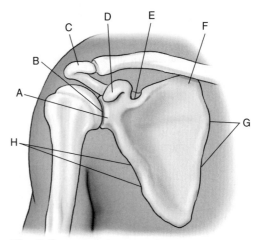

Fig. 5-3. Frontal view, scapula.

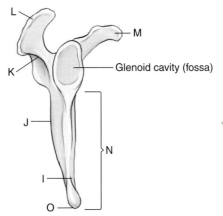

Fig. 5-4. Lateral view, scapula.

13. Identify the structures labeled on Fig. 5-5.

   A. _____

   B. _____ joint

   C. _____

   D. _____

   E. _____

   F. _____

   G. Is this an **internal** or **external** rotation AP projection of the proximal humerus and shoulder?

   _____

   H. Does Fig. 5-5 represent an **AP** or a **lateral** perspective of the proximal humerus?

   _____

   I. Are the epicondyles of the distal humerus **parallel** or **perpendicular** to the IR on this projection?

   _____

Identify the structures labeled on Fig. 5-6.

   J. _____

   K. _____

   L. _____

   M. _____

   N. What is the correct term to describe the projection shown

   in Fig. 5-6? _____

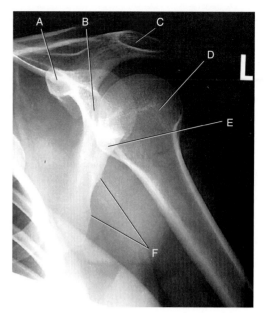

Fig. 5-5. Radiograph.

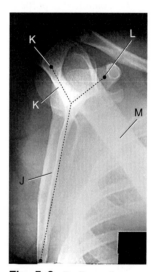

Fig. 5-6. Radiograph.

14. Identify the structures labeled on Fig. 5-7.

A. _____

B. _____

C. _____

D. _____

E. What is the name of the projection shown in Fig. 5-7?

_____

F. How much (at what angle) should the affected arm be abducted from the body for this projection?

_____

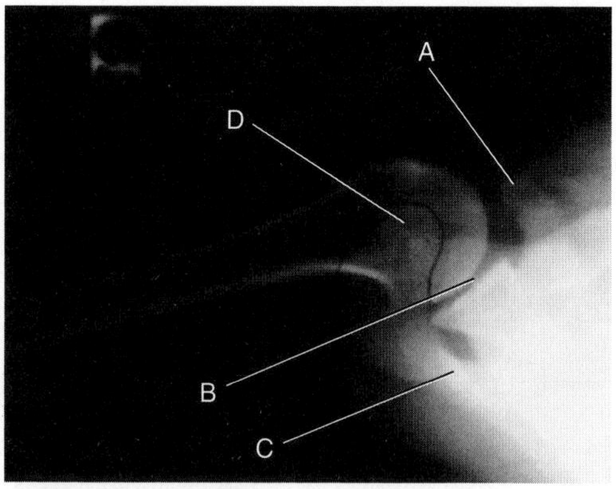

Fig. 5-7. Radiograph.

PART II: RADIOGRAPHIC POSITIONING
REVIEW EXERCISE B: Positioning of the Humerus and Shoulder Girdle (see textbook pp. 179-204)

1. Identify the correct proximal humerus rotation for the each of the following.

_____ 1. Greater tubercle profiled laterally

_____ 2. Humeral epicondyles angled 45° to image receptor (IR)

_____ 3. Epicondyles perpendicular to IR

_____ 4. Supination of hand

_____ 5. Palm of hand against thigh

_____ 6. Epicondyles parallel to IR

_____ 7. Lesser tubercle profiled medially

_____ 8. Proximal humerus in a lateral position

_____ 9. Proximal humerus in position for an anteroposterior (AP) projection

A. External rotation

B. Internal rotation

C. Neutral rotation

2. Identify the proximal humerus rotation represented on the radiographs in Figs. 5-8 to 5-10.

A. Fig. 5-8 represents _____ rotation.

B. Fig. 5-9 represents _____ rotation.

C. Fig. 5-10 represents _____ rotation.

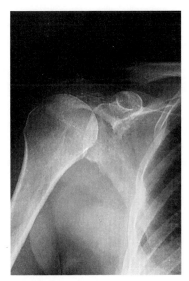

Fig. 5-8. Proximal humerus.

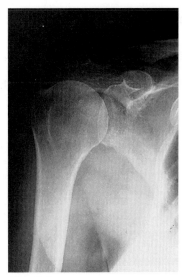

Fig. 5-9. Proximal humerus.

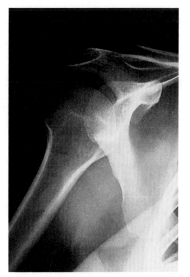

Fig. 5-10. Proximal humerus.

3. Indicate whether each of the following positioning and technical considerations is true or false for the shoulder girdle.

   A. True/False: The use of a grid is not required for shoulder studies that measure less than 10 cm.

   B. True/False: The kV range for adult shoulder projections is between 80 and 90 kV for analog and 100 to 110 kV for digital imaging systems

   C. True/False: Low mA with short exposure times should be used for adult shoulder studies.

   D. True/False: Large focal spot setting should be selected for most adult shoulder studies.

   E. True/False: A high-speed screen-IR system is recommended for analog shoulder studies when using a grid.

   F. True/False: A 72-inch (183-cm) source-image distance (SID) is recommended for most shoulder girdle studies.

   G. True/False: The use of contact shields over the breast, lung, and thyroid regions is recommended for most shoulder projections.

4. Which one of the following kV ranges (analog) should be used for a shoulder series on an average adult?

   A. 70 to 80 kV   C. 80 to 90 kV

   B. 55 to 60 kV   D. 65 to 75 kV

5. If physical immobilization is required, which individual should be asked to restrain a child for a shoulder series?

   A. Parent or guardian   C. Radiography student

   B. Radiologic technologist   D. Nurse aide

6. True/False: CT arthrography of the shoulder joint often requires the use of iodinated contrast media injected into the joint space.

7. True/False: Magnetic resonance imaging (MRI) is an excellent modality for demonstrating bony injuries of the shoulder girdle.

8. True/False: Nuclear medicine bone scans can demonstrate signs of osteomyelitis and cellulitis.

9. True/False: Radiography is more sensitive than nuclear medicine for demonstrating physiologic aspects of the shoulder girdle.

10. True/False: Sonography (ultrasound) can provide a functional (dynamic) evaluation of joint movement that MRI cannot.

11. Match each of the following clinical indications to its correct definition.

_____ 1. Compression between the greater tuberosity and soft tissues on the coracoacromial ligamentous and osseous arch

_____ 2. Injury of the anteroinferior glenoid labrum

_____ 3. Inflammatory condition of the tendon

_____ 4. Superior displacement of the distal clavicle

_____ 5. Compression fracture of the articular surface of the humeral head

_____ 6. Traumatic injury to one or more of the supportive muscles of the shoulder girdle

_____ 7. Atrophy of skeletal tissue

A. Acromioclavicular joint dislocation

B. Bankart lesion

C. Hill-Sachs defect

D. Impingement syndrome

E. Osteoporosis

F. Rotator cuff tear

G. Tendonitis

12. Match the following radiographic appearances to the correct pathology.

_____ 1. Subacromial spurs

_____ 2. Fluid-filled joint space

_____ 3. Thin bony cortex

_____ 4. Abnormal widening of acromioclavicular joint space

_____ 5. Calcified tendons

_____ 6. Avulsion fracture of the glenoid rim

_____ 7. Narrowing of joint space

_____ 8. Closed joint space

_____ 9. Compression fracture of humeral head

A. Rheumatoid arthritis

B. Bankart lesion

C. Hill-Sachs defect

D. Osteoarthritis

E. Bursitis

F. Osteoporosis

G. Impingement syndrome

H. Acromioclavicular joint separation

I. Tendonitis

13. Which one of the following clinical indications requires a decrease in manual exposure factors?

A. Impingement syndrome

B. Bursitis

C. Bankart lesion

D. Osteoporosis

14. Which two routine shoulder projections are routinely taken for a shoulder (with no traumatic injury) and proximal humerus?

A. _____   B. _____

15. Specifically, where is the central ray placed for an AP projection of the shoulder?

_____

16. Which lateral projection can be performed to demonstrate the *entire* humerus for a patient with a midhumeral fracture?

_____

17. To best demonstrate a possible Hill-Sachs defect, which additional positioning technique can be added to the inferosuperior axial projection?

    A. Angle central ray 10° to 15° caudad   C. Angle central ray 3° to 5° caudad

    B. Rotate affected arm externally approximately 45°   D. Place humeral epicondyles parallel to IR

18. What type of central ray angulation is required for the inferosuperior axial projection for the shoulder?

    A. 25° to 30° medially   C. 25° anterior and 25° medially

    B. 35° to 45° medially   D. Central ray perpendicular to IR

19. The _____ projection of the shoulder produces an image of the glenoid process in profile.

    This projection is also referred to as the _____ method.

20. Which one of the following projections produces a tangential projection of the intertubercular groove?

    A. Fisk modification   C. Hobbs modification

    B. Grashey method   D. Lawrence method

21. The supine version of the tangential projection for the intertubercular groove requires that the central ray be

    angled _____ posteriorly from the horizontal plane.

22. Which one of the following projections is best for demonstrating a possible dislocation of the proximal humerus?

    A. Posterior oblique (Grashey method)   C. Inferosuperior axial (Clements modification) projection

    B. Fisk modification   D. Scapular Y projection

23. The _____ projection is the special projection of the shoulder that best demonstrates the acromiohumeral space for possible subacromial spurs, which create shoulder impingement symptoms.

    This projection is also referred to as the _____ method.

24. Which of the following nontrauma projections can be performed erect to provide a lateral view of the proximal humerus in relationship to the glenohumeral joint?

    A. Tangential projection (Fisk modification)

    B. AP projection-neutral rotation

    C. PA transaxillary projection (Hobbs modification)

    D. Posterior oblique position (Grashey method)

25. How much is the CR angled for the inferosuperior axial projection (Clements modification) if the patient cannot fully abduct the arm 90°?

    A. 5° to 15°   C. 25° to 30°

    B. 45°   D. 20°

26. What CR angle is required for the AP axial projection (Alexander method) for AC joints?

    A. 25° cephalad   C. 5° to 10° caudad

    B. 45° caudad   D. 15° cephalad

27. True/False: The PA transaxillary projection (Hobbs modification) requires no CR angle.

28. True/False: The transthoracic lateral projection can be performed for possible fractures or dislocations of the proximal humerus.

29. True/False: The use of a breathing technique can be performed for the transthoracic lateral humerus projection.

30. True/False: The affected arm must be placed into external rotation for the transthoracic lateral projection.

31. True/False: A central ray angle of 10° to 15° caudad may be used for the transthoracic lateral projections if the patient is unable to elevate the uninjured arm and shoulder sufficiently.

32. True/False: The scapular Y lateral (anterior oblique) position requires the body to be rotated 30° to 40° anteriorly toward the affected side.

33. Which two landmarks are placed perpendicular to the IR for the scapular Y lateral projection?

_____

34. Which special projection of the shoulder requires that the affected side be rotated 45° toward the cassette and uses

    a 45° caudad central ray angle? _____

35. A posterior dislocation of the humerus projects the humeral head _____ (**superior** or **inferior**) to the glenoid cavity with the special projection described in the previous question.

36. A thin-shouldered patient requires _____ (more or less) CR angle for an AP axial clavicle projection than a large-shouldered patient.

37. What must be ruled out before performing the weight-bearing study for acromioclavicular joints?

_____

38. Match each of the following projections with its corresponding method name. Method names may be used more than once.

    _____ 1. Inferosuperior axial   A. Neer method

    _____ 2. Posterior oblique for glenoid cavity   B. Grashey method

    _____ 3. Tangential for intertubercular (bicipital) groove   C. Lawrence method

    _____ 4. Supraspinatus outlet tangential   D. Fisk modification

    _____ 5. Transthoracic lateral   E. Garth method

    _____ 6. AP apical oblique axial

39. Where is the CR centered for the AP scapula projection?

_____

40. What type of CR angle is required for the lateral scapula position?

    A. 10° to 15° cephalad   C. 10° to 15° caudad

    B. 5° to 15° caudad   D. None

REVIEW EXERCISE C: Problem Solving for Technical and Positioning Errors

1. The following factors were used to produce a radiograph of an AP projection of the shoulder: 85 kV, 20 mAs, high-speed screens, 40-inch (102-cm) SID, grid, and suspended respiration. The resultant radiograph demonstrated poor radiographic contrast between bony and soft tissue structures. Which of these factors can be altered during the repeat exposure to improve radiographic quality?

2. A radiograph of an AP axial clavicle projection reveals that the clavicle is projected below the superior border of the scapula. What can the technologist do to correct this problem during the repeat exposure?

3. A radiograph of an AP scapula reveals that the scapula is within the lung field and difficult to see. Which two things can the technologist do to improve the visibility of the scapula during the repeat exposure?

4. A radiograph of an AP projection (with external rotation) of a shoulder (with no traumatic injury) reveals that neither the greater nor lesser tubercles are profiled. What must be done to correct this during the repeat exposure?

5. A radiograph of a lateral scapula position reveals that it is not a true lateral projection. (Considerable separation exists between the axillary and vertebral borders.) The projection was taken using the following factors: erect position, 40-inch (102-cm) SID, 45° rotation toward cassette from posteroanterior (PA), central ray centered to midscapula, and no central ray angulation. Based on these factors, how can this position be improved during the repeat exposure?

6. A radiograph of the AP oblique (Grashey method) taken as a 35° oblique projection reveals that the borders of the glenoid cavity are not superimposed. The patient has large, rounded shoulders. What must be done to get better superimposition of the cavity during the repeat exposure?

7. **Situation:** A patient with a possible right shoulder dislocation enters the emergency room. The technologist attempts to perform an erect transthoracic lateral projection, but the patient is unable to raise the left arm and shoulder high enough. The resultant radiograph reveals that the shoulders are superimposed, and the right shoulder and humeral head are not well visualized. What can be done to improve this image during the repeat exposure?

8. **Situation:** A patient with a possible fracture of the right proximal humerus from an automobile accident enters the emergency room. The patient has other injuries and is unable to stand or sit erect. Which positioning routine should be used to determine the extent of the injury?

9. **Situation:** A patient with a clinical history of chronic shoulder dislocation comes to the radiology department. The orthopedic physician suspects that a Hill-Sachs defect may be present. Which specific position(s) may be used to best demonstrate this pathologic feature?

_____

10. **Situation:** A patient with a possible Bankart lesion comes to the radiology department. List three projections that can be performed that may demonstrate signs of this injury.

   A. _____

   B. _____

   C. _____

11. **Situation:** A patient with a possible rotator cuff tear comes to the radiology department. Which one of the following imaging modalities would best demonstrate this injury?

   A. Arthrography   C. Nuclear medicine

   B. MRI   D. Radiography

12. **Situation:** A patient with a clinical history of tendon injury in the shoulder region comes to the radiology department. The orthopedic physician needs a _functional_ study of the shoulder joint performed to determine the extent of the tendon injury. Which of the following modalities would best demonstrate this injury?

   A. Arthrography   C. Ultrasound

   B. MRI   D. Nuclear medicine

13. A radiograph of an AP projection with external rotation of the shoulder does not demonstrate either the greater or lesser tubercle in profile. What is the most likely cause for this radiographic outcome?

_____

14. A radiograph of a transthoracic lateral projection demonstrates considerable superimposition of lung markings and ribs over the region of the proximal shoulder. What can the technologist do to minimize this problem during the repeat exposure?

_____

15. **Situation:** A patient enters the ER with a definite fracture to the midhumerus. Because of other trauma the patient is unable to stand. Which lateral projection would demonstrate the entire humerus?

_____

16. **Situation:** The AP apical oblique axial projection (Garth method) is performed on a patient with a shoulder injury. The resultant radiograph demonstrates the proximal humeral head projected below the glenoid cavity. What type of trauma or pathology is indicated with this radiographic appearance?

_____

REVIEW EXERCISE D: Critique Radiographs of the Humerus and Shoulder Girdle (see textbook p. 205)

The following questions relate to the radiographs found at the end of Chapter 5 of the textbook. Evaluate these radiographs for the radiographic criteria categories (1 through 5) that follow. Describe the corrections needed to improve the overall image. The major, or "repeatable" errors are specific errors that indicate the need for a repeat exposure, regardless of the nature of the other errors.

A. AP clavicle (Fig. C5-96)

Description of possible error:

    1. Anatomy demonstrated: _____

    2. Part positioning: _____

    3. Collimation and central ray: _____

    4. Exposure: _____

    5. Anatomic side markers: _____

Repeatable error(s): _____

B. AP shoulder—external rotation (Fig. C5-97)

Description of possible error:

    1. Anatomy demonstrated: _____

    2. Part positioning: _____

    3. Collimation and central ray: _____

    4. Exposure: _____

    5. Anatomic side markers: _____

Repeatable error(s): _____

C. AP scapula (Fig. C5-98)

Description of possible error:

    1. Anatomy demonstrated: _____

    2. Part positioning: _____

    3. Collimation and central ray: _____

    4. Exposure: _____

    5. Anatomic side markers: _____

Repeatable error(s): _____

D. AP humerus (Fig. C5-99)

Description of possible error:

1. Anatomy demonstrated: _____

2. Part positioning: _____

3. Collimation and central ray: _____

4. Exposure: _____

5. Anatomic side markers: _____

Repeatable error(s): _____

Which projection (AP, lateral, or oblique) and which rotation of the proximal humerus are evident (internal, external,

or neutral)? _____

PART III: LABORATORY EXERCISES

You must gain experience in positioning each part of the humerus and shoulder girdle before performing the following exams on actual patients. You can get experience in positioning and radiographic evaluation of these projections by performing exercises using radiographic phantoms and practicing on other students (although you will not be taking actual exposures).

The following suggested activities assume that your teaching institution has an energized lab and radiographic phantoms. If not, perform Laboratory Exercises B and C, the radiographic evaluation, and the physical positioning exercises. (Check off each step and projection as you complete it.)

Laboratory Exercise A: Energized Laboratory

1. Using the thorax radiographic phantom, produce radiographs of the following basic routines:

_____ AP shoulder   _____ Posterior oblique (Grashey method)

_____ AP and AP axial clavicle   _____ AP and lateral scapula

Laboratory Exercise B: Radiographic Evaluation

1. Evaluate and critique the radiographs produced in the preceding, additional radiographs provided by your instructor, or both. Evaluate each radiograph for the following points:

_____ Evaluate the completeness of the study. (Are all of the pertinent anatomic structures included on the radiograph?)

_____ Evaluate for positioning or centering errors (e.g., rotation, off centering).

_____ Evaluate for correct exposure factors and possible motion. (Are the density-brightness and contrast of the images acceptable?)

_____ Determine whether markers and an acceptable degree of collimation and/or area shielding are seen on the images.

Laboratory Exercise C: Physical Positioning

On another person, simulate performing all of the following basic and special projections of the humerus and shoulder girdle. Include the six steps listed in the following and described in the textbook. (Check off each step when completed satisfactorily.)

Step 1. Appropriate size and type of image receptor with correct markers

Step 2. Correct central ray placement and centering of part to central ray and/or IR

Step 3. Accurate collimation

Step 4. Area shielding of patient where advisable

Step 5. Use of proper immobilizing devices when needed

Step 6. Approximate correct exposure factors, breathing instructions where applicable, and "making" exposure

Projections	*Step 1*	*Step 2*	*Step 3*	*Step 4*	*Step 5*	*Step 6*
● Humerus (AP and lateral)	_____	_____	_____	_____	_____	_____
● Transthoracic lateral for humerus	_____	_____	_____	_____	_____	_____
● Shoulder series (nontrauma) (AP internal and external rotation)	_____	_____	_____	_____	_____	_____
● Inferosuperior axial (Lawrence)	_____	_____	_____	_____	_____	_____
● Posterior oblique (Grashey)	_____	_____	_____	_____	_____	_____
● Tangential (Fisk) for intertubercular groove	_____	_____	_____	_____	_____	_____
● Anterior oblique–Scapular Y	_____	_____	_____	_____	_____	_____
● Transthoracic lateral (Lawrence)	_____	_____	_____	_____	_____	_____
● AP apical oblique axial (Garth)	_____	_____	_____	_____	_____	_____
● AP and AP axial clavicle	_____	_____	_____	_____	_____	_____
● AP and lateral scapula	_____	_____	_____	_____	_____	_____
● Acromioclavicular joints (with and without weights)	_____	_____	_____	_____	_____	_____

SELF-TEST

This self-test should be taken only after completing all of the readings, review exercises, and laboratory activities for a particular section. The purpose of this test is not only to provide a good learning exercise but also to serve as a strong indicator of what your final unit evaluation exam will cover. It is strongly suggested that if you do not get at least a 90% to 95% grade on each self-test, you should review those areas in which you missed questions before going to your instructor for the final unit evaluation exam.

1. Select the term(s) that correctly describe(s) the shoulder joint.

   A. Humeroscapular   C. Glenohumeral

   B. Scapulohumeral   D. B and C

2. Which specific joint is found on the lateral end of the clavicle?

   A. Scapulohumeral   C. Acromioclavicular

   B. Sternoclavicular   D. Glenohumeral

3. Which of the following is *not* an angle found on the scapula?

   A. Inferior angle   C. Lateral angle

   B. Medial angle   D. Superior angle

4. Which one of the following structures of the scapula extends most anteriorly?

   A. Glenoid cavity   C. Scapular spine

   B. Acromion   D. Coracoid process

5. True/False: The male clavicle is shorter and less curved than the female clavicle.

6. Which bony structure separates the supraspinous and infraspinous fossae?

   A. Scapular spine   C. Acromion

   B. Glenoid cavity   D. Superior border of scapula

7. Which one of the following structures is considered to be the most posterior?

   A. Scapular notch   C. Acromion

   B. Coracoid process   D. Glenoid process

8. What is the type of joint movement for the scapulohumeral joint?

   A. Plane   C. Ellipsoidal

   B. Spheroidal   D. Trochoidal

9. Identify the labeled structures on Fig. 5-11. (Terms may be used more than once.)

_____ A.   1. Spine of scapula

_____ B.   2. Lesser tubercle

_____ C.   3. Coracoid process

_____ D.   4. Lateral (axillary) border of scapula

_____ E.   5. Scapulohumeral joint

_____ F.   6. Clavicle

_____ G.   7. Intertubercular groove

_____ H.   8. Acromion of scapula

_____ I.   9. Neck of scapula

_____ J.   10. Greater tubercle

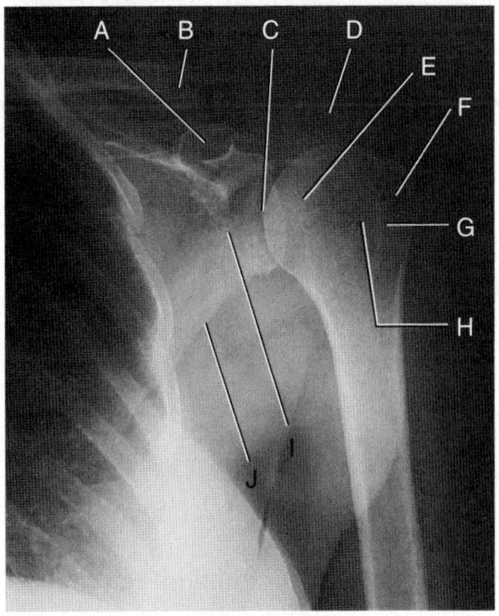

Fig. 5-11. Shoulder projection.

K. Does Fig. 5-11 represent an AP projection with: (A) an internal, (B) an external, or (C) a neutral rotation of

   the humerus? _____

Identify the labeled structures on Fig. 5-12. (Terms may be used more than once.)

_____ L.   11. Lateral extremity of clavicle

_____ M.   12. Head of humerus

_____ N.   13. Glenoid cavity

_____ O.

_____ P.

_____ Q.

_____ R.

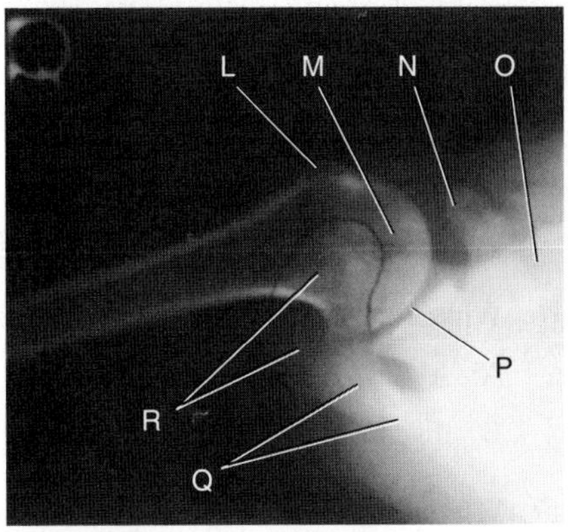

Fig. 5-12. Shoulder projection.

S. What is the correct term and method for the projection
   seen on Fig. 5-12?

   (a) Inferosuperior axial projection

   (b) Transthoracic lateral—Lawrence method

   (c) Posterior oblique—Grashey method

   (d) PA Transaxillary projection—Hobbs modification

10. Which one of the following analog technical considerations does not apply for adult shoulder radiography?

   A. Non-grid

   B. High-speed IR

   C. 40- to 44-inch (102- to 113-cm) SID

   D. 70- to 80-kV

11. True/False: Even though the amount of radiation exposure is minimal for most shoulder projections, gonadal shielding should be used for children and adults of childbearing age.

12. True/False: The greatest technical concern during a pediatric shoulder study is voluntary motion.

13. Which one of the following imaging modalities or procedures best demonstrates osteomyelitis?
    A. Ultrasound
    B. MRI
    C. CT arthrography
    D. Nuclear medicine

14. Which one of the following imaging modalities or procedures provides a functional, or dynamic, study of the shoulder joint?
    A. Ultrasound
    B. Radiography
    C. Nuclear medicine
    D. MRI

15. Match each of the following clinical indications to its correct definition.

    _____ 1. Disability of the shoulder joint caused by chronic inflammation in and around the joint

    _____ 2. Injury to the anteroinferior glenoid labrum

    _____ 3. Chronic systemic disease with arthritic inflammatory changes throughout the body

    _____ 4. Superior displacement of distal clavicle

    _____ 5. Compression fracture of humeral head

    _____ 6. Traumatic injury to one or more muscles of the shoulder joint

    _____ 7. Reduction in the quantity of bone

    A. Rotator cuff tear
    B. Osteoporosis
    C. Rheumatoid arthritis
    D. Idiopathic chronic adhesive capsulitis
    E. Bankart lesion
    F. Acromioclavicular joint dislocation
    G. Hill-Sachs defect

16. Which one of the following projections and/or positions best demonstrates signs of impingement syndrome?
    A. AP and lateral shoulder external rotation
    B. Inferosuperior axial
    C. Inferosuperior axial with exaggerated rotation
    D. Tangential projection (Neer method)

17. Which one of the following pathologic conditions often produces narrowing of the joint space?
    A. Osteoarthritis
    B. Bursitis
    C. Osteoporosis
    D. Idiopathic chronic adhesive capsulitis

18. Which one of the following pathologic conditions may require a reduction in manual exposure factors?
    A. Bursitis
    B. Rheumatoid arthritis
    C. Rotator cuff tear
    D. Bankart lesion

19. Which routine projection of the shoulder requires that the humeral epicondyles be parallel to the IR?
    A. External rotation
    B. Neutral rotation
    C. Internal rotation
    D. Posterior oblique–Grashey method

20. Where is the central ray centered for an AP projection–external rotation of the shoulder?
    A. Acromion
    B. 1 inch (2.5 cm) superior to coracoid process
    C. 1 inch (2.5 cm) inferior to coracoid process
    D. 2 inches (5 cm) inferior to acromioclavicular joint

21. Which position of the shoulder and proximal humerus projects the lesser tubercle in profile medially?

    A. External rotation   C. Internal rotation

    B. Neutral rotation   D. Exaggerated rotation

22. What central ray angle should be used for the inferosuperior axial projection for the scapulohumeral joint space?

    A. 15° medially   C. 25° anteriorly and medially

    B. 25° to 30° medially   D. 35° to 45° medially

23. To best demonstrate the Hill-Sachs defect on the inferosuperior axial projection, which additional positioning maneuver must be used?

    A. Angle central ray 35° medially   C. Use exaggerated internal rotation

    B. Use exaggerated external rotation   D. Abduct arm 120° rotation from midsagittal plane (MSP)

24. How are the humeral epicondyles aligned for a rotational lateromedial projection of the humerus?

    A. 45° to IR   C. Parallel to IR

    B. Perpendicular to IR   D. 20° angle to IR

25. Which special projection of the shoulder places the glenoid cavity in profile for an "open" scapulohumeral joint?

    A. Garth method   C. Fisk modification

    B. Transthoracic lateral—Lawrence method   D. Grashey method

26. For the erect version of the tangential projection for the intertubercular groove, the patient leans forward

    _____ from vertical.

    A. 5° to 7°   C. 10° to 15°

    B. 20° to 25°   D. 35° to 45°

27. What is the major advantage of the supine, tangential version of the intertubercular groove projection over the erect version?

    A. Less radiation exposure   C. Less risk for motion

    B. Reduced OID   D. Ability to use automatic exposure control (AEC)

28. Which one of the following projections best demonstrates the supraspinatus outlet region?

    A. Tangential projection (Neer method)   C. Inferosuperior axial

    B. Fisk method   D. PA transaxillary projection (Hobbs modification)

29. With which one of the following projections can a breathing technique be employed?

    A. Grashey method   C. Scapular Y lateral

    B. Transthoracic lateral for humerus   D. Garth method

30. What central ray angulation is required for the tangential projection-supraspinatus outlet (Neer method)?

    A. 10° to 15° caudad   C. 25° anteriorly and medially

    B. 45° caudad   D. None; central ray is perpendicular

31. Which clinical indication is best demonstrated with the Garth method?

    A. Bursitis
    B. Rheumatoid arthritis
    C. Scapulohumeral dislocations
    D. Signs of shoulder impingement

32. Which anatomy of the shoulder is best demonstrated with a PA transaxillary projection (Hobbs modification)?

    A. Scapulohumeral joint space
    B. Coracoacromial arch
    C. Coracoid process
    D. Scapula in profile

33. If the patient cannot fully abduct the affected arm 90° for the inferosuperior axial projection (Clements

    modification), the technologist can angle the CR _____° toward the axilla.

    A. 5° to 15°
    B. 20° to 25°
    C. 25° to 30°
    D. 45°

34. Which one of the following projections requires the CR to be centered 2 inches (5 cm) inferior and medial from the superolateral border of the shoulder?

    A. Tangential projection (Fisk modification)
    B. Inferosuperior axial (Clements projection)
    C. Posterior oblique (Grashey method)
    D. Scapula Y lateral projection

35. Which anatomy is best demonstrated with the Alexander method?

    A. Scapulohumeral joint
    B. Coracoid process
    C. Proximal humerus
    D. AC joints

36. Which type of injury must be ruled out before the weight-bearing phase of an AC joint study?

    A. Shoulder separation
    B. Fractured clavicle
    C. Bursitis of the scapulohumeral joint
    D. Bankart lesion

37. What is the <u>minimum</u> amount of weight a large adult should have strapped to each wrist for the weight-bearing phase of an AC joint study?

    A. 5 to 7 lb
    B. 8 to 10 lb
    C. 12 to 15 lb
    D. 20 to 30 lb

38. True/False: A posteroanterior (PA) axial projection of the clavicle requires a 35° to 45° caudal central ray angle.

39. True/False: A 72-inch (183-cm) SID is recommended for acromioclavicular joint studies.

40. Which two positioning landmarks are aligned perpendicularly to the IR for the lateral scapula projection?

    A. Scapular spine and greater tubercle
    B. Superior angle and AC joint
    C. AC joint and greater tubercle
    D. Acromion and coracoid process

41. A radiograph of a posterior oblique (Grashey method) reveals that the anterior and posterior glenoid rims are not superimposed. The following positioning factors were used: erect position, body rotated 25° to 30° toward the affected side, central ray perpendicular to scapulohumeral joint space, and affected arm slightly abducted in neutral rotation. Which one of the following modifications will superimpose the glenoid rims during the repeat exposure?

    A. Angle central ray 10° to 15° caudad
    B. Rotate body less toward affected side
    C. Place affected arm in external rotation position
    D. Rotate body more toward affected side

42. **Situation:** A patient with a possible shoulder dislocation enters the emergency room. A neutral AP projection of the shoulder has been taken, confirming a dislocation. Which additional projection should be taken?

A. Inferosuperior axial (Clements modification)

B. Alexander method

C. Garth method

D. AP, external rotation

43. A radiograph of an AP axial clavicle taken on an asthenic type patient reveals that the clavicle is projected in the lung field below the top of the shoulder. The following positioning factors were used: erect position, central ray angled 15° cephalad, 40-inch (102-cm) SID, and respiration suspended at end of expiration. Which one of the following modifications should be made during the repeat exposure?

A. Increase central ray angulation

B. Suspend respiration at end of inspiration

C. Reverse central ray angulation

D. Use 72-inch (183-cm) SID

44. **Situation:** A patient with a possible right shoulder separation enters the emergency room. Which one of the following routines should be used?

A. Acromioclavicular joint series: Non–weight-bearing and weight-bearing projections

B. AP neutral projection and Garth method

C. AP neutral and transthoracic lateral projections

D. AP internal and external projections

45. **Situation:** A patient comes to the radiology department with a history of tendonitis of the bicep tendon. Which of the following projections will best demonstrate calcification of the tendon within the intertubercular groove?

A. Garth method

B. Grashey method

C. PA transaxillary projection (Hobbs modification)

D. Tangential projection—Fisk modification

46. An AP apical oblique axial (Garth method) radiographic image demonstrates poor visibility of the shoulder joint. The technologist used the following factors: Patient erect, facing the x-ray tube, 45° of rotation of affected shoulder toward the IR, 45° cephalad angle, and the CR centered to the scapulohumeral joint. What of the following factors would have contributed to this poor Garth position?

A. Wrong direction of CR angle

B. Incorrect CR centering

C. Position must be performed recumbent

D. Shoulder rotated in wrong direction

47. **Situation:** A patient is referred to radiology for a nontrauma shoulder series. The routine calls for a PA transaxillary projection (Hobbs modification) be included. But the patient is unable to stand and is confined to a wheelchair. What should the technologist do at this point?

A. Ask another technologist to hold the patient erect for the projection.

B. Perform the projection with the patient's upper chest prone on the table.

C. Perform a recumbent posterior oblique (Grashey method) instead.

D. Eliminate projection from positioning routine.

48. **Situation:** A patient enters ER with a proximal and midhumeral fracture. The patient is in extreme pain. Which one of the following positioning routines would demonstrate the entire humerus without excessive movement of the limb?

   A. AP and mediolateral humerus

   B. AP and transthoracic lateral (Lawrence method)

   C. AP and transthoracic lateral of humerus

   D. AP and scapular Y lateral

49. For the following critique questions, see Fig. C5-96, an AP clavicle radiograph, on p. 205 in your textbook.

   A. Which positioning error(s) is (are) visible on this AP left clavicle radiograph? (More than one answer may be selected.)

   (a) All essential anatomic structures are not demonstrated.

   (b) Central ray is centered incorrectly.

   (c) Collimation is not evident.

   (d) Exposure factors are incorrect.

   (e) No anatomic marker is visible on the radiograph.

   (f) Slight rotation toward the right is evident.

   (g) Slight rotation toward the left is evident.

   B. Which error(s) identified in the preceding is (are) considered "repeatable"?

   _____

   C. Which of the following modifications must be made during the repeat exposure? (More than one answer may be selected.)

   (a) Increase collimation.

   (b) Center central ray correctly.

   (c) Decrease exposure factors.

   (d) Increase exposure factors.

   (e) Place anatomic marker on image receptor (IR) before exposure.

   (f) Ensure that no rotation occurs to the right or left.

50. For the following critique questions, refer to the AP scapula radiograph, Fig. C5-98, on p. 205 in your textbook.

   A. Which positioning error(s) is (are) visible on this radiograph? (More than one answer may be selected.)

   (a) All essential anatomic structures are not demonstrated.

   (b) Central ray is centered incorrectly.

   (c) Collimation is not evident.

   (d) Exposure factors are incorrect.

   (e) No anatomic marker is visible on radiograph.

   (f) Excessive rotation toward the right is evident.

   (g) Excessive rotation toward the left is evident.

   B. Which error(s) identified in the preceding is (are) considered "repeatable"?

   _____

C. Which of the following modifications must be made during the repeat exposure? (More than one answer may be selected.)

(a) Increase collimation.

(b) Center central ray more inferiorly.

(c) Decrease exposure factors.

(d) Increase exposure factors.

(e) Place anatomic marker on IR before exposure.

(f) Rotate body slightly toward the left.

(g) Rotate elbow slightly toward the right.

6 Lower Limb

CHAPTER OBJECTIVES

After you have successfully completed the activities in this chapter, you will be able to:

_____ 1. Identify the bones and specific features of the toes, foot, ankle, lower leg, knee, patella, and distal femur.

_____ 2. On drawings and radiographs, identify specific anatomic features of the foot, ankle, leg, knee, patella, and distal femur.

_____ 3. Identify specific joints of the foot, ankle, leg, and knee according to the correct classification and movement type.

_____ 4. Match specific clinical indications of the lower limb to the correct definition.

_____ 5. Match specific clinical indications of the lower limb to the correct radiographic appearance.

_____ 6. Describe the basic and special projections of the toes, foot, ankle, calcaneus, knee, patella, intercondylar fossa, and femur, including central ray placement and angulation, correct image receptor size and placement, part positioning, technical factors, and evaluation criteria.

_____ 7. List the various patient dose ranges for each projection of the lower limb.

_____ 8. Given various hypothetic situations, identify the correct modification of a position and/or exposure factors to improve the radiographic image.

_____ 9. Given various hypothetic situations, identify the correct position for a specific pathologic form or condition.

_____ 10. Given radiographs of specific lower limb projections, identify specific positioning and exposure factor errors.

Positioning and Radiographic Critique

_____ 1. Using a peer, perform basic and special projections of the lower limb.

_____ 2. Using foot and knee phantoms, produce satisfactory radiographs of the lower limb (if equipment is available).

_____ 3. Critique and evaluate lower limb radiographs based on the five divisions of radiographic criteria: (1) anatomy demonstrated, (2) position, (3) collimation and central ray, (4) exposure, and (5) anatomic side markers.

_____ 4. Distinguish between acceptable and unacceptable lower limb radiographs based on exposure factors, motion, collimation, positioning, or other errors.

LEARNING EXERCISES

Complete the following review exercises after reading the associated pages in the textbook as indicated by each exercise. Answers to each review exercise are given at the end of the review exercises.

PART I: RADIOGRAPHIC ANATOMY

REVIEW EXERCISE A: Radiographic Anatomy of the Foot and Ankle (see textbook pp. 208-213)

1. Fill in the number of bones for the following:

   A. Phalanges _____   C. Tarsals _____

   B. Metatarsals _____   D. Total _____

2. What are two differences in the phalanges of the foot as compared with the phalanges of the hand?

   A. _____

   B. _____

3. Which tuberosity of the foot is palpable and a common site of foot trauma?

   _____

4. Where are the sesamoid bones of the foot most commonly located? _____

5. What is the largest and strongest tarsal bone? _____

6. What is the name of the joint found between the talus and calcaneus? _____

7. List the three specific articular facets found in the joint described in the previous question.

   A. _____   B. _____   C. _____

8. The small opening, or space, found in the middle of the joint identified in question 6 is called the:

   _____.

9. Match each of the following characteristics to the correct tarsal bone. (Answers may be used more than once.)

   _____ 1. Forms an aspect of the ankle joint   A. Calcaneus

   _____ 2. The smallest of the cuneiforms   B. Talus

   _____ 3. Found on the medial side of the foot between the talus C. Cuboid

   _____ 4. The largest of the cuneiforms   D. Navicular

   _____ 5. Articulates with the second, third, and fourth metatarsal   E. Lateral cuneiform

   _____ 6. The most superior tarsal bone   F. Intermediate cuneiform

   _____ 7. Articulates with the first metatarsal   G. Medial cuneiform

   _____ 8. Common site for bone spurs

   _____ 9. A tarsal found anterior to the calcaneus and lateral to
              the lateral cuneiform

   _____ 10. The second largest tarsal bone

10. Identify the labeled structures found in Figs. 6-1 and 6-2.

A. _____

B. _____

C. _____

D. _____

E. _____

F. _____

G. _____

H. _____

I. _____

J. _____

K. _____

L. _____

M. Fig. 6-1 represents a radiograph of which projection

of the foot? _____

N. _____

O. _____

P. _____

Q. _____

R. _____

S. _____

T. Fig. 6 -2 represents a radiograph of which projection?

_____

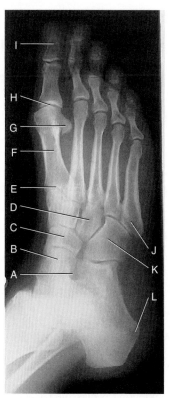

Fig. 6-1. Anatomy of the foot.

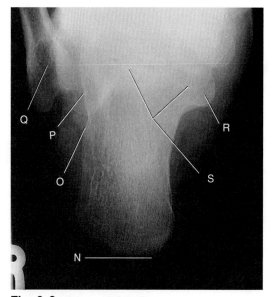

Fig. 6-2. Anatomy of the foot.

11. True/False: The cuboid articulates with the four bones of the foot.

12. The calcaneus articulates with the talus and the:

   A. Navicular   C. Medial cuneiform

   B. Cuboid   D. Lateral cuneiform

13. List the two arches of the foot.

   A. _____   B. _____

14. Which three bones make up the ankle joint?

   A. _____   B. _____   C. _____

15. The three bones of the ankle form a deep socket into which the talus fits. This socket is called the

   _____.

16. The distal tibial joint surface forming the roof of the distal ankle joint is called the:

   A. Tibial plafond   C. Tibial plateau

   B. Articular facet   D. Ankle mortise

17. True/False: The medial malleolus is approximately ½ inch (1 cm) posterior to the lateral malleolus.

18. The ankle joint is classified as a synovial joint with _____ type movement.

19. Identify the structures labeled on Figs. 6-3 and 6-4.

Fig. 6-3

   A. _____

   B. _____

   C. _____

   D. _____

   E. _____

Fig. 6-4

   F. _____

   G. _____

   H. _____

   I. _____

   J. _____

   K. _____

   L. _____

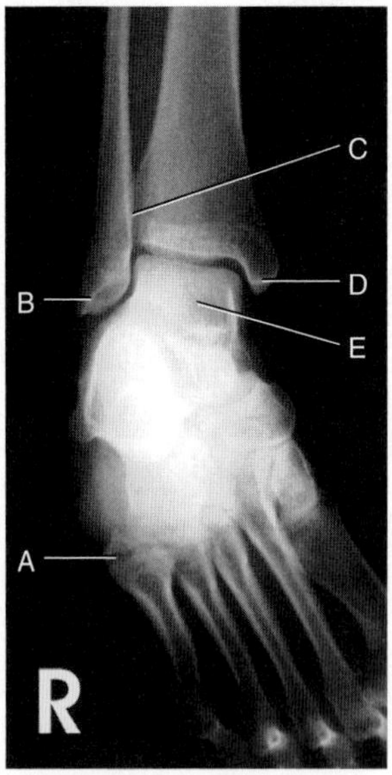

Fig. 6-3. Anatomy of the ankle.

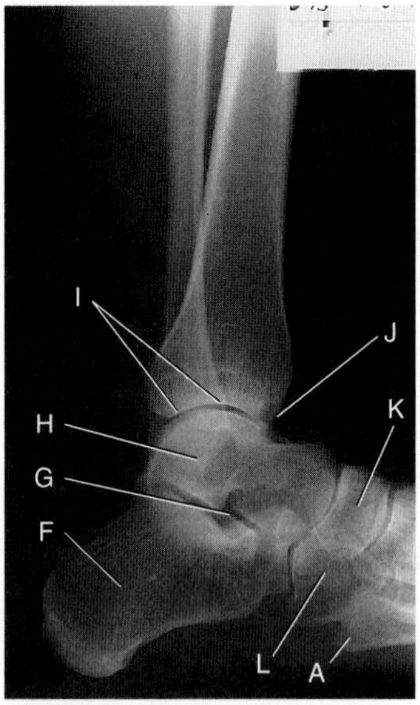

Fig. 6-4. Anatomy of the ankle.

   M. Fig. 6-3 represents a radiograph of which projection of the ankle? _____

REVIEW EXERCISE B: Radiographic Anatomy of the Lower Leg, Knee, and Distal Femur (see textbook pp. 214-218)

1. The _____ is the weight-bearing bone of the lower leg.

2. What is the name of the large prominence located on the midanterior surface of the proximal tibia that serves as a distal attachment for the patellar tendon? _____

3. What is the name of the small prominence located on the posterolateral aspect of the medial condyle of the femur that is an identifying landmark to determine possible rotation of a lateral knee? _____

4. A small, triangular depression located on the tibia that helps form the distal tibiofibular joint is called the

   _____.

5. The articular facets of the proximal tibia are also referred to as the _____.

6. The articular facets slope _____ ° posteriorly.
   A. 25   C. 35
   B. 45   D. 10 to 15

7. The most proximal aspect of the fibula is the _____.

8. The extreme distal end of the fibula forms the _____.

9. What is the name of the largest sesamoid bone in the body? _____

10. What are two other names for the patellar surface of the femur?

    A. _____   B. _____

11. What is the name of the depression located on the posterior aspect of the distal femur? _____

12. Why must the central ray be angled 5° to 7° cephalad for a lateral knee position? _____

13. The slightly raised area located on the posterolateral aspect of the medial femoral condyle is called the:
    A. Trochlear tubercle   C. Adductor tubercle
    B. Anterior crest   D. Tibial tuberosity

14. What are the two palpable bony landmarks found on the distal femur?

    A. _____   B. _____

15. The general region of the posterior knee is called the _____.

16. True/False: Flexion of 20° of the knee forces the patella firmly against the patellar surface of the femur.

17. True/False: The patella acts like a pivot to increase the leverage of a large muscle found in the anterior thigh.

18. True/False: The posterior surface of the patella is normally rough.

19. For which large muscle does the patella serve as a pivot to increase the leverage? _____.

20. List the correct terms for the following joints:

    A. Between the patella and distal femur _____

    B. Between the two condyles of the femur and tibia _____

21. List the four major ligaments of the knee.

    A. _____   C. _____

    B. _____   D. _____

22. The crescent-shaped fibrocartilage disks that act as shock absorbers in the knee joint are called _____.

23. List the two bursae found in the knee joint.

    A. _____   B. _____

24. Match each of the following structures to the correct bone (answers may be used more than once).

    _____   1. Tibial plafond   A. Tibia

    _____   2. Medial malleolus   B. Fibula

    _____   3. Lateral epicondyle   C. Distal femur

    _____   4. Patellar surface   D. Patella

    _____   5. Articular facets

    _____   6. Fibular notch

    _____   7. Styloid process

    _____   8. Base

    _____   9. Intercondyloid eminence

    _____   10. Neck

25. Match each of the following articulations to the correct joint classification or movement type (answers may be used more than once).

_____ 1. Ankle joint

_____ 2. Patellofemoral

_____ 3. Proximal tibiofibular

_____ 4. Tarsometatarsal

_____ 5. Knee joint (femorotibial)

_____ 6. Distal tibiofibular

A. Synarthrodial (gomphoses type)

B. Ginglymus (hinge)

C. Sellar (saddle)

D. Plane (gliding)

E. Amphiarthrodial (syndesmosis type)

F. Bicondylar

26. Identify the labeled structures on Figs. 6-5 through 6-7.

Fig. 6-5

A. _____

B. _____

C. _____

D. _____

E. _____

F. _____

G. _____

H. _____

I. _____

Fig. 6-6

J. _____

K. _____

L. _____

M. _____

N. _____

O. _____ (° angle)

P. _____

Q. _____

R. _____

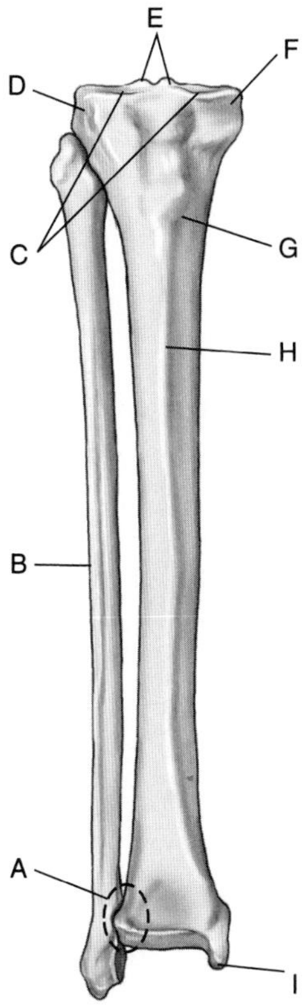

Fig. 6-5. Frontal view of tibia and fibula.

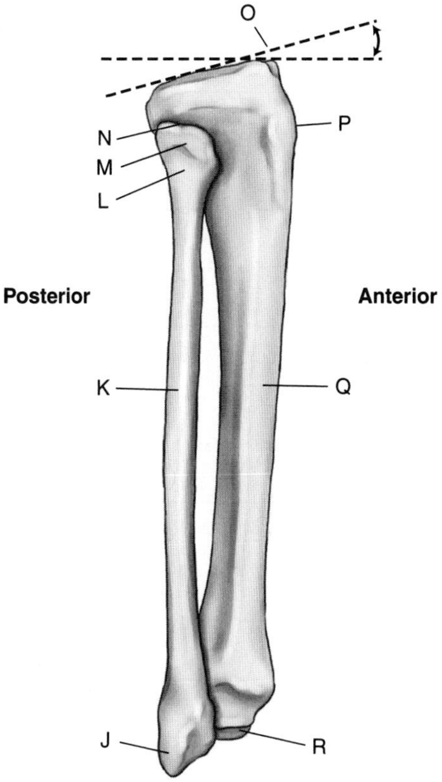

Fig. 6-6. Lateral view of tibia and fibula.

Fig. 6-7

S. _____

T. _____

U. _____

V. _____

W. _____

X. Which projection does the radiograph in

Fig. 6-7 represent? _____

27. Identify the bony structures labeled on Figs. 6-8 and 6-9.

Fig. 6-8

A. _____

B. _____

C. _____

D. _____

E. _____

F. _____

G. _____

H. _____

Fig. 6-9

I. _____

J. _____

K. _____

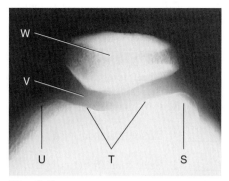

Fig. 6-7. Anatomy of the knee and patella.

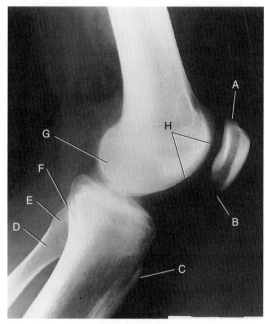

Fig. 6-8. True lateral radiograph of the knee.

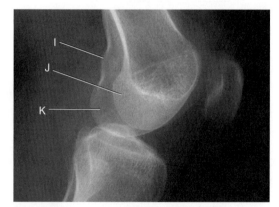

Fig. 6-9. Lateral radiograph of the knee.

28. Match the following foot and ankle movements to the correct definition.

_____ A. Inward turning or bending of ankle   1. Inversion (varus)

_____ B. Decreasing the angle between the dorsum   2. Plantar flexion
            pedis and anterior lower leg

_____ C. Extending the ankle or pointing the foot   3. Eversion (valgus)
            and toe downward

_____ D. Outward turning or bending of ankle   4. Dorsiflexion

PART II: RADIOGRAPHIC POSITIONING
REVIEW EXERCISE C: Positioning of the Foot and Ankle (see textbook pp. 219-239)

1. True/False: The recommended source image receptor distance (SID) for lower limb radiography is 40 inches (102 cm).

2. True/False: Multiple images can be placed on the same IR when using analog imaging systems.

3. True/False: With careful and close collimation, gonadal shielding does not have to be used during lower limb radiography.

4. True/False: With digital radiography, the anatomy should be centered to the IR.

5. True/False: A kV range between 50 and 70 should be used for analog lower limb radiography.

6. True/False: A kV range for digital imaging is typically lower as compared with film-screen ranges.

7. Match the following clinical indications to the correct definition.

_____ A. An inflammatory condition involving the anterior, proximal tibia   1. Exostosis

_____ B. Also known as osteitis deformans   2. Lisfranc joint injury

_____ C. Malignant tumor of the cartilage   3. Bone cyst

_____ D. Inherited type of arthritis that commonly affects males   4. Reiter's syndrome

_____ E. Benign, neoplastic bone lesion caused by overproduction of   5. Osteoid osteoma
          bone at a joint

                                                         6. Ewing's sarcoma

_____ F. Benign bone lesion usually developing in teens or young adults   7. Gout

_____ G. Most prevalent primary bone malignancy in pediatric patients   8. Paget's disease

_____ H. Benign, neoplastic bone lesion filled with clear fluid   9. Osgood-Schlatter disease

_____ I. Injury to a large ligament located between the bases of the first and   10. Chondrosarcoma
          second metatarsal

_____ J. Condition affecting the sacroiliac joints and lower limbs of
          young men, especially the posterosuperior margin of the calcaneus

8. The formal name for "runner's knee" is _____.

9. What is another term for osteomalacia? _____

10. Match the following radiographic appearances to the correct clinical indication.

_____ A. Asymmetric erosion of joint spaces with calcaneal erosion   1. Osteoid osteoma

_____ B. Uric acid deposits in joint spaces   2. Ewing's sarcoma

_____ C. Well-circumscribed lucency   3. Gout

_____ D. Small, round/oval density with lucent center   4. Osgood-Schlatter disease

_____ E. Narrowed, irregular joint surfaces with sclerotic articular surfaces   5. Osteoarthritis

_____ F. Fragmentation or detachment of the tibial tuberosity   6. Osteomalacia

_____ G. Ill-defined area of bone destruction with surrounding "onion peel"   7. Reiter's syndrome

_____ H. Decreased bone density and bowing deformities of weight-bearing limbs   8. Bone cyst

11. Why is the central ray angled 10° to 15° toward the calcaneus for an anteroposterior (AP) projection of the toes?

_____

12. Where is the central ray centered for an AP oblique projection of the foot? _____

13. Which projection is best for demonstrating the sesamoid bones of the foot? _____

14. The foot should be dorsiflexed so that the plantar surface of the foot is _____° from vertical for the sesamoid projection.

15. Why should the central ray be perpendicular to the metatarsals for an AP projection of the foot?

_____

16. If a foreign body is lodged in the plantar surface of the foot, which type of central ray angle should be used for the AP projection?

A. 10° posterior   C. 10° anterior

B. 15° posterior   D. None. Use a perpendicular central ray.

17. Rotation can be determined on a radiograph of an AP foot projection by the near-equal distance between the

_____ metatarsals.

18. Which oblique projection of the foot best demonstrates the majority of the tarsal bones?

_____

19. Which oblique projection of the foot best demonstrates the navicular and the first and second cuneiforms with

minimal superimposition? _____

20. Which projection will place the foot into a true lateral position: mediolateral or lateromedial?

_____

21. Which type of study should be performed to best evaluate the status of the longitudinal arches of the foot?

_____

22. How should the central ray be angled from the long axis of the foot for the plantodorsal axial projection of the calcaneus? _____

23. Which calcaneal structure should appear medially on a well-positioned plantodorsal axial projection?

_____

24. Where is the central ray placed for a mediolateral projection of the calcaneus? _____

25. Which joint surface of the ankle is *not* typically visualized with a correctly positioned AP projection of the ankle?
    A. Medial surface of joint   C. Lateral surface of joint
    B. Superior surface of joint   D. All of the listed surfaces of the joint *are* visualized.

26. Why should AP, 45° oblique, and lateral ankle radiographs include the proximal metatarsals?

_____

27. How much (if any) should the foot and ankle be rotated for an AP mortise projection of the ankle?

_____

28. Which projection of the ankle best demonstrates a possible fracture of the lateral malleolus?

_____

29. With a true lateral projection of the ankle, the lateral malleolus is:
    A. Projected over the anterior aspect of the distal tibia
    B. Projected over the posterior aspect of the distal tibia
    C. Directly superimposed over the distal tibia
    D. Directly superimposed over the medial malleolus

30. Which projections of the ankle require forced inversion and eversion movements?

_____

REVIEW EXERCISE D: Positioning of the Tibia, Fibula, Knee, and Distal Femur (see textbook pp. 242-257)

1. What is the basic positioning routine for a study of the tibia and fibula? _____

2. Why is it important to include the knee joint for an initial study of tibia trauma, even if the patient's symptoms involve the middle and distal aspect?

_____

3. To include both joints for a lateral projection of the tibia and fibula for an adult, the technologist may place the

   cassette _____ in relation to the part.
   A. Parallel   C. Diagonal
   B. Perpendicular   D. Transverse

4. What is the recommended central ray angulation for an AP projection of the knee for a patient with thick thighs and buttocks (i.e., measuring greater than 24 cm)?
   A. 3° to 5° caudad   C. Central ray perpendicular to IR
   B. 3° to 5° cephalad   D. Central ray perpendicular to patellar plane

5. Where is the central ray centered for an AP projection of the knee?
   A. ½ inch (1.25 cm) distal to apex of patella   C. Midpatella
   B. 1 inch (2.5 cm) proximal to apex of patella   D. Level of tibial tuberosity

6. Which basic projection of a knee best demonstrates the proximal fibula free of superimposition?
   A. True AP   C. AP oblique, 45° medial rotation
   B. True lateral   D. AP oblique, 45° lateral rotation

7. For the AP oblique projection of the knee, the _____ rotation (medial [internal] or lateral [external]) best visualizes the lateral condyle of the tibia and the head and neck of the fibula.

8. What is the recommended central ray placement for a lateral knee position on a tall, slender male patient with a narrow pelvis (without support of the lower leg)?
   A. 5° to 10° caudad   C. Central ray perpendicular to IR
   B. 5° cephalad   D. Central ray perpendicular to patellar plane

9. How much flexion is recommended for a lateral projection of the knee?
   A. No flexion   C. 30° to 35°
   B. 20° to 30°   D. 45°

10. Which positioning error(s) is present if the distal borders of the femoral condyles are not superimposed on a

    radiograph of a lateral knee on an average size knee? _____

11. Which positioning error is present if the posterior portions of the femoral condyles are not superimposed on a

    lateral knee radiograph? _____

12. Which anatomic structure of the femur can be used to determine which rotation error (over-rotation or under-rotation) is present on a slightly rotated lateral knee radiograph?

    _____

13. Which special projection of the knee best evaluates the knee joint for cartilage degeneration or deformities?

    _____

14. What is the best modality to examine ligament injuries to the knee?
    A. CT   C. MRI
    B. Nuclear medicine   D. Ultrasound

15. Which one of the following special projections of the knee best demonstrates the intercondylar fossa?

    A. Holmblad   C. AP weight-bearing, bilateral projections

    B. Merchant   D. Settegast

16. How much flexion of the lower leg is required for the PA axial projection (Camp-Coventry method) when the central ray is angled 40° caudad? _____

17. Why is the posteroanterior (PA) axial projection for the intercondylar fossa recommended instead of an AP axial projection? _____

18. What type of CR angulation is required for the PA axial weight-bearing projection (Rosenberg method)?

    A. None CR is perpendicular   C. 10° cephalad

    B. 10° caudad   D. 5° to 7° cephalad

19. How much flexion of the knees is required for the PA axial weight-bearing projection (Rosenberg method)?

    A. 20° to 30°   C. 5° to 10°

    B. 35° to 40°   D. 45°

20. How much knee flexion is required for the PA axial projection (Holmblad method)?

    A. 45°   C. 60° to 70°

    B. 35°   D. None. Lower limb is fully extended

21. What type of CR angle is required for the PA axial (Holmblad method)?

    A. 10° caudad   C. 15° to 20° cephalad

    B. 10° cephalad   D. None. CR is perpendicular to IR

22. True/False: To place the interepicondylar line parallel to the image receptor for a PA projection of the patella, the lower limb must be rotated approximately 5° internally.

23. How much part flexion is recommended for a lateral projection of the patella?

_____

24. How much central ray angle from the long axis of the femora is required for the tangential (Merchant method) bilateral projection? _____

25. How much part flexion is required for the following methods?

    A. Hughston method _____

    B. Settegast method _____

26. What type of CR angle is required for the superoinferior sitting tangential method for the patella?

    A. 40° cephalad   C. Depends on degree of flexion

    B. 5° to 10° caudad   D. None. CR is perpendicular to IR

27. Match each of the following descriptions of positioning for projections of the knee and/or patella to its correct name or term. (Use each answer only once.)

_____ 1. Can be performed using a wheelchair or lowered radiographic table

_____ 2. Patient prone; requires 90° knee flexion

_____ 3. Patient prone with 40° to 50° knee flexion and with equal 40° to 50° caudad CR angle

_____ 4. IR is placed on a foot stool to minimize the OID

_____ 5. Patient prone with 55° knee flexion and 15° to 20° CR angle from long axis of lower leg.

_____ 6. Patient supine with cassette resting on midthighs

_____ 7. Patient supine with 40° knee flexion and with 30° caudad CR angle from horizontal

A. Inferosuperior for patellofemoral joint

B. Merchant method

C. Hughston method

D. Camp-Coventry method

E. Settegast method

F. Holmblad method (variation)

G. Hobbs modification

28. Which of the following special projections of the knee must be performed erect?

A. Rosenberg method   C. Settegast method

B. Camp-Coventry method   D. Hughston method

29. True/False: The recommended SID is 48 inches (123 cm) to 72 inches (183 cm) for the tangential (bilateral Merchant) projection.

30. How much knee flexion is required for the horizontal beam lateral patella projection?

A. 5° or 10°   C. 25° or 30°

B. 15° to 20°   D. None

REVIEW EXERCISE E: Problem Solving for Technical and Positioning Errors

1. **Situation:** A radiograph of an AP projection of the foot reveals that the metatarsophalangeal joints are not open and the metatarsals are somewhat foreshortened. What positioning error was involved, and what modification should be made to improve this image on the repeat exposure?

_____

2. **Situation:** A radiograph of an AP oblique-medial rotation projection of the foot reveals that the proximal third to fifth metatarsals are superimposed. What type of positioning error led to this radiographic outcome?

_____

3. **Situation:** A radiograph of a plantodorsal axial projection of the calcaneus reveals considerable foreshortening of the calcaneus. What type of positioning modification is needed on the repeat exposure?

_____

4. **Situation:** A radiograph of an AP projection of the ankle reveals that the lateral surface of the ankle joint is totally open. (It should not be open on a true AP projection.) The technologist is positive that the ankle was in the correct, true AP position with the long axis of the foot perpendicular to the IR. What else could have led to this joint space being open?

_____

5. **Situation:** A radiograph of an intended AP mortise projection reveals that the lateral malleolus is superimposed over the talus, and the distal tibiofibular joint is not well demonstrated. What is the most likely reason for this radiographic outcome?

_____

6. **Situation:** A radiograph of an AP knee projection demonstrates that the femorotibial joint space is not open at all. The patient is young and has no history of degenerative disease. What type of positioning modification may improve the outcome of this projection?

_____

7. **Situation:** A radiograph of an AP oblique with medial rotation of the knee to demonstrate the proximal fibula reveals that there is total superimposition of the proximal tibia and the fibula. What must be modified to correct this projection?

_____

8. **Situation:** A radiograph of a lateral recumbent knee reveals that the posterior border of the medial femoral condyle (identified by the adductor tubercle) is not superimposed but is slightly posterior to the lateral condyle. The fibular head is also completely superimposed by the tibia. What type of positioning error led to this radiographic outcome?

_____

9. **Situation:** A patient with trauma to the medial aspect of the foot comes to the emergency room. A heavy object was dropped on the foot near the base of the first metatarsal. Basic foot projections do not clearly demonstrate this region. What other projection of the foot could be used to better delineate this area?

_____

10. **Situation:** A radiograph of an AP and lateral tibia and fibula reveals that the ankle joint is not included on the AP projection, but both the knee and the ankle are included on the lateral projection. What should the technologist do in this situation?

_____

11. **Situation:** A radiograph obtained by using the PA axial (Camp-Coventry method) reveals that the distal femoral condyles, articular facets, and intercondylar fossa are asymmetric. What possible positioning errors may have produced this distortion of the anatomy?

_____

12. **Situation:** A radiograph of a lateral patella reveals that the patella is drawn tightly against the intercondylar sulcus. Which positioning modification should be performed to improve the quality of the image during the repeat exposure?

_____

13. **Situation:** A patient with a history of degenerative disease of the left knee joint comes to the radiology department. The orthopedic surgeon orders a radiographic study to determine the extent of damage to the joint space. Which projection(s) should be performed?

_____

14. **Situation:** A patient with a possible Lisfranc joint injury. Which radiographic position(s) best demonstrate this

type of injury?_____

15. **Situation:** A patient with a history of pain in the feet comes to the radiology department. The referring physician orders a study to evaluate the longitudinal arches of the feet. Which positioning routine should be used?

_____

16. **Situation:** A patient with bony, loose bodies (or "joint mice") within the knee joint comes to radiology for a knee series. The AP and lateral knee projections fail to demonstrate any loose bodies. What additional knee projection can be taken to better demonstrate them?

_____

17. **Situation:** A young male patient comes to the radiology department with a clinical history of Osgood-Schlatter disease. Which single projection of the basic knee series will best demonstrate this condition?

_____

18. **Situation:** A radiograph of a mediolateral knee projection demonstrates that the medial femoral condyle is projected inferior to the lateral condyle. What can the technologist do to correct this problem during the repeat exposure?

_____

19. **Situation:** A physician orders a bilateral, tangential projection of the patella and patellofemoral joint space. But the patient is restricted to a wheelchair and cannot lie on the radiographic table because of chronic pain. Which projection could be performed with the patient remaining in the wheelchair?

_____

20. **Situation:** A tangential (inferosuperior) projection of the patellofemoral joint space reveals that the patella is seated into the intercondylar sulcus and the joint space is not demonstrated. What possible positioning errors may have produced this radiographic outcome?

_____

The following questions relate to the radiographs found at the end of Chapter 6 of the textbook. Evaluate these radiographs for the radiographic criteria categories (1 through 5) that follow. Describe the corrections needed to improve the overall image. The major, or "repeatable," errors are specific errors that indicate the need for a repeat exposure, regardless of the nature of the other errors.

Comparing these radiographs with the correctly positioned and exposed radiographs in this chapter of the textbook will help you evaluate each of them for errors.

A. Bilateral tangential patella (Fig. C6-141)

Description of possible error:

    1. Anatomy demonstrated: _____

    2. Part positioning: _____

    3. Collimation and central ray: _____

    4. Exposure: _____

    5. Anatomic side markers: _____

Repeatable error(s): _____

B. Plantodorsal (axial) calcaneus (Fig. C6-142)

Description of possible error:

    1. Anatomy demonstrated: _____

    2. Part positioning: _____

    3. Collimation and central ray: _____

    4. Exposure: _____

    5. Anatomic side markers: _____

Repeatable error(s): _____

C. AP mortise ankle (Fig. C6-143)

Description of possible error:

    1. Anatomy demonstrated: _____

    2. Part positioning: _____

    3. Collimation and central ray: _____

    4. Exposure: _____

    5. Anatomic side markers: _____

Repeatable error(s): _____

D. AP lower leg (Fig. C6-144)

Description of possible error:

1. Anatomy demonstrated: _____

2. Part positioning: _____

3. Collimation and central ray: _____

4. Exposure: _____

5. Anatomic side markers: _____

Repeatable error(s): _____

E. Lateral knee (Fig. C6-145)

Description of possible error:

1. Anatomy demonstrated: _____

2. Part positioning: _____

3. Collimation and central ray: _____

4. Exposure: _____

5. Anatomic side markers: _____

Repeatable error(s): _____

F. AP medial oblique knee (Fig. C6-146)

Description of possible error:

1. Anatomy demonstrated: _____

2. Part positioning: _____

3. Collimation and central ray: _____

4. Exposure: _____

5. Anatomic side markers: _____

Repeatable error(s): _____

PART III: LABORATORY ACTIVITIES

You must gain experience in positioning each part of the lower limb before performing the following exams on actual patients. You can get experience in positioning and radiographic evaluation of these projections by performing exercises using radiographic phantoms and practicing on other students (although you will not be taking actual exposures).

The following suggested activities assume that your teaching institution has an energized lab and radiographic phantoms. If not, perform Laboratory Exercises B and C, the radiographic evaluation, and the physical positioning exercises. (Check off each step and projection as you complete it.)

Laboratory Exercise A: Energized Laboratory

1. Using the foot/ankle radiographic phantom, produce radiographs of the basic routines for the following:

   _____ Foot

   _____ Ankle

   _____ Calcaneus

2. Using the knee radiographic phantom, produce radiographs of the following basic routines:

   _____ AP

   _____ AP oblique, medial rotation

   _____ Lateral (horizontal beam lateral if flexed knee is not available)

Laboratory Exercise B: Radiographic Evaluation

1. Evaluate and critique the radiographs produced in the preceding, additional radiographs provided by your instructor, or both. Evaluate each radiograph for the following points:

   _____ Evaluate the completeness of the study. (Are all of the pertinent anatomic structures included on the radiograph?)

   _____ Evaluate for positioning or centering errors (e.g., rotation, off-centering).

   _____ Evaluate for correct exposure factors and possible motion. (Are the density and contrast of the images acceptable?)

   _____ Determine whether anatomic side markers and an acceptable degree of collimation and/or area shielding are seen on the images.

Laboratory Exercise C: Physical Positioning

On another person, simulate performing all basic and special projections of the lower limb as follows. Include the six steps listed below and described in the textbook. (Check off each step when completed satisfactorily.)

Step 1. Appropriate size and type of image receptor with correct markers

Step 2. Correct central ray placement and centering of part to central ray and/or image receptor

Step 3. Accurate collimation

Step 4. Area shielding of patient where advisable

Step 5. Use of proper immobilizing devices when needed

Step 6. Approximate correct exposure factors, breathing instructions where applicable, and "making" exposure

Projections	*Step 1*	*Step 2*	*Step 3*	*Step 4*	*Step 5*	*Step 6*
● Positioning routine for a specific toe	____	____	____	____	____	____
● Basic foot routine	____	____	____	____	____	____
● Special projection for sesamoid bones	____	____	____	____	____	____
● Basic projections of the calcaneus	____	____	____	____	____	____
● Weight-bearing foot projections	____	____	____	____	____	____
● Basic ankle routine, including mortise and 45° oblique projections	____	____	____	____	____	____
● AP and lateral tibia and fibula	____	____	____	____	____	____
● Basic knee routine	____	____	____	____	____	____
● Special projections for intercondylar fossa	____	____	____	____	____	____
● Weight-bearing AP knee projections	____	____	____	____	____	____
● Special projections for patellofemoral joint space	____	____	____	____	____	____

SELF-TEST

This self-test should be taken only after completing all of the readings, review exercises, and laboratory activities for a particular section. The purpose of this test is not only to provide a good learning exercise but also to serve as a strong indicator of what your final evaluation exam will be. It is strongly suggested that if you do not get at least a 90% to 95% grade on this self-test, you should review those areas in which you missed questions before going to your instructor for the final evaluation exam for this chapter.

1. Which of the following is not an aspect of the metatarsal?

   A. Head   C. Body

   B. Tail   D. Base

2. True/False: The distal portion of the fifth metatarsal is a common fracture site.

3. Where are the sesamoid bones of the foot most commonly located?

   A. Plantar surface near head of first metatarsal

   B. Plantar surface at first tarsometatarsal joint

   C. Dorsum aspect near base of first metatarsal

   D. Plantar surface near cuboid bone

4. What is the name of the tarsal bone found on the medial side of the foot between the talus and three cuneiforms?

   A. Calcaneus   C. Cuboid

   B. Lateral malleolus   D. Navicular

5. Which tarsal bone is considered to be the smallest?

   A. Medial cuneiform   C. Intermediate cuneiform

   B. Navicular   D. Lateral cuneiform

6. What is another term for the talocalcaneal joint?

   A. Tarsometatarsal joint   C. Mortise joint

   B. Subtalar joint   D. Tibiocalcaneal joint

7. The distal tibial joint surface is called the:

   A. Medial malleolus   C. Lateral malleolus

   B. Tibial plafond   D. Anterior tubercle

8. True/False: The mortise of the ankle should be totally open and visible on a correctly positioned anteroposterior (AP) projection of the ankle.

9. Match each of the following structures or characteristics to the correct bone of the foot or ankle. (Use each choice only once.)

_____ 1. Trochlear process   A. Metatarsal

_____ 2. Lateral malleolus   B. Talus

_____ 3. The second largest tarsal bone   C. Tibia

_____ 4. Found between the navicular and base of first metatarsal   D. Calcaneus

_____ 5. Base   E. Sinus tarsi

_____ 6. Found between the calcaneus and talus   F. Medial cuneiform

_____ 7. Anterior tubercle   G. Fibula

10. Match the structures labeled on Fig. 6-10. (Use each choice only once.)

_____ A.   1. Talus

_____ B.   2. First metatarsal

_____ C.   3. Lateral malleolus

_____ D.   4. Distal tibiofibular joint

_____ E.   5. Medial malleolus

F. What projection does this radiograph represent?

A. AP mortise ankle   C. AP ankle

B. AP stress ankle—inversion   D. AP stress ankle—eversion

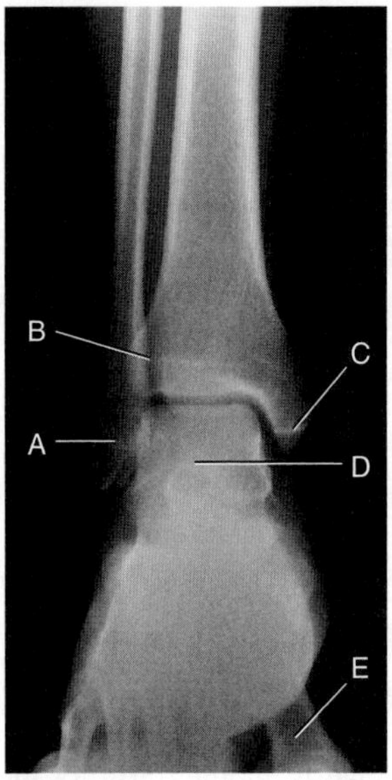

Fig. 6-10. Anatomy of the ankle.

11. Match the structures labeled on the radiographs in Figs. 6-11 through 6-13. (Answers may be used more than once.)

_____ A.

_____ B.

_____ C.

_____ D.

_____ E.

_____ F.

_____ G.

_____ H.

_____ I.

_____ J.

_____ K.

1. Distal phalanx, second digit

2. Proximal phalanx, first digit

3. Interphalangeal joint

4. Head of second metatarsal

5. Metatarsophalangeal joint of first digit

6. Base of first metatarsal

7. Proximal phalanx, second digit

8. Head of first metatarsal

9. Distal phalanx, first digit

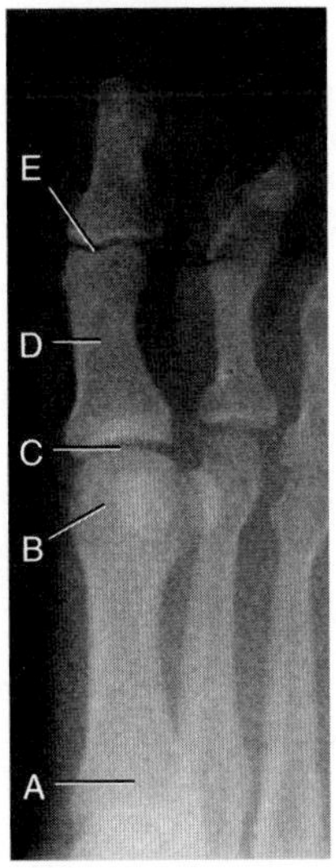

Fig. 6-11. Anatomy of the metatarsal bones and digits.

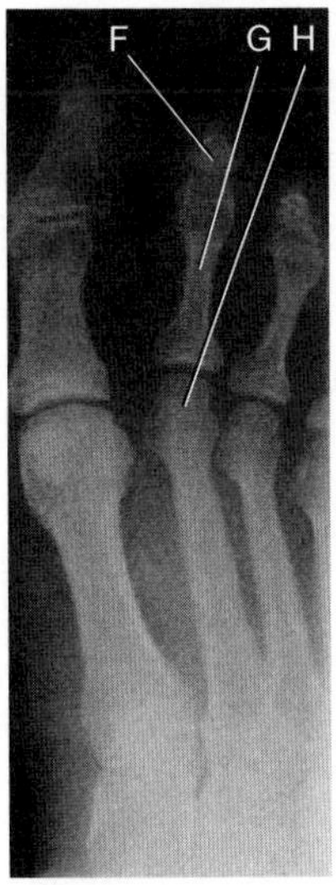

Fig. 6-12. Anatomy of the metatarsal bones and digits.

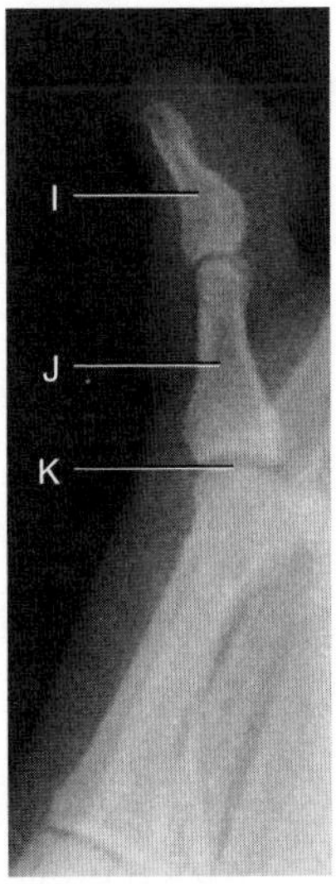

Fig. 6-13. Anatomy of the metatarsal bones and digits.

12. Which of the radiographs in the previous question represents an AP oblique projection of the toes?

A. Fig. 6-11

B. Fig. 6-13

C. Fig. 6-12

D. None of the above

13. What is the correct central ray centering placement for an AP projection of the toes?

A. Affected MTP joint

B. Affected DIP joint

C. Affected PIP joint

D. Head of affected metatarsal

14. Which type of central ray angle is required for an AP projection of the toes?

A. None (central ray is perpendicular)

B. 10° to 15° posterior

C. 5° posterior

D. 20° to 25° posterior

15. Which of the following projections is used for the sesamoid bones of the foot?

A. AP and lateral weight-bearing

B. Camp-Coventry

C. Tangential

D. AP mortise

16. How much foot rotation is required for the AP oblique, medial rotation projection of the foot?

A. 3° to 5°

B. 45°

C. 15° to 20°

D. 30° to 40°

17. What is another term for the AP projection of the foot?

    A. Mortise projection
    B. Plantodorsal projection
    C. Weight-bearing study
    D. Dorsoplantar projection

18. What CR angle is generally required for the AP projection of the foot?

    A. 10° posterior
    B. 10° anterior
    C. 15° posterior
    D. None (central ray is perpendicular)

19. Which projection of the foot best demonstrates the cuboid?

    A. AP
    B. AP oblique—lateral rotation
    C. AP oblique—medial rotation
    D. Lateromedial

20. What is another term for the intercondyloid eminence?

    A. Tibial plateaus
    B. Intercondylar fossa
    C. Tibial tuberosity
    D. Intercondylar tubercles

21. What is the name of the deep depression found on the posterior aspect of the distal femur?

    A. Intercondylar fossa
    B. Intercondylar sulcus
    C. Patellar surface
    D. Articular facets

22. A line drawn across the most distal aspect of the medial and lateral femoral condyles would be

    _____ from being at a right angle (90°) to the long axis of the femur.

    A. 5° to 7°
    B. 3° to 5°
    C. 0°
    D. 10° to 20°

23. True/False: The angle referred to in question 22 would be less on a tall, slender person.

24. The upper, or superior, portion of the patella is called the:

    A. Apex
    B. Base
    C. Styloid process
    D. Patellar head

25. Which two ligaments of the knee joint help stabilize the knee from the anterior and posterior perspective?

    A. Collaterals
    B. Patellar
    C. Cruciates
    D. Quadriceps femoris

26. Which structures serve as shock absorbers within the knee joint?

    A. Articular facets
    B. Infrapatellar and suprapatellar bursae
    C. Menisci
    D. Infrapatellar fat pads

27. Match the structures labeled on Figs. 6-14 and 6-15. (Use each choice only once.)

_____ A.

_____ B.

_____ C.

_____ D.

_____ E.

_____ F.

_____ G.

_____ H.

_____ I.

_____ J.

1. Medial condyle of tibia

2. Neck of fibula

3. Head of fibula

4. Articular facets

5. Patella

6. Lateral condyle of femur

7. Proximal tibiofibular joint

8. Intercondyloid eminence

9. Femorotibial joint space

10. Lateral condyle of tibia

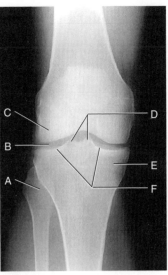

Fig. 6-14. AP radiograph of the knee.

28. Which knee projection does Fig. 6-15 represent?

A. AP

B. AP oblique—medial rotation

C. AP oblique—lateral rotation

D. AP weight-bearing

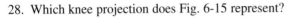

Fig. 6-15. Radiograph of the knee.

29. Match the parts labeled on Figs. 6-16 and 6-17. (Answers may be used more than once.)

_____ A.

_____ B.

_____ C.

_____ D.

_____ E.

_____ F.

_____ G.

_____ H.

_____ I.

_____ J.

1. Adductor tubercle

2. Head of fibula

3. Medial femoral condyle

4. Anterior aspect of medial condyle

5. Lateral femoral condyle

6. Anterior aspect of lateral femoral condyle

7. Tibial tuberosity

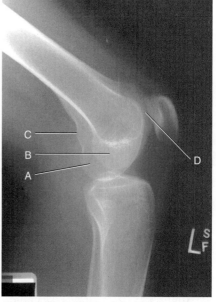

Fig. 6-16. Anatomy of the knee.

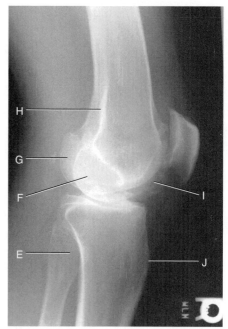

Fig. 6-17. Anatomy of the knee.

30. What is the *primary* positioning error present on Fig. 6-16 (mediolateral projection)?

    A. Overangulation of central ray

    B. Under-rotation toward image receptor

    C. Over-rotation of knee toward image receptor

    D. Underangulation of central ray

31. True/False: The mediolateral knee position in Fig. 6-16 is excessively flexed.

32. What is the *primary* positioning error in Fig. 6-17 (mediolateral projection)?

    A. Overangulation of central ray

    B. Under-rotation toward image receptor

    C. Over-rotation of knee toward image receptor

    D. Underangulation of central ray

33. Which one of the following conditions may cause the tibial tuberosity to be pulled away from the tibial shaft?

    A. Gout

    B. Reiter's syndrome

    C. Osteomalacia

    D. Osgood-Schlatter disease

34. Which of the following pathologic conditions involves a large band ligament found in the foot?

    A. Reiter's syndrome

    B. Paget's disease

    C. Exostosis

    D. Lisfranc injury

35. Which one of the following conditions may produce the radiographic appearance of a destructive lesion with irregular periosteal reaction?

    A. Osteogenic sarcoma

    B. Gout

    C. Bone cyst

    D. Osteoid osteoma

36. What is the common term for chondromalacia patellae?

    A. Brittle bone disease

    B. Runner's knee

    C. Degenerative joint disease

    D. Giant cell tumor

37. Where is the central ray placed for a plantodorsal axial projection of the calcaneus?

    A. Calcaneal tuberosity

    B. Sustentaculum tali

    C. Base of third metatarsal

    D. 1 inch (2.5 cm) inferior to medial malleolus

38. Which ankle projection is best for demonstrating the mortise of the ankle?

    A. AP

    B. AP oblique (15° to 20° medial rotation)

    C. AP oblique (15° to 20° lateral rotation)

    D. Mediolateral

39. Which imaginary plane should be placed parallel to the IR for an AP projection of the knee?

    A. Intermalleolar

    B. Midcoronal

    C. Midsagittal

    D. Interepicondylar

40. Which joint space should be open or almost open for a well-positioned AP oblique knee projection with medial rotation?

    A. Both sides of knee joint

    B. Proximal tibiofibular

    C. Distal tibiofibular

    D. Patellofemoral

41. True/False: A 5° to 7° cephalad angle of the central ray for a lateral projection of the knee helps superimpose the distal borders of the medial and lateral condyles of the femur when the lower leg has not been supported.

42. Why is a PA projection of the patella preferred to an AP projection?

    A. Less object image receptor distance (OID)   C. Less magnification of patella

    B. Less distortion of patella   D. All of these

43. **Situation:** A projection is performed for the patellofemoral joint with the patient supine and the knee flexed 40°. The central ray is angled 30° caudad from horizontal. The cassette is resting on the lower legs supported by a special cassette-holding device. Which one of the following methods has been described?

    A. Camp-Coventry   C. Hughston

    B. Settegast   D. Bilateral Merchant

44. What is the major *disadvantage* of the Settegast method?

    A. Requires use of specialized equipment   C. Requires overflexion of knee

    B. Requires AP positioning   D. Requires the use of a long OID

45. **Situation:** A radiograph of an AP knee reveals that the joint spaces are not equally open and the proximal fibula is superimposed over the tibia. Which specific positioning error leads to this radiographic outcome?

    A. Underangulation of central ray   C. Overangulation of central ray

    B. Lateral rotation of lower limb   D. Medial rotation of lower limb

46. **Situation:** A radiograph of the Camp-Coventry method was produced, but the intercondylar fossa is not open and is foreshortened. The following positioning factors were used: prone position, lower leg flexed 45°, and central ray angled 30° caudad and centered to the popliteal crease. Which of the following should be done during the repeat exposure to produce a more diagnostic image?

    A. Decrease lower leg flexion to 30°   C. Increase CR angle to 45° caudad

    B. Rotate lower limb 5° internally   D. Increase flexion of lower limb to 50° to 60°

47. **Situation:** A radiograph of a plantodorsal axial projection of the calcaneus reveals that the calcaneus is foreshortened. The following positioning factors were used: supine position, foot dorsiflexed perpendicular to image receptor, and central ray angled 30° cephalad and centered to base of third metatarsal. Which of the following should be done during the repeat exposure to produce a more diagnostic image?

    A. Increase central ray angulation to 40°   C. Reduce dorsiflexion of foot

    B. Reverse direction of central ray angulation   D. Center central ray to sustentaculum tali

48. **Situation:** A bilateral patellofemoral joint space study is ordered. The patient is paraplegic and cannot stand. Which of the following projections is best suited for this patient?

    A. Hobbs modification   C. Bilateral Merchant method

    B. Bilateral inferosuperior axial   D. Bilateral Settegast method

49. **Situation:** A radiograph of an AP mortise projection of the ankle reveals that the lateral joint space is not open with the lateral malleolus superimposed over the talus. The talus is distorted. What positioning error leads to this outcome?

    A. Insufficient medial rotation   C. Excessive dorsiflexion of the foot

    B. Excessive medial rotation   D. Excessive plantar flexion of the foot

50. **Situation:** A patient is referred to radiology for a possible Lisfranc injury. Which of the following positioning routines best demonstrates this condition?

    A. Weight-bearing knee study   C. Knee routine to include intercondylar fossa projection

    B. AP and lateral lower leg   D. Weight-bearing foot study

7 Femur and Pelvic Girdle

CHAPTER OBJECTIVES

After you have successfully completed the activities in this chapter, you will be able to:

_____ 1. Identify the bones and specific features of the femur and pelvic girdle on drawings and radiographs.

_____ 2. Identify the location of the major landmarks of the pelvis and hip and describe two methods of locating the femoral head and neck on an anteroposterior (AP) hip and pelvis radiograph.

_____ 3. List the structural and functional differences of the greater and lesser pelvis and the structural difference between the male and female pelvis.

_____ 4. List the correct classification and movement type for the pelvic joints.

_____ 5. Identify the specific pediatric and geriatric applications for pelvis and hip radiographic examinations as described in the textbook.

_____ 6. Match specific clinical indications of the pelvic girdle to the correct definition.

_____ 7. Match specific clinical indications of the pelvic girdle to the correct radiographic appearance.

_____ 8. Determine whether a pelvis or hip is in a true AP position based on the established radiographic criteria.

_____ 9. Given various hypothetic clinical situations, identify the correct modification of a position and/or exposure factors to improve the radiographic image.

_____ 10. Given radiographs of specific femur, hip, and pelvis projections, identify positioning and exposure factor errors.

POSITIONING AND RADIOGRAPHIC CRITIQUE

_____ 1. Using a peer, position for the basic and special projections of the femur and pelvic girdle.

_____ 2. Using a pelvic radiographic phantom, produce satisfactory radiographs of specific positions (if equipment is available).

_____ 3. Critique and evaluate pelvic girdle radiographs based on the five divisions of radiographic criteria: (1) anatomy demonstrated, (2) position, (3) collimation and central ray, (4) exposure, and (5) anatomic side markers.

_____ 4. Distinguish between acceptable and unacceptable pelvic girdle radiographs based on exposure factors, motion, collimation, positioning, or other errors.

LEARNING EXERCISES

Complete the following review exercises after reading the associated pages in the textbook as indicated by each exercise. Answers to each review exercise are given at the end of the review exercises.

PART I: RADIOGRAPHIC ANATOMY
REVIEW EXERCISE A: Radiographic Anatomy of the Femur, Hips, and Pelvis (see textbook pp. 262-268)

1. The largest and strongest bone of the body is the _____.

2. A small depression located in the center of the femoral head is the _____.

3. The lesser trochanter is located on the _____ (medial or lateral) aspect of the proximal femur.

   It projects _____ (anteriorly or posteriorly) from the junction between the neck and shaft.

4. Because of the alignment between the femoral head and pelvis, the lower limb must be rotated

   _____° internally to place the femoral neck parallel to the plane of the image receptor to achieve a true anteroposterior (AP) projection.

5. True/False: The terms *pelvis* and *pelvic girdle* are not synonymous.

   A. List the four bones that make up the pelvis. _____

   B. List the two bones that make up the pelvic girdle. _____

   C. List two additional terms used for the bones identified in B.

   (a) _____

   (b) _____

6. List the three divisions of the hip bone.

   A. _____   B. _____   C. _____

7. All three divisions of the hip bone eventually fuse at the _____ at the age of

   _____.

8. What are the two important radiographic landmarks found on the ilium?

   A. _____   B. _____

9. Which bony landmark is found on the most inferior aspect of the posterior pelvis?

   _____

10. What is the name of the joint found between the superior rami of the pubic bones?

    _____

11. The _____ of the pelvis is the largest foramen in the skeletal system.

12. The upper margin of the greater trochanter is approximately (A) _____° above the level of the superior border of the symphysis pubis, and the ischial tuberosity is about (B)

_____° below.

13. An imaginary plane that divides the pelvic region into the greater and lesser pelvis is called

the _____.

14. List the alternate terms for the greater and lesser pelvis.

    A. Greater pelvis _____   B. Lesser pelvis _____

15. List the major function of the greater pelvis and the lesser pelvis.

    A. Greater pelvis _____   B. Lesser pelvis _____

16. List the three aspects of the lesser pelvis, which also describe the birth route during the delivery process.

    A. _____

    B. _____

    C. _____

17. Match the following structures or characteristics to the correct hip bone. (Answers may be used more than once.)

    _____ 1. Possesses a large tuberosity found at the most inferior   A. Ilium
             aspect of the pelvis
                                                                                 B. Ischium
    _____ 2. Lesser sciatic notch
                                                                                 C. Pubis
    _____ 3. Ala

    _____ 4. Posterior superior iliac spine (PSIS)

    _____ 5. Possesses a slightly movable joint

    _____ 6. Anterior superior iliac spine (ASIS)

    _____ 7. Forms the anterior, inferior aspect of the lower pelvic girdle

    _____ 8. Articulates with the sacrum to form the SI joints

18. In the past, which radiographic examination was performed to measure the fetal head in comparison with the

maternal pelvis to predict possible birthing problems? _____

19. What imaging modality has replaced the procedure identified in question 18? _____

20. Indicate whether the following radiographic characteristics apply to a male (M) or female (F) in relation to an AP projection of the pelvis.

_____ 1. Wide, more flared ilia   M. Male

_____ 2. Pubic arch angle of 110°   F. Female

_____ 3. A heart-shaped inlet

_____ 4. Narrow ilia that are less flared

_____ 5. Pubic arch angle of 75°

_____ 6. Larger and more round-shaped inlet

21. List the joint classification, mobility type, and movement type for the joints of the pelvis. Write *N/A* (not applicable) if the mobility or movement type does not apply.

	Classification	*Mobility Type*	*Movement Type*
A. Hip	_____	_____	_____
B. Sacroiliac	_____	_____	_____
C. Symphysis pubis	_____	_____	_____
D. Acetabulum (union)	_____	_____	_____

22. Identify the structures labeled on Figs. 7-1 and 7-2. Where indicated, use the following abbreviations to identify with which bone of the pelvis each labeled part is associated: *IL*, ilium; *IS*, ischium; *P*, pubis.

Structure   **Bone**

A. _____   _____

B. _____   _____

C. _____   _____

D. _____   _____

E. _____   _____

F. _____   _____

G. _____   _____

H. _____   _____

I. _____   _____

J. _____   _____

K. _____   _____

L. _____   _____

M. _____   _____

N. _____   _____

O. _____   _____

P. _____   _____

Q. _____   _____

R. _____   _____

S. _____   _____

T. _____   _____

U. _____   _____

V. _____   _____

W. _____   _____

X. _____   _____

Y. _____   _____

Z. _____   _____

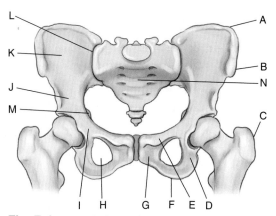

Fig. 7-1. Frontal view, pelvis.

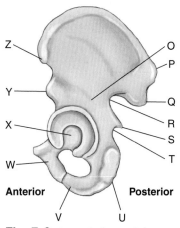

Fig. 7-2. Lateral view, pelvis.

PART II: RADIOGRAPHIC POSITIONING

REVIEW EXERCISE B: Positioning of the Femur, Hips, and Pelvis (see textbook pp. 269-286)

1. Which two bony landmarks need to be palpated for hip localization?

   A. _____   B. _____

2. From the midpoint of the imaginary line created by the two landmarks identified in the previous question, where

   would the femoral neck be located? _____

3. A second method for locating the femoral head is to palpate the _____ and go _____

   inches (_____ cm) medial at the level of the _____, which is _____

   inches (_____ cm) distal to the original palpation point.

4. To achieve a true AP position of the proximal femur, the lower limb must be rotated

   _____ internally.

5. Which structures on an AP pelvis or hip radiograph indicate whether the proximal head and neck are in position

   for a true AP projection? _____

6. Which physical sign **may** indicate that a patient has a hip fracture? _____

7. Which projection should be taken first and reviewed by a radiologist before attempting to rotate the hip into a

   lateral position (if trauma is suspected)? _____

8. Gonadal shielding should be used for all patients of reproductive age, unless _____.

9. Should a gonadal shield be used for a hip study on a young female? _____

   If yes, describe how it should be placed on the patient. _____

10. Should a gonadal shield be used for a hip study on a young male? _____

    If yes, describe how it should be placed on the patient. _____

11. What is the advantage of using 90 kV rather than a lower kV range for hip and pelvis studies on younger patients

    with an analog imaging system? _____

12. What is the disadvantage of using 90 kV for hip and pelvis studies, especially on older patients with some bone

    mass loss with an analog imaging system? _____

13. Which one of the following conditions is a common clinical indication for performing pelvic and hip examinations
    on a pediatric (newborn) patient?

    A. Osteoporosis   C. Ankylosing spondylitis

    B. Developmental dysplasia of hip (DDH)   D. Osteoarthritis

14. True/False: Geriatric patients are often more prone to hip fractures because of their increased incidence of
    osteoporosis.

15. Which one of the following imaging modalities can be used on a newborn to assess hip joint stability during movement of the lower limbs?

   A. Sonography

   B. Computed tomography

   C. Magnetic resonance imaging

   D. Nuclear medicine

16. Which one of the following imaging modalities is most sensitive in diagnosing early signs of metastatic carcinoma of the pelvis?

   A. Sonography

   B. Computed tomography

   C. Magnetic resonance imaging

   D. Nuclear medicine

17. Match each of the following clinical indications to the correct definition. (Use each choice only once.)

   _____ A. A degenerative joint disease

   _____ B. Most common fracture in older patients because of high incidence of osteoporosis or avascular necrosis

   _____ C. A malignant tumor of the cartilage of hip

   _____ D. A disease producing extensive calcification of the longitudinal ligament of the spinal column

   _____ E. A fracture resulting from a severe blow to one side of the pelvis

   _____ F. Malignancy spread to bone via the circulatory and lymphatic systems or direct invasion

   _____ G. Now referred to as developmental dysplasia of the hip

   1. Metastatic carcinoma

   2. Ankylosing spondylitis

   3. Congenital dislocation

   4. Chondrosarcoma

   5. Proximal hip fracture

   6. Pelvic ring fracture

   7. Osteoarthritis

18. Which of the following devices will improve overall visibility of the proximal hip demonstrated on an axiolateral (inferosuperior) projection?

   A. Small focal spot

   B. 6:1 grid

   C. Compensating filter

   D. Shadow shield

19. Which of the following modalities will best demonstrate a possible pelvic ring fracture?

   A. CT

   B. Nuclear medicine

   C. MRI

   D. Sonography

20. True/False: Both joints must be included on an AP and lateral projection of the femur even if a fracture of the proximal femur is evident.

21. Where is the central ray placed for an AP pelvis projection? _____

22. The central ray for the AP pelvis projection is approximately _____ inch(es) (cm) inferior to the level of the ASIS.

23. Which specific positioning error is present when the left iliac wing is elongated on an AP pelvis radiograph?

   _____

24. Which specific positioning error is present when the left obturator foramen is more open than the right side on an

AP pelvis radiograph? _____

25. Indicate whether each of the following projections is used for patients with traumatic (T) injuries or nontraumatic (NT) injuries.

    _____ A. Axiolateral, inferosuperior (Danelius-Miller) projection   T. Traumatic

    _____ B. Unilateral frog-leg (modified Cleaves method)   NT. Not traumatic

    _____ C. AP bilateral "frog-leg" (modified Cleaves method)

    _____ D. Modified axiolateral (Clements-Nakayama method)

    _____ E. AP axial for pelvic "outlet"

26. Which of the following projections is recommended to demonstrate the superoposterior wall of the acetabulum?

    A. AP axial "inlet"   C. Axiolateral inferosuperior

    B. PA axial oblique   D. Modified axiolateral

27. When gonadal shielding is not used, _____ (males or females) receive a greater gonadal dose with an AP pelvis projection.

28. How many degrees are the femurs abducted (from the vertical plane) for the bilateral frog-leg projection?

_____

29. Where is the central ray placed for a bilateral frog-leg (modified Cleaves method) projection?

_____

30. Which size of analog cassette should be used for an adult bilateral frog-leg projection?

_____

31. Where is the central ray placed for an AP unilateral frog-leg projection? _____

32. Which central ray angle is required for the "outlet" projection (Taylor method) for a female patient?

    A. 15° to 25° caudad   C. 20° to 35° cephalad

    B. 30° to 45° cephalad   D. None (central ray is perpendicular)

33. Which type of pathology is best demonstrated with the posterior oblique (Judet method)?

    A. Acetabular fractures   C. Proximal femur fractures

    B. Anterior pelvic bone fractures   D. Femoral neck fractures

34. How much obliquity of the body is required for the posterior oblique projection (Judet method)?

    A. None (central ray is perpendicular)   C. 30°

    B. 20°   D. 45°

35. What type of CR angle is used for a PA axial oblique (Teufel) projection?

    A. 15° cephalad   C. 5° caudad

    B. 15° to 20° cephalad   D. 12° cephalad

36. How is the pelvis (body) positioned for a PA axial oblique (Teufel) projection?

    A. PA with 45° rotated away from affected side

    B. Prone or erect PA—no rotation

    C. PA 35° to 40° toward affected side

    D. AP with 40° away from affected side

37. True/False: Any orthopedic device or appliance of the hip should be seen in its entirety on an AP hip radiograph.

38. The axiolateral (inferosuperior) projection is designed for _____ (traumatic or nontraumatic) situations.

39. How is the unaffected leg positioned for the axiolateral hip projection? _____

40. Which one of the following factors does *not* apply to an axiolateral (inferosuperior) projection of the hip on a male patient?

    A. IR parallel to femoral neck   C. Use of gonadal shielding

    B. 80 to 90 kV   D. Use of a stationary grid

41. True/False: An AP pelvis projection using 90 kV and 8 mAs results in less patient dose than a projection using 80 kV and 12 mAs (for both males and females).

42. True/False: The unaffected foot during an axiolateral (inferosuperior) projection can be burned if allowed to rest on the collimator.

43. The modified axiolateral requires the CR to be angled _____° posteriorly from horizontal.

44. Which special projection of the hip demonstrates the anterior and posterior rims of the acetabulum and the ilioischial and iliopubic columns? (Include the projection name and the method name.)

    A. _____

    B. Which central ray angle (if any) is used for this projection? _____

45. What is the name of a special projection of the pelvis used to assess trauma to pubic and ischial structures? (Include the projection name and the method name.) _____

46. Match each of the following projections with its corresponding proper name. (Use each choice only once.)

    _____ 1. Axiolateral (inferosuperior)   A. Judet

    _____ 2. Modified axiolateral   B. Taylor

    _____ 3. Bilateral or unilateral frog-leg   C. Clements-Nakayama

    _____ 4. PA axial oblique for acetabulum   D. Danelius-Miller

    _____ 5. AP axial for pelvic "outlet" bones   E. Teufel

    _____ 6. Posterior oblique for acetabulum   F. Modified Cleaves

47. What is the optimal amount of hip abduction applied for the unilateral "frog-leg" projection to demonstrate the femoral neck without distortion?

    A. 45° from vertical   C. 10° from vertical

    B. 90° from vertical   D. 20° to 30° from vertical

48. True/False: The Lauenstein/Hickey method for the unilateral "frog-leg" projection will produce distortion of the femoral neck.

49. How much is the IR tilted for the modified axiolateral projection of the hip? _____

50. True/False: Gonadal shielding can be used for males for the axiolateral (inferosuperior) projection of the hip.

REVIEW EXERCISE C: Problem Solving for Technical and Positioning Errors

1. **Situation:** A radiograph of an AP pelvis projection reveals that the lesser trochanters are readily demonstrated on the medial side of the proximal femurs. The patient is ambulatory but has a history of early osteoarthritis in both hips. Which positioning modification needs to be made to prevent this positioning error?

   _____

   _____

2. **Situation:** A radiograph of an AP pelvis reveals that the right iliac wing is foreshortened as compared with the left side. Which specific positioning error has been made?

   _____

   _____

3. **Situation:** A radiograph of a unilateral frog-leg (modified Cleaves) projection produces distortion of the femoral neck. Based on the AP hip projection, the radiologist suspects a nondisplaced fracture of the femoral neck. What can the technologist do to better define this region?

   _____

   _____

4. **Situation:** A radiograph of an axiolateral (inferosuperior) projection reveals that the posterior aspect of the acetabulum and femoral head were cut off of the bottom of the image. The emergency room physician requests that the position be repeated. What can be done to avoid this problem on the repeat exposure?

   _____

   _____

5. **Situation:** A radiograph of an AP axial projection for anterior pelvic bones reveals that the pubic and ischial bones are not elongated sufficiently. The following analog factors were used for this study: 86 kV, 7 mAs, Bucky, 20° to 30° central ray cephalad angle, and 40-inch (102-cm) source image receptor distance (SID). The female patient was placed in a supine position on the table. What must be changed to improve the quality of the image during the repeat exposure?

   _____

   _____

6. **Situation:** A patient enters the ER with a pelvis injury resulting from a motor vehicle accident. The initial AP pelvis projection demonstrates a possible defect or fracture of the left acetabulum. No other fractures are detected and the patient is able to move comfortably. What additional projections can be taken to demonstrate a possible acetabular fracture?

   _____

   _____

7. **Situation:** A radiograph of an AP pelvis reveals that overall the image is underexposed (underpenetrated). The following analog factors were used: 80-kV, 40-inch (102-cm) SID, Bucky, and AEC with the center chamber activated. Which one of these factors should be changed to produce increased image density?

_____

_____

8. **Situation:** A radiograph from a modified axiolateral projection reveals excessive grid lines on the image, which also appears underexposed. What can be done to avoid this problem during the repeat exposure?

_____

_____

9. **Situation:** A portable AP and lateral hip study is ordered for a patient who is in recovery following hip replacement surgery. The radiograph of the AP hip reveals that the upper portion of the acetabular prosthesis is slightly cut off but is included on the lateral projection. Should the technologist repeat the AP projection? Why or why not?

_____

_____

10. **Situation:** A patient with hip pain from a fall enters the emergency room. The physician orders a left hip study. When moved to the radiographic table, the patient complains loudly about the pain in the left hip. Which positioning routine should be used for this patient?

_____

_____

11. **Situation:** A patient has just been moved to his hospital room after a bilateral hip replacement surgery. The surgeon has ordered a postoperative hip routine for both hips. Which specific positioning routine should be used? (The patient can be brought to the radiology department.)

_____

_____

12. **Situation:** A patient with a possible pelvic ring fracture from a trauma enters the emergency room. The AP pelvis projection, which was taken to determine whether the right acetabulum is fractured, is inconclusive. Which other radiographic projection can be taken to better visualize the acetabulum? What other imaging modality can be used to determine the presence of a pelvic ring fracture?

_____

_____

13. **Situation:** A physician orders a study for inlet and outlet projections of the pelvis. Which projections could be performed to meet this request?

_____

14. **Situation:** A technologist notices that his AP pelvis projections often demonstrate a moderate degree of rotation. What positioning technique can the technologist perform to eliminate (or at least minimize) rotation on his AP pelvis projections?

_____

_____

15. **Situation:** A very young child comes to the radiology department with a clinical history of DDH. What is the most common positioning routine for this condition?

_____

_____

REVIEW EXERCISE D: Critique Radiographs of the Femur and Pelvis (see textbook p. 287)

The following questions relate to the radiographs found at the end of Chapter 7 of the textbook. Evaluate these radiographs for the radiographic criteria categories (1 through 5) that follow. Describe the corrections needed to improve the overall image. The major, or "repeatable," errors are specific errors that indicate the need for a repeat exposure, regardless of the nature of the other errors.

A. AP pelvis (Fig. C7-77)

Description of possible error:

 1. Anatomy demonstrated: _____

 2. Part positioning: _____

 3. Collimation and central ray: _____

 4. Exposure: _____

 5. Markers: _____

Repeatable error(s): _____

B. AP Pelvis (Fig. C7-78)

Description of possible error:

 1. Anatomy demonstrated: _____

 2. Part positioning: _____

 3. Collimation and central ray: _____

 4. Exposure: _____

 5. Markers: _____

Repeatable error(s): _____

C. Unilateral "frog-leg" projection (performed cystography) (Fig. C7-79)

Description of possible error:

1. Anatomy demonstrated: _____

2. Part positioning: _____

3. Collimation and central ray: _____

4. Exposure: _____

5. Markers: _____

Repeatable error(s): _____

D. Bilateral frog-leg (2-year-old) (Fig. C7-80)

Description of possible error:

1. Anatomy demonstrated: _____

2. Part positioning: _____

3. Collimation and central ray: _____

4. Exposure: _____

5. Markers: _____

Repeatable error(s): _____

PART III: LABORATORY EXERCISES

You must gain experience in positioning each part of the proximal femur and pelvis before performing the following exams on actual patients. You can get experience in positioning and radiographic evaluation of these projections by performing exercises using radiographic phantoms and practicing positioning on other students (although you will not be taking actual exposures).

The following suggested activities assume that your teaching institution has an energized lab and radiographic phantoms. If not, perform Laboratory Exercises B and C, the radiographic evaluation and the physical positioning exercises. (Check off each step and projection as you complete it.)

Laboratory Exercise A: Energized Laboratory

1. Using the pelvic radiographic phantom, produce radiographs of the following basic routines:

_____ AP pelvis projection

_____ Posterior oblique positions for acetabulum, Judet method

_____ AP axial projection, Taylor method

Laboratory Exercise B: Radiographic Evaluation

1. Evaluate and critique the radiographs produced above, additional radiographs provided by your instructor, or both. Evaluate each radiograph for the following points:

_____ Evaluate the completeness of the study. (Are all of the pertinent anatomic structures included on the radiograph?)

_____ Evaluate for positioning or centering errors (e.g., rotation, off centering).

_____ Evaluate for correct exposure factors and possible motion. (Are the density, brightness, and contrast of the images acceptable?)

_____ Determine whether markers and an acceptable degree of collimation and/or area shielding are visible on the images.

Laboratory Exercise C: Physical Positioning

On another person, simulate performing all basic and special projections of the proximal femur and pelvic girdle as follows. Include the six steps listed in the following and described in the textbook. (Check off each step when completed satisfactorily.)

Step 1. Appropriate size and type of image receptor with correct markers

Step 2. Correct central ray placement and centering of part to central ray and/or image receptor

Step 3. Accurate collimation

Step 4. Area shielding of patient where advisable

Step 5. Use of proper immobilizing devices when needed

Step 6. Approximate correct exposure factors, breathing instructions when applicable, and initiating exposure

Projections	Step 1	Step 2	Step 3	Step 4	Step 5	Step 6
• AP and lateral femur	_____	_____	_____	_____	_____	_____
• AP pelvis	_____	_____	_____	_____	_____	_____
• AP hip, unilateral	_____	_____	_____	_____	_____	_____
• Unilateral frog-leg	_____	_____	_____	_____	_____	_____
• Bilateral frog-leg	_____	_____	_____	_____	_____	_____
• Axiolateral (inferosuperior) projection	_____	_____	_____	_____	_____	_____
• Modified axiolateral	_____	_____	_____	_____	_____	_____
• Anterior oblique for acetabulum	_____	_____	_____	_____	_____	_____
• AP axial for "outlet"	_____	_____	_____	_____	_____	_____

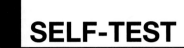 **SELF-TEST**

MY SCORE = _____%

This self-test should be taken only after completing all of the readings, review exercises, and laboratory activities for a particular section. The purpose of this test is not only to provide a good learning exercise but also to serve as a strong indicator of what your final evaluation exam for this chapter will cover. It is strongly suggested that if you do not get at least a 90% to 95% grade on each self-test, you should review those areas in which you missed questions before going to your instructor for the final evaluation exam.

1. List the four bones of the pelvis.

   A. _____   C. _____

   B. _____   D. _____

2. List the three divisions of the hip bone.

   A. _____   B. _____   C. _____

3. *Innominate bone* is another name for:

   A. One half of pelvic girdle   C. Ossa coxae

   B. Hip bone   D. All of the above

4. What is the largest foramen in the body? _____

5. Which one of the following landmarks is not a palpable bony landmark?

   A. Greater trochanter   C. Ischial tuberosity

   B. Lesser trochanter   D. Anterior superior iliac spine (ASIS)

6. What are the two aspects of the ischium?

   A. _____   B. _____

7. What is the name of the imaginary plane that separates the false from the true pelvis?

   _____

8. Match the following structures or characteristics to the correct division of the pelvis.

   _____ 1. Lesser pelvis   A. False pelvis

   _____ 2. Supports the lower abdominal organs   B. True pelvis

   _____ 3. Formed primarily by the ala of the ilium

   _____ 4. Cavity

   _____ 5. Greater pelvis

   _____ 6. Forms the actual birth canal

   _____ 7. Found below the pelvic brim

Chapter **7** **Femur and Pelvic Girdle: Self-Test**

9. The pubic arch angle on an average male pelvis is an _____ (acute or obtuse) angle

   that is _____ (greater than or less than) 90°.

10. Identify the labeled structures found on the following radiographs.

   A. _____

   B. _____

   C. _____

   D. _____

   E. _____

   F. _____

   G. _____

   H. _____

   I. _____

   J. Is Fig. 7-3 a male or

      female pelvis? _____

   K. _____

   L. _____

   M. _____

   N. _____

   O. Which projection of the hip is

      represented on Fig. 7-4? _____

   P. _____

   Q. _____

   R. _____

   S. _____

   T. _____

   U. _____

   V. _____

   W. Which projection of the hips is represented

      on Fig. 7-5? _____

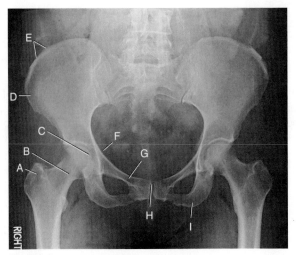

Fig. 7-3. AP pelvis radiograph.

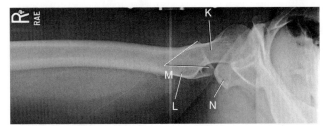

Fig. 7-4. Lateral hip radiograph.

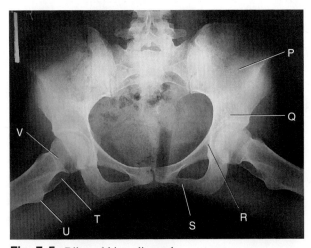

Fig. 7-5. Bilateral hip radiograph.

11. Indicate whether the following radiographic characteristics are those of a male (M) or female (F) pelvis.

_____ 1. Heart-shaped (oval) inlet   F. Female

_____ 2. Acute pubic arch (less than 90°)   M. Male

_____ 3. Iliac wings that are more flared

_____ 4. Obtuse pubic arch (greater than 90°)

_____ 5. Larger and more rounded inlet

_____ 6. Iliac wings that are less flared

12. Which one of the following structures is considered to be the most posterior?

   A. Ischial spines   C. Symphysis pubis

   B. ASIS   D. Acetabulum

13. The small depression near the center of the femoral head where a ligament is attached is called the

   _____.

14. Which of the following joints are a synovial joint but with amphiarthrodial mobility?

   A. Union of acetabula   C. Sacroiliac joints

   B. Hip joint   D. Symphysis pubis

15. Which of the following devices should be used for an axiolateral (inferosuperior) projection of the hip to equalize density (brightness) of the hip region?

   A. Grid   C. Small focal spot

   B. High-speed IR   D. Compensating filter

16. Which of the following modalities is used to assess joint stability during movement of the lower limbs on infants?

   A. Sonography   C. CT

   B. MR   D. Weight-bearing pelvis radiographic projections

17. A geriatric patient with an externally rotated lower limb may have:

   A. A normal hip joint   C. Fractured proximal femur

   B. Osteoarthritis   D. Slipped capital femoral epiphysis (SCFE)

18. Which one of the following pathologic indications may result in the early fusion of the sacroiliac (SI) joints?

   A. Chondrosarcoma   C. Developmental dysplasia of the hip

   B. Metastatic carcinoma   D. Ankylosing spondylitis

19. Match each of the following radiographic appearances with the correct clinical indications. (Use each choice only once.)

_____ 1. Usually consists of numerous small lytic lesions

_____ 2. Increased hip joint space and misalignment

_____ 3. Bilateral radiolucent lines across bones and misalignment of SI joints

_____ 4. Early fusion of SI joints and "bamboo spine"

_____ 5. Epiphyses appear shorter and epiphyseal plate wider

_____ 6. Hallmark sign of spurring and narrowing of joint space

A. Pelvic ring fracture

B. DDH

C. Osteoarthritis

D. SCFE

E. Ankylosing spondylitis

F. Metastatic carcinoma

20. Which one of the following radiographic signs indicates that the proximal femurs are in position for a true AP projection?

A. Appearance of the greater trochanter in profile

B. Limited visibility of fovea capitis

C. Limited visibility of the lesser trochanter in profile

D. Symmetric appearance of iliac wings

21. What is another term for the outlet of the true pelvis?

A. Ischial spines

B. Inferior aperture

C. Pelvic brim

D. Cervix

22. The typical physical sign for a possible hip fracture is the _____ of the involved foot.

A. External rotation

B. Abduction

C. Internal rotation

D. Adduction

23. Which one of the following projections or methods is often performed to evaluate a pediatric patient for congenital hip dislocation?

A. Bilateral modified Cleaves

B. Clements-Nakayama

C. Taylor method

D. Judet method

24. What type of central ray angle is required when using the AP axial for outlet (Taylor method) for a male patient?

A. None (central ray is perpendicular)

B. 10° to 15° caudad

C. 20° to 35° cephalad

D. 30° to 45° cephalad

25. How much is the pelvis and/or thorax rotated for a PA axial oblique (Teufel method) for acetabulum?

A. 15° toward affected side

B. 30° to 35° away from affected side

C. 20° away from affected side

D. 35° to 40° toward affected side

26. What type of CR angle is required for the PA axial oblique (Teufel method) for acetabulum?

A. 12° cephalad

B. 20° caudad

C. 15° cephalad

D. 25° cephalad

27. True/False: The unilateral frog-leg projection (modified Cleaves method) is intended for nontraumatic hip situations.

28. True/False: Centering for the AP pelvis projection is 1 inch, or 2.5 cm, superior to the symphysis pubis.

29. True/False: The modified axiolateral (Clements-Nakayama method) is classified as a nontraumatic lateral hip projection.

30. What type of CR angle is required for the Judet method?

   A. 12° cephalad   C. 15° cephalad

   B. 5° to 10° caudad   D. None. CR is perpendicular.

31. Which one of the following projections or methods is used to evaluate the pelvic inlet for possible fracture?

   A. Danelius-Miller   C. Taylor

   B. AP axial projection   D. Clements-Nakayama

32. **Situation:** An initial AP pelvis radiograph reveals possible fractures involving the lower anterior pelvis. The emergency room physician asks for another projection to better demonstrate this area of the pelvis. The patient is traumatized and must remain in a supine position. Which projection should be taken?

   _____

33. **Situation:** A radiograph of an axiolateral (inferosuperior) projection of a hip demonstrates a soft tissue density that is visible across the affected hip and acetabulum. This artifact is obscuring the image of the proximal femur. What is the most likely cause of the artifact, and how can it be prevented from showing up on the repeat exposure?

   _____

   _____

34. **Situation:** A unilateral frog-leg (modified Cleaves) demonstrates foreshortening of the femoral necks. The physician is unsure if there is a defect within the anatomic neck. What can be done to minimize distortion of the neck during a repeat exposure?

   _____

   _____

35. **Situation:** A radiograph of an AP hip reveals that the lesser trochanter is not visible. Should the technologist

   repeat the projection? _____ If yes, what should be modified to improve the image during the repeat exposure?

   _____

   _____

36. **Situation:** A young patient with a clinical history of SCFE comes to the radiology department. Which projection(s) are most often taken for this condition?

   _____

   _____

37. **Situation:** A radiograph produced using the AP axial (Taylor method) demonstrates that the anterior pelvic bones of a female patient are foreshortened. The following positioning factors were used: supine position, 40-inch (102-cm) SID, and central ray angled 30° caudad and centered 1 to 2 inches (3 to 5 cm) distal to symphysis pubis. Which one of the following modifications should be made during the repeat exposure?

A. Increase central ray angle

C. Center central ray at level of ASIS

B. Reverse central ray angle

D. Place patient prone on table

38. **Situation:** A radiograph of an AP projection of the pelvis demonstrates that the left obturator foramen is narrowed and the right one is open. What is the specific positioning error present on this radiograph?

_____

_____

39. **Situation:** A patient enters the emergency room with a possible pelvic ring fracture. The AP pelvis projection is inclusive on the extent and location of the fracture(s). What additional pelvis projection(s) can be taken on this patient to demonstrate possible pelvic fractures? (More than one correct answer is possible.)

_____

_____

40. **Situation:** A radiograph of the Teufel method (PA axial oblique) demonstrates distortion of the acetabulum. During positioning, the patient was rotated 35° to 40° toward the affected side and CR was angled 20° cephalad. What modifications are needed during the repeat exposure?

_____

_____

8 Cervical and Thoracic Spine

CHAPTER OBJECTIVES

After you have successfully completed the activities in this chapter, you will be able to:

_____ 1. Using drawings and radiographs, identify specific anatomic structures of the cervical and thoracic spine.

_____ 2. Identify specific features of the cervical and thoracic vertebrae that distinguish them from other aspects of the vertebral column.

_____ 3. Identify the location, angulation, classification, and type of movement for specific joints of the cervical and thoracic spine.

_____ 4. List additional terms for the first, second, and seventh cervical vertebrae.

_____ 5. Identify topographic landmarks that can be palpated to locate specific thoracic and cervical vertebrae.

_____ 6. Match specific clinical indications of the cervical and thoracic spine to the correct definition.

_____ 7. Identify which radiographic projection and/or procedure best demonstrates specific pathologic indications.

_____ 8. Identify structures that are best demonstrated with each position of the cervical and thoracic spine.

_____ 9. Identify basic and special projections of the cervical and thoracic spine and list the correct size and type of image receptor (IR) and the central ray location, direction, and angulation for each position.

_____ 10. Given various hypothetic situations, identify the correct modification of a position and/or exposure factors to improve the radiographic image.

_____ 11. Given radiographs of specific cervical and thoracic spine projections, identify positioning and exposure factor errors.

POSITIONING AND RADIOGRAPHIC CRITIQUE

_____ 1. Using a peer, position for basic and special projections of the cervical and thoracic spine.

_____ 2. Using appropriate radiographic phantoms, produce satisfactory radiographs of specific positions (if equipment is available).

_____ 3. Critique and evaluate cervical and thoracic spine radiographs based on the five divisions of radiographic criteria: (1) anatomy demonstrated, (2) position, (3) collimation and central ray, (4) exposure, and (5) anatomic side markers.

_____ 4. Distinguish between acceptable and unacceptable spine radiographs based on exposure factors, motion, collimation, positioning, or other errors.

LEARNING EXERCISES

Complete the following review exercises after reading the associated pages in the textbook as indicated by each exercise. Answers to each review exercise are given at the end of the review exercises.

PART I: RADIOGRAPHIC ANATOMY
REVIEW EXERCISE A: Radiographic Anatomy of the Cervical and Thoracic Spine (see textbook pp. 290-301)

1. List the number of bones found in each division in the adult vertebral column.

   A. Cervical _____   D. Sacrum _____

   B. Thoracic _____   E. Coccyx _____

   C. Lumbar _____   F. Total _____

Refer to Fig. 8-1 to answer questions 2 through 4.

2. List the two primary or posterior convex curves seen in the vertebral column.

   A. _____

   B. _____

3. Indicate which two portions of the vertebral column are classified as secondary or compensatory curves.

   A. _____

   B. _____

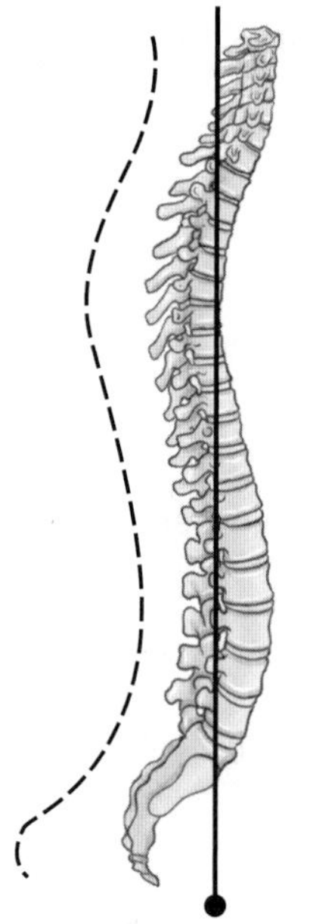

Posterior   Centerline of gravity   **Anterior**

Fig. 8-1. Lateral view, spinal column.

4. Match the correct aspect(s) of the vertebral column with the following characteristics. (There may be more than one correct answer.)

   _____ 1. Convex curve (with respect to posterior)   A. Cervical spine

   _____ 2. Concave curve (with respect to posterior)   B. Thoracic spine

   _____ 3. Secondary curve   C. Lumbar spine

   _____ 4. Primary curve   D. Sacrum

   _____ 5. Develops as child learns to hold head erect

5. An abnormal, or exaggerated, "sway back" lumbar curvature is called _____.

6. An abnormal lateral curvature seen in the thoracolumbar spine is called _____.

7. The two main parts of a typical vertebra are the _____ and the

   _____.

8. The _____ are two bony aspects of the vertebral arch that extend posteriorly from each pedicle to join at the midline.

9. The _____ foramina are created by two small notches on the superior and inferior aspects of the pedicles.

10. The opening, or passageway, for the spinal cord is the _____.

11. The spinal cord begins with the (A) _____ of the brain and extends down to the

    (B) _____ vertebra, where it tapers and ends. This tapered ending is called the

    (C) _____.

12. Which structures pass through the intervertebral foramina? _____

13. Identify the following structures labeled on these drawings of typical thoracic vertebrae (Fig. 8-2).

Superior view

A. _____

B. _____

C. _____

D. _____

E. _____

F. _____

Lateral view

G. _____

H. _____

I. _____

J. _____

K. _____

Lateral oblique view

L. _____

M. _____ joint

N. _____

O. _____

P. _____

Q. The joints between the ribs and vertebrae

at N are called _____.

R. The joints between the ribs and vertebrae

at P are called _____.

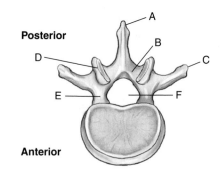

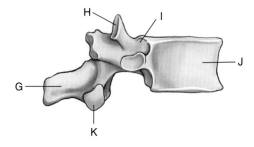

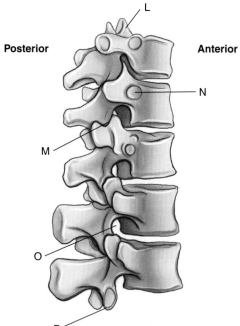

Fig. 8-2. Typical thoracic vertebrae.

14. Which of the following is found between the superior and inferior articular processes?

    A. Intervertebral joints   C. Zygapophyseal joints

    B. Articular joints   D. Intervertebral facets

15. True/False: Only T1, T11, and T12 have *full* facets for articulation with ribs.

16. True/False: The zygapophyseal joints of *all* cervical vertebrae are visualized only in a true lateral position.

17. List the outer and inner aspects of the intervertebral disk.

    A. Outer aspect _____   B. Inner aspect _____

18. The condition involving a "slipped disk" is correctly referred to as _____.

19. List the alternative names for the following cervical vertebrae.

    A. C1: _____

    B. C2: _____

    C. C7: _____

20. List three features that make the cervical vertebrae unique.

    A. _____

    B. _____

    C. _____

21. A short column of bone found between the superior and articular processes in a typical cervical vertebra is called

    _____.

22. What is the term for the same structure, identified in the previous question, for the C1 vertebra?

    _____

23. The zygapophyseal joints for the second through seventh cervical vertebrae are at a _____ ° angle to

    the midsagittal plane; the thoracic vertebrae are at a _____ ° angle to the midsagittal plane.

24. What is the name of the joint found between the superior articular processes of C1 and the occipital condyles of

    the skull? _____

25. The modified body of C2 is called the _____ or _____.

26. A lack of symmetry of the zygapophyseal joints between C1 and C2 may be caused by injury or may be associated

    with_____.

27. What is the unique feature of all thoracic vertebrae that distinguishes them from other vertebrae?

    _____

28. Which specific thoracic vertebrae are classified as typical thoracic vertebrae (i.e., they least resemble cervical or

lumbar vertebrae)? _____

29. Identify the labeled structures on the radiographs of the cervical spine in Figs. 8-3 and 8-4. (Indicate the specific structure and the vertebra of which it is a part.)

Structure	*Vertebra*
A. _____	_____
B. _____	_____
C. _____	_____
D. _____	_____
E. _____	_____
F. _____	_____
G. _____	_____
H. _____	_____

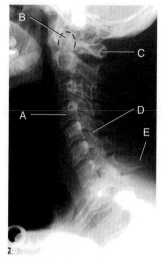

Fig. 8-3. Lateral view, cervical spine.

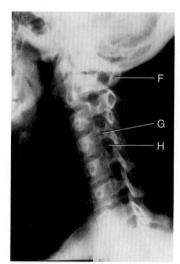

Fig. 8-4. 45° oblique view, cervical spine.

30. For the central ray to pass through and "open" the intervertebral spaces on a 45° posterior oblique projection of

the cervical vertebrae, what central ray angle (if any) is required? _____

PART II: RADIOGRAPHIC POSITIONING

REVIEW EXERCISE B: Positioning of the Cervical and Thoracic Spine (see textbook pp. 302-320)

1. Name the following parts of the sternum or associated topographic landmarks.

   A. Upper portion of sternum: _____

   B. Superior margin of this upper section (landmark): _____

   C. Center portion of sternum: _____

   D. Joint between top and center portions (landmark): _____

   E. Most inferior aspect of sternum (landmark): _____

2. Match the following topographic landmarks to the correct vertebral level. (Use each choice only once.)

   _____ 1. Gonion   A. C7-T1

   _____ 2. Xiphoid process (tip)   B. T2-T3

   _____ 3. Thyroid cartilage   C. C1

   _____ 4. Jugular notch   D. T4-T5

   _____ 5. Sternal angle   E. T9-T10

   _____ 6. Mastoid tip   F. C4-C6

   _____ 7. Vertebra prominens   G. T7

   _____ 8. 3 to 4 inches (8 to 10 cm) below jugular notch   H. C3

3. In addition to the gonads, which other radiosensitive organs are of greatest concern during cervical and thoracic spine radiography?

   _____

4. List the two advantages of using higher kV exposure factors (analog imaging) for spine radiography, especially on an anteroposterior (AP) thoracic spine radiograph.

   A. _____   B. _____

5. True/False: When using digital imaging for spine radiography, it is important to use close collimation, grids, and lead masking.

6. True/False: If close collimation is used during conventional (analog) radiography of the spine, the use of lead masking (blockers) is generally not required.

7. True/False: To a certain degree, magnetic resonance imaging (MRI) and computed tomography (CT) are replacing myelography as the imaging modalities of choice for the diagnosis of a ruptured intervertebral disk.

8. True/False: Nuclear medicine is often performed to diagnose bone tumors of the spine.

9. To ensure that the intervertebral joint spaces are open for lateral thoracic spine projections, it is important to:

   A. Keep the vertebral column parallel to the image receptor (IR)

   B. Use a small focal spot

   C. Use a breathing technique

   D. Angle the central ray caudad

10. For lateral and oblique projections of the cervical spine, it is important to minimize magnification and maximize detail by: (More than one answer may be used.)

    A. Keeping vertebral column parallel to image receptor

    B. Using a small focal spot

    C. Increasing source image receptor distance (SID)

    D. Using a breathing technique

11. Match each of the following clinical indications of the spine to the correct definition. (Use each choice only once.)

    _____ A. Fracture through the pedicles and anterior arch of C2 with forward displacement upon C3

    _____ B. Inflammation of the vertebrae

    _____ C. Abnormal or exaggerated convex curvature of the thoracic spine

    _____ D. Comminuted fracture of the vertebral body with posterior fragments displaced into the spinal canal

    _____ E. Avulsion fracture of the spinous process of C7

    _____ F. Abnormal lateral curvature of the spine

    _____ G. A form of rheumatoid arthritis

    _____ H. Impact fracture from axial loading of the anterior and posterior arch of C1

    _____ I. Mild form of scoliosis and kyphosis developing during adolescence

    _____ J. Produces the "bow tie" sign

    1. Ankylosing spondylitis

    2. Clay shoveler's fracture

    3. Unilateral subluxation

    4. Kyphosis

    5. Scheuermann disease

    6. Scoliosis

    7. Jefferson fracture

    8. Teardrop burst fracture

    9. Hangman's fracture

    10. Spondylitis

12. List the **conventional** radiographic examination and/or projections performed for the following clinical indications.

   A. Scoliosis: _____

   B. Teardrop burst fracture: _____

   C. Jefferson fracture: _____

   D. Scheuermann disease: _____

   E. Unilateral subluxation of cervical spine: _____

   F. HNP: _____

13. What are the major differences between spondylosis and spondylitis?

   _____

14. True/False: Many geriatric patients have a fear of falling off the radiographic table.

15. What is the name of the radiographic procedure that requires the injection of contrast media into the subarachnoid

   space? _____

16. Which imaging modality is ideal for detecting early signs of osteomyelitis?

   _____

17. Which two landmarks must be aligned for an AP "open mouth" projection? _____

18. True/False: The tip of the odontoid process does not have to be demonstrated on the AP "open mouth" projection because it is best seen on the lateral projection.

19. What is the purpose of the 15° to 20° angle for the AP axial projection of the cervical spine?

   _____

20. For an AP axial of the cervical spine, a plane through the tip of the mandible and

   _____ should be parallel to the angled central ray.

   A. Mastoid process   C. Base of skull
   B. Gonion   D. External auditory meatus (EAM)

21. True/False: Less CR angle is required for the AP axial projection of the cervical spine if the examination is performed supine rather than erect.

22. What are two important benefits of an SID longer than 40 to 44 inches (102 to 112 cm) for the lateral cervical spine projection?

   A. _____   B. _____

23. What central ray angulation must be used with a posterior oblique projection of the cervical spine?

   _____

24. Which foramina are demonstrated with a left posterior oblique (LPO) position of the cervical spine?

_____

25. Which foramina are demonstrated with a left anterior oblique (LAO) position of the cervical spine?

_____

26. In addition to extending the chin, which additional positioning technique can be performed to ensure that the mandible is not superimposed over the upper cervical vertebrae for the oblique projections?

_____

27. What is the recommended SID for a lateral projection of the cervical spine?

_____

28. The lateral projection of the cervical spine should be taken during _____ (inspiration, expiration, or suspended respiration). Why?

_____

29. Which specific projection must be taken first if trauma to the cervical spine is suspected and the patient is in a

supine position on a backboard? _____

30. The proper name of the method for performing the cervicothoracic lateral (swimmer's) position is the

_____.

31. Where should the central ray be placed for a cervicothoracic lateral (swimmer's) position?

_____

32. Which region of the spine must be demonstrated with a cervicothoracic lateral (swimmer's) position?

_____

33. Which one of the following projections is considered a "functional study" of the cervical spine?
    A. AP "wagging jaw" projection   C. Fuchs or Judd method
    B. AP "open mouth" position   D. Hyperextension and hyperflexion lateral positions

34. When should the Judd or Fuchs method be performed? _____

35. Which AP projection of the cervical spine demonstrates the entire upper cervical spine with one single projection?

_____

36. Which two things can be done to produce equal density along the entire thoracic spine for the AP projection

(especially for a patient with a thick chest)? _____

37. What is the purpose of using an orthostatic (breathing) technique for a lateral projection of the thoracic spine?

_____

38. Which zygapophyseal joints are demonstrated in a right anterior oblique (RAO) projection of the thoracic spine?

_____

39. Which one of the following projections delivers the greatest skin dose to the patient?

A. AP thoracic spine projection

B. Lateral cervical spine projection

C. Cervicothoracic lateral position

D. Fuchs or Judd method

40. True/False: The thyroid dose used during a posterior oblique cervical spine projection is more than 10 times greater than the dose used for an anterior oblique projection of the cervical spine.

41. Which of the following structures is best demonstrated with an AP axial vertebral arch projection?

A. Spinous processes of lumbar spine

B. Articular pillars (lateral masses) of cervical spine

C. Zygapophyseal joints of thoracic spine

D. Cervicothoracic spine region

42. What central ray angle must be used with the AP axial—vertebral arch projection?

A. 15° to 20° cephalad

B. 5° to 10° cephalad

C. 20° to 30° caudad

D. None (central ray is perpendicular to IR)

43. What ancillary device should be placed behind the patient on the tabletop for a recumbent lateral projection of the

thoracic spine? _____

44. Which skull positioning line is aligned perpendicular to the IR for a PA (Judd) projection for the odontoid process?

_____

45. Which zygapophyseal joints are best demonstrated with an LPO position of the thoracic spine?

_____

46. How much rotation of the body is required for an oblique position of the thoracic spine from a true lateral position?

_____

REVIEW EXERCISE C: Problem Solving for Technical and Positioning Errors

1. A radiograph of an AP "open mouth" projection of the cervical spine reveals that the base of the skull is superimposed over the upper odontoid process. Which **specific** positioning error is present on this radiograph?

_____

2. A radiograph of an AP axial projection of the cervical spine reveals that the intervertebral disk spaces are not open. The following positioning factors were used: extension of the skull, central ray angled 10° cephalad, central ray centered to the thyroid cartilage, and no rotation or tilt of the spine. Which of these factors must be modified to produce a more diagnostic image?

_____

3. A radiograph of a right posterior oblique (RPO) cervical spine projection reveals that the lower intervertebral foramina are *not* open. The upper intervertebral foramina are well visualized. What positioning error most likely led to this radiographic outcome?

   _____

4. A radiograph on a lateral projection of the cervical spine reveals that C7 is not clearly demonstrated. The following factors were used: erect position, 44-inch (112-cm) SID, arms down by the patient's side, and exposure made during inspiration. Which two of these factors should be changed to produce a more diagnostic image during the repeat exposure?

   _____

5. A radiograph of an AP "wagging jaw" (Ottonello method) projection taken at 75 kV, 20 mAs, and 0.5 second demonstrates that part of the image of the mandible is still visible and obscuring the upper cervical spine. Which modification needs to be made to produce a more diagnostic image during the repeat exposure?

   _____

6. A radiograph of a lateral thoracic spine reveals that lung markings and ribs make it difficult to visualize the vertebral bodies. The following factors were used: recumbent position, 40-inch (102-cm) SID, short exposure time, and exposure made during full expiration. Which one of these factors must be modified to produce a more diagnostic image during the repeat exposure?

   _____

7. A radiograph of an AP projection of the thoracic spine reveals that the upper thoracic spine is greatly overexposed but the lower vertebrae are well visualized. The head of the patient was placed at the anode end of the table. What can be modified during the repeat exposure to produce a more diagnostic image?

   _____

8. A radiograph of a cervicothoracic lateral position demonstrates superimposition of the humeral heads over the upper thoracic spine. Because of an arthritic condition, the patient is unable to rotate the shoulders any farther apart. What can the technologist do to further separate the shoulders during the repeat exposure?

   _____

9. **Situation:** A patient with a possible cervical spine injury enters the emergency room. The patient is on a backboard. Which projection of the cervical spine should be taken first?

   _____

10. **Situation:** A patient who has been in a motor vehicle accident (MVA) enters the emergency room. The basic projections of the cervical spine reveal no subluxation (partial dislocation) or fracture. The physician wants the spine evaluated for whiplash injury. Which additional projections would best demonstrate this type of injury?

    _____

11. **Situation:** A patient comes to the radiology department for a cervical spine series. An AP "open mouth" radiograph indicates that the base of the skull and lower edge of the front incisors are superimposed, but the top of the dens is not clearly demonstrated. What should the technologist do to demonstrate the upper portion of the dens? (A horizontal beam lateral projection has ruled out a C-spine fracture or subluxation.)

    _____

12. **Situation:** A patient comes to the radiology department for a routine cervical spine series. The lateral projection demonstrates only the C1 to C6 region. The radiologist wants to see C7-T1. What additional projection can be taken to demonstrate this region of the spine?

_____

13. **Situation:** A patient enters the ER with a possible cervical spine fracture, but the initial projections do not demonstrate any gross fracture or subluxation. After reviewing the initial radiographs, the ER physician suspects either a congenital defect or fracture of the articular pillars of C4. He wants an additional projection taken to better see this aspect of the vertebrae. What additional projection can be taken to demonstrate the articular pillars of C4?

_____

14. **Situation:** A patient comes to the ER with a possible Jefferson fracture. Other than a lateral projection or a CT scan, what specific radiographic projection will best demonstrate this type of fracture?

_____

15. **Situation:** A patient comes to the radiology department with a clinical history of Scheuermann disease. Which radiographic procedure is often performed for this condition?

_____

REVIEW EXERCISE D: Critique Radiographs of the Cervical and Thoracic Spine (see textbook p. 320)

The following questions relate to the radiographs found at the end of Chapter 8 of the textbook. Evaluate these radiographs for the radiographic criteria categories (1 through 5) that follow. Describe the corrections needed to improve the overall image. The major, or "repeatable," errors are specific errors that indicate the need for a repeat exposure, regardless of the nature of the other errors.

A. AP open mouth (Fig. C8-91)

Description of possible error:

    1. Anatomy demonstrated: _____

    2. Part positioning: _____

    3. Collimation and central ray: _____

    4. Exposure: _____

    5. Anatomic side markers: _____

Repeatable error(s): _____

B. AP open mouth (Fig. C8-92)

Description of possible error:

1. Anatomy demonstrated: _____

2. Part positioning: _____

3. Collimation and central ray: _____

4. Exposure: _____

5. Anatomic side markers: _____

Repeatable error(s): _____

C. AP axial projection (Fig. C8-93)

Description of possible error:

1. Anatomy demonstrated: _____

2. Part positioning: _____

3. Collimation and central ray: _____

4. Exposure: _____

5. Anatomic side markers: _____

Repeatable error(s): _____

D. Right posterior oblique (Fig. C8-94)

Description of possible error:

1. Anatomy demonstrated: _____

2. Part positioning: _____

3. Collimation and central ray: _____

4. Exposure: _____

5. Anatomic side markers: _____

Repeatable error(s): _____

E. Lateral (trauma) (Fig. C8-95)

Description of possible error:

    1. Anatomy demonstrated: _____

    2. Part positioning: _____

    3. Collimation and central ray: _____

    4. Exposure: _____

    5. Anatomic side markers: _____

Repeatable error(s): _____

F. AP for odontoid process—Fuchs method (Fig. C8-96)

Description of possible error:

    1. Anatomy demonstrated: _____

    2. Part positioning: _____

    3. Collimation and central ray: _____

    4. Exposure: _____

    5. Anatomic side markers: _____

Repeatable error(s): _____

G. AP thoracic spine (Fig. C8-97)

Description of possible error:

    1. Anatomy demonstrated: _____

    2. Part positioning: _____

    3. Collimation and central ray: _____

    4. Exposure: _____

    5. Anatomic side markers: _____

Repeatable error(s): _____

PART III: LABORATORY EXERCISES

You must gain experience in positioning each part of the cervical and thoracic spine before performing the following exams on actual patients. You can get experience in positioning and radiographic evaluation of these projections by performing exercises using radiographic phantoms and practicing positioning on other students (although you will not be taking actual exposures).

The following suggested activities assume that your teaching institution has an energized lab and radiographic phantoms. If not, perform Laboratory Exercises B and C, the radiographic evaluation and the physical positioning exercises. (Check off each step and projection as you complete it.)

Laboratory Exercise A: Energized Laboratory

1. Using the radiographic phantom, produce radiographs of the following basic routines.

   A. AP, lateral, and oblique cervical spine   B. AP, lateral, and oblique thoracic spine

Laboratory Exercise B: Radiographic Evaluation

1. Evaluate and critique the radiographs produced above, additional radiographs provided by your instructor, or both. Evaluate each radiograph for the following points.

   _____ Evaluate the completeness of the study. (Are all of the pertinent anatomic structures included on the radiograph?)

   _____ Evaluate for positioning or centering errors (e.g., rotation, off centering).

   _____ Evaluate for correct exposure factors and possible motion. (Are the density and contrast of the images acceptable?)

   _____ Determine whether anatomic side markers and an acceptable degree of collimation and/or area shielding are visible on the images.

Laboratory Exercise C: Physical Positioning

On another person, simulate performing all basic and special projections of the cervical and thoracic spine as follows. Include the six steps listed in the following and described in the textbook. (Check off each step when completed satisfactorily.)

Step 1. Appropriate size and type of image receptor with correct markers

Step 2. Correct central ray placement and centering of part to central ray and/or image receptor

Step 3. Accurate collimation

Step 4. Area shielding of patient where advisable

Step 5. Use of proper immobilizing devices when needed

Step 6. Approximate correct exposure factors, breathing instructions where applicable, and initiating exposure

Projections	Step 1	Step 2	Step 3	Step 4	Step 5	Step 6
● Cervical spine series (AP axial, AP C1-2, oblique, lateral)	_____	_____	_____	_____	_____	_____
● Thoracic spine series (AP and lateral)	_____	_____	_____	_____	_____	_____
● Swimmer's lateral	_____	_____	_____	_____	_____	_____
● Hyperextension and flexion laterals	_____	_____	_____	_____	_____	_____
● AP "wagging jaw" projection	_____	_____	_____	_____	_____	_____
● AP (Fuchs) projection for dens	_____	_____	_____	_____	_____	_____
● PA (Judd) projection for dens	_____	_____	_____	_____	_____	_____
● Thoracic spine oblique projections	_____	_____	_____	_____	_____	_____

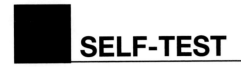

SELF-TEST

This self-test should be taken only after completing all of the readings, review exercises, and laboratory activities for a particular section. The purpose of this test is not only to provide a good learning exercise but also to serve as a strong indicator of what your final evaluation exam for this chapter will cover. It is strongly suggested that if you do not get at least a 90% to 95% grade on each self-test, you should review those areas in which you missed questions before going to your instructor for the final evaluation exam.

1. At which vertebral level does the solid spinal cord terminate? _____

2. How many segments make up the sacrum in the neonate? _____

3. Which of the following divisions of the spine is described as possessing a primary curve? (There may be more than one correct answer.)

   A. Thoracic   C. Lumbar

   B. Cervical   D. Sacral

4. True/False: The lumbar possesses a concave posterior spinal curvature.

5. An abnormal or exaggerated thoracic spinal curvature with increased convexity is called _____.

6. An abnormal or exaggerated lateral spinal curvature is called _____.

7. What is the correct term for the condition involving a "slipped disk"? _____

8. Which foramina are created by the superior and inferior vertebral notches? _____

9. Which joints are found between the superior and inferior articular processes? _____

10. Which one of the following structures makes up the inner aspect of the intervertebral disk?

    A. Annulus fibrosus   C. Annulus pulposus

    B. Nucleus pulposus   D. Nucleus fibrosus

11. True/False: The carotid artery and certain nerves pass through the cervical transverse foramina.

12. True/False: The thoracic spine possesses facets for rib articulations and bifid spinous processes.

13. The intervertebral foramina for the cervical spine lie at a _____° angle to the midsagittal plane.

14. Which ligament holds the dens against the anterior arch of C1? _____

15. The large joint space between C1 and C2 is called the _____.

16. Two partial facets found on the thoracic vertebrae are called _____.

17. Which of the following thoracic vertebrae do not possess a facet for the costotransverse joint? (There may be more than one correct answer.)

A. T1   B. T7   C. T11   D. T12

18. What are two distinctive features of all cervical vertebrae that make them different from any other vertebrae?

A. _____   B. _____

19. What is the one feature of all thoracic vertebrae that makes them different from all other vertebrae?

_____

20. Which position of the thoracic spine best demonstrates the intervertebral foramina?

_____

21. Identify the following structures labeled on Figs. 8-5, 8-6, and 8-7 (include the specific vertebra of which each structure is a part).

Structure	*Vertebra*

Fig. 8-5

A. _____   _____

B. _____   _____

C. _____   _____

D. _____   _____

E. _____   _____

F. _____   _____

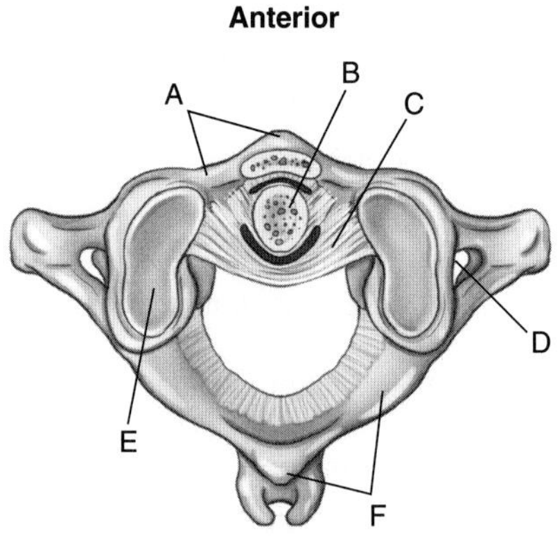

Fig. 8-5. Superior view.

Fig. 8-6

G. _____   _____

H. _____   _____

I. _____   _____

J. _____   _____

K. _____   _____

L. _____   _____

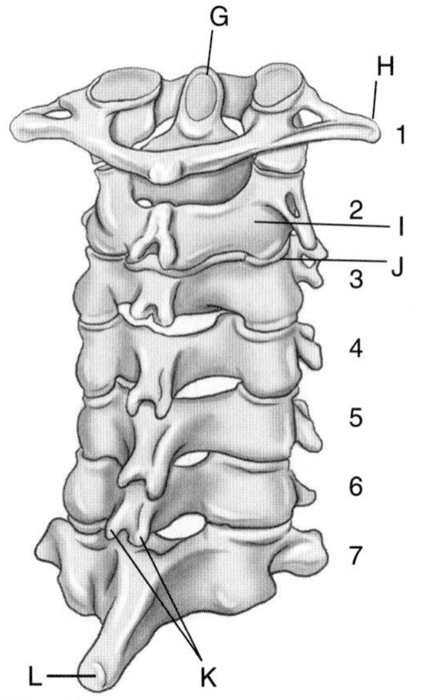

Fig. 8-6. Posterolateral view, cervical spine.

Fig. 8-7

M. _____   _____

N. _____   _____

O. _____   _____

P. _____   _____

Q. _____   _____

R. _____   _____

S. Which vertebrae are represented by this drawing?

_____

T. How can these specific vertebrae be identified?

_____

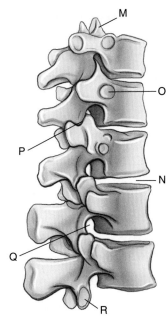

Fig. 8-7. Lateral oblique view.

22. Identify the following structures and vertebrae labeled on this AP "open mouth" cervical spine radiograph (Fig. 8-8).

Structure	*Vertebra*
A. _____	_____
B. _____	_____
C. _____	_____
D. _____	_____
E. _____	_____
F. _____	_____
G. _____	_____

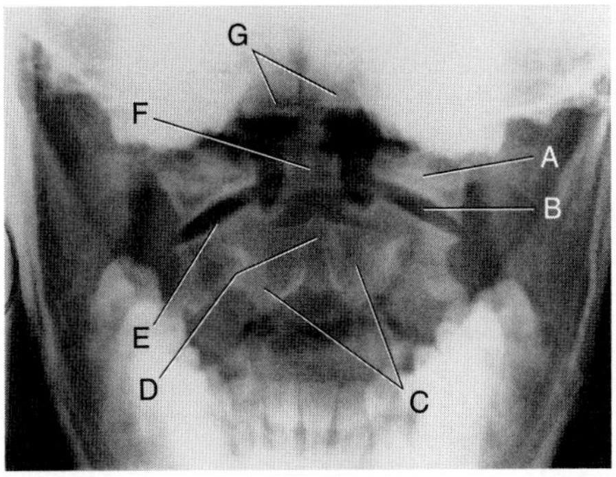

Fig. 8-8. AP "open mouth" cervical spine radiograph.

23. Which position or projection of the cervical spine best demonstrates the zygapophyseal joints (between C3 to C7)?

_____

24. Which specific joint spaces are visualized with a left anterior oblique (LAO) projection of the thoracic spine?

_____

25. Match each of the following topographic landmarks to the correct vertebral level (using each choice only once).

———— 1. Vertebra prominens   A. T2-T3

———— 2. Jugular notch   B. C7-T1

———— 3. 3 to 4 inches (8 to 10 cm) below jugular notch   C. T7

———— 4. Gonion   D. C3

———— 5. Sternal angle   E. C4-C6

———— 6. Thyroid cartilage   F. T4-T5

26. Which of the following imaging modalities is **not** normally performed to rule out a herniated nucleus pulposus (HNP)?

A. Computed tomography (CT)   C. Magnetic resonance imaging (MRI)

B. Myelography   D. Nuclear medicine

27. An avulsion fracture of the spinous processes of C6 through T1 is called a:

A. Hangman's fracture   C. Jefferson fracture

B. Clay shoveler's fracture   D. Teardrop burst fracture

28. Scheuermann disease is a form of:

A. Scoliosis and/or kyphosis   C. Arthritis

B. Subluxation   D. Fracture

29. True/False: HNP most frequently develops at the L2-L3 vertebral level.

30. Which two things can be done to minimize the effects of scatter radiation on lateral projections of the thoracic and lumbar spine?

A. _____   B. _____

31. Which position or projection best demonstrates the zygapophyseal joints between C1 and C2?

_____

32. How much and in which direction (caudad or cephalad) should the central ray be angled for each of the following projections?

A. An AP axial projection of the cervical spine: _____

B. An anterior oblique projection of the cervical spine: _____

C. A posterior oblique projection of the cervical spine: _____

33. Which one of the following projections of the cervical spine demonstrates the left intervertebral foramen?

A. Left posterior oblique (LPO)   C. Lateral projection

B. Left anterior oblique (LAO)   D. Right anterior oblique (RAO)

34. In addition to using a long SID, list the two positioning techniques you can use to lower the shoulders to visualize C7-T1 for a lateral projection of the cervical spine.

A. _____ B. _____

35. Which position or projection demonstrates the lower cervical and upper thoracic spine (C4 to T3) in a lateral

perspective? (Fracture/subluxation has been ruled out.) _____

36. List the two positions or projections that will project the dens in the center of the foramen magnum.

A. _____ B. _____

37. **Situation:** A lateral cervical spine radiograph demonstrates that the zygapophyseal joint spaces are not superimposed. Which type of positioning error(s) may lead to this radiographic outcome?

_____

38. **Situation:** A radiograph of a lateral thoracic spine projection reveals that the intervertebral foramina and intervertebral joint spaces are not clearly demonstrated. Which type of problems can lead to this radiographic outcome?

_____

39. **Situation:** A patient who was involved in a motor vehicle accident (MVA) 3 days ago is experiencing severe neck pain and comes to the radiology department for a cervical spine series. The patient is not wearing a cervical collar. Should the technologist take a horizontal beam lateral projection and have it cleared before proceeding with the study? Explain.

_____

40. **Situation:** A patient with a possible Jefferson fracture enters the ER. Which specific radiographic position best demonstrates this type of fracture?

_____

41. **Situation:** A radiograph of an AP open mouth projection of the cervical spine demonstrates the upper incisors superimposed over the top of the dens. What specific positioning error is present on this radiograph?

_____

42. **Situation:** A patient comes to the radiology department for a follow-up study for a clay shoveler's fracture. Which spine projections will best demonstrate this type of fracture?

_____

43. **Situation:** A patient comes to the radiology department for a follow-up study 6 months after having spinal fusion surgery of the lower cervical spine (C5-C6). The surgeon wants to check for anteroposterior mobility of the fused spine. Beyond the basic cervical spine projections, what additional projections can be taken to assess mobility of the spine?

_____

44. Which one of the following technical factors is most important in producing a high-quality CR image?

A. Decrease SID whenever possible   C. Decrease kV as much as possible

B. Minimize the use of grids   D. Collimate as close as possible

45. Which of the following imaging modalities is recommended for a "teardrop burst" fracture?

A. CT   C. Nuclear medicine

B. MRI   D. Sonography

9 Lumbar Spine, Sacrum, and Coccyx

CHAPTER OBJECTIVES

After you have successfully completed the activities in this chapter, you will be able to:

_____ 1. On drawings and radiographs, identify specific anatomic structures of the lumbar spine, sacrum, and coccyx.

_____ 2. Identify the anatomic structures that make up the "Scottie dog" sign.

_____ 3. Identify the classification and type of movement of the joints found in the lumbar spine.

_____ 4. List topographic landmarks that can be palpated to locate specific aspects of the lumbar spine, sacrum, and coccyx.

_____ 5. Define specific types of pathologic features of the spine as described in the textbook.

_____ 6. Identify radiographic appearances related to these specific types of pathologic spine features.

_____ 7. Identify basic and special projections of the lumbar spine, sacrum, coccyx, and sacroiliac joints, including the correct size and type of image receptor (IR), central ray location, direction, and angulation of the central ray for each projection.

_____ 8. Identify which structures are best seen with specific projections of the lumbar spine.

_____ 9. Identify the approximate difference in patient doses between anteroposterior (AP) compared with posteroanterior (PA) projections and anterior compared with posterior oblique positions of the lumbar spine.

_____ 10. Given various hypothetic situations, identify the correct modification of a position and/or exposure factors to improve the radiographic image.

_____ 11. Given radiographs of specific lumbosacral spine projections or positions, identify positioning and exposure factor errors.

POSITIONING AND RADIOGRAPHIC CRITIQUE

_____ 1. Using a peer, position for basic and special projections of the lumbosacral spine.

_____ 2. Using a lumbar spine radiographic phantom, produce satisfactory radiographs of specific positions (if equipment is available).

_____ 3. Critique and evaluate lumbar spine and SI joint radiographs based on the five divisions of radiographic criteria: (1) anatomy demonstrated, (2) position, (3) collimation and central ray, (4) exposure, and (5) anatomic side markers.

_____ 4. Distinguish between acceptable and unacceptable lumbosacral spine radiographs based on exposure factors, motion, collimation, positioning, or other errors.

Complete the following review exercises after reading the associated pages in the textbook as indicated by each exercise. Answers to each review exercise are given at the end of the review exercises.

PART I: RADIOGRAPHIC ANATOMY
REVIEW EXERCISE A: Radiographic Anatomy of the Lumbar Spine, Sacrum, and Coccyx (see textbook pp. 324-328)

1. A portion of the lamina located between the superior and inferior articular processes is called the

   _____.

2. The superior and inferior vertebral notches join together to form the:

   A. Vertebral foramen   C. Pedicle

   B. Intervertebral foramina   D. Lamina

3. Which radiographic position best demonstrates the structure identified in the previous question?

   _____

4. Identify the parts of a typical lumbar vertebra as labeled on Fig. 9-1.

   A. _____

   B. _____

   C. _____

   D. _____

   E. _____

   F. The central ray projection labeled *F* in this drawing best demonstrates the

      _____

      _____

   G. The central ray projection labeled *G* best demonstrates the

      _____

      _____

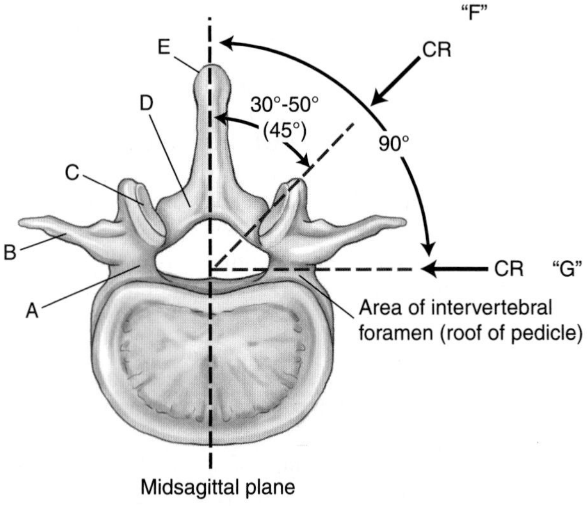

Fig. 9-1. Typical L3 vertebra.

5. Would the degree of angle to demonstrate the structures identified in *F* in the previous question be greater or

   lesser for the lower lumbar vertebrae as compared with the upper? _____

6. The small foramina found in the sacrum are called _____.

7. The anterior and superior aspect of the sacrum that forms the posterior wall of the pelvic inlet is called the

_____.

8. What is another term for the sacral horns? _____

9. The sacroiliac joints lie at an oblique angle of _____° to the coronal plane.

10. What is the formal term for the "tail bone"? _____

11. What is the name for the superior broad aspect of the coccyx? _____

12. List the structure classification and movement classification and type for the following joints of the vertebrae.

	Classification	*Mobility Type*	*Movement Type*
A. Zygapophyseal	_____	_____	_____
B. Intervertebral	_____	_____	_____

13. Identify the following structures labeled on the radiographs of the lumbar spine (Figs. 9-2 and 9-3).

A. _____

B. _____

C. _____

D. _____

E. _____

F. _____ joint

G. _____

H. _____

I. _____

J. _____

K. _____

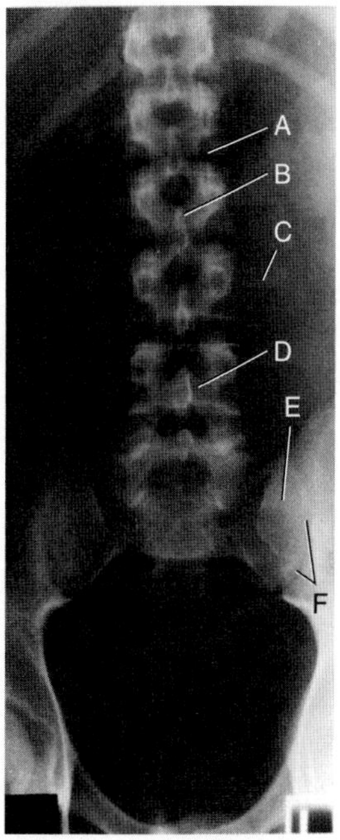

Fig. 9-2. Anteroposterior.

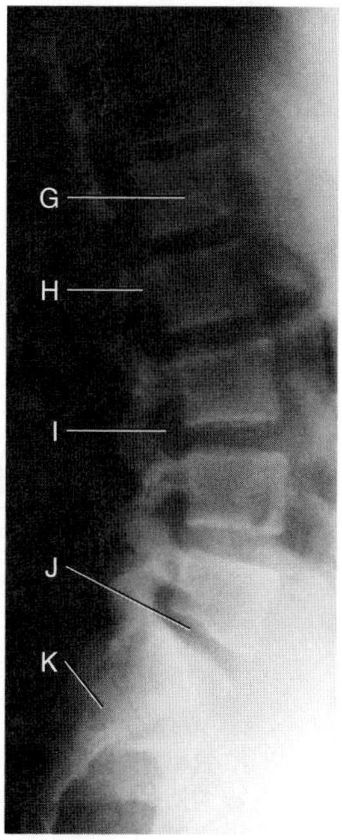

Fig. 9-3. Lateral.

Identify parts of the "Scottie dog" image, which should be visible on an oblique lumbar spine (Figs. 9-4 and 9-5).

L. _____

M. _____ joint

N. _____

O. _____

P. _____

Q. _____

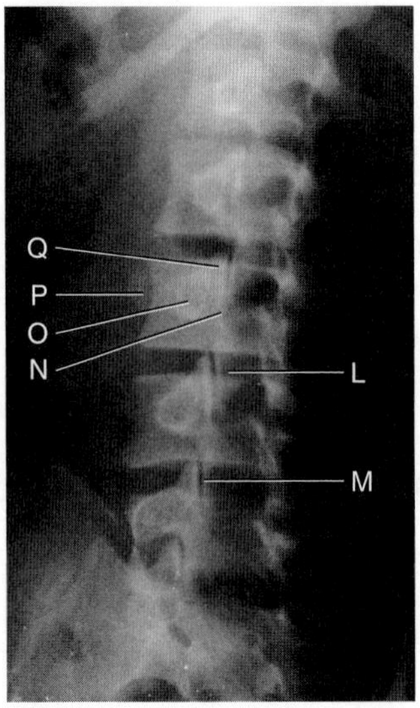

Fig. 9-4. Oblique. 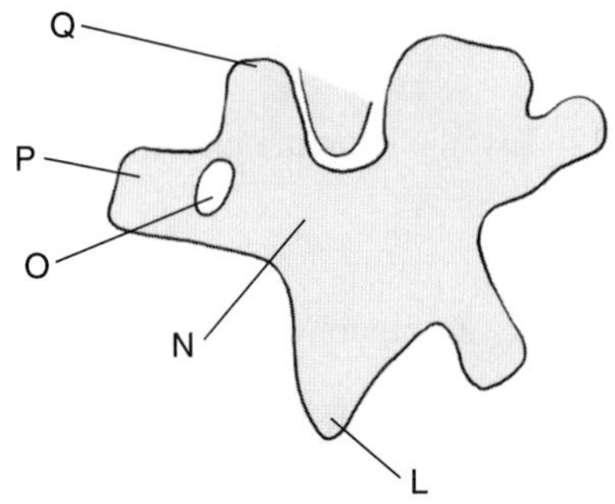   **Fig. 9-5.** "Scottie dog."

14. List the specific joints or foramina that are demonstrated with the following lumbar spine positions.

A. Left posterior oblique (LPO): _____   D. Right posterior oblique (RPO): _____

B. Right anterior oblique (RAO): _____   E. Left anterior oblique (LAO): _____

C. Lateral: _____

15. The degree of obliquity required for an oblique projection at the T12-L1 level is approximately

_____, whereas the L5-S1 level spine requires a(n)

_____ oblique. Therefore, a(n) _____ oblique is

performed for the general lumbar spine.

PART II: RADIOGRAPHIC POSITIONING
REVIEW EXERCISE B: Positioning of the Lumbar Spine, Sacrum, Coccyx, and SI Joints (see textbook pp. 330-350)

1. Match each of the following topographic landmarks to the correct vertebral level. (Use each choice only once.)

_____ 1. ASIS   A. L2-L3

_____ 2. Xiphoid process   B. L4-L5

_____ 3. Lower costal margin   C. S1-S2

_____ 4. Iliac crest   D. Tip of coccyx

_____ 5. Symphysis pubis   E. T9-T10

2. True/False: The use of higher kV and lower mA seconds (mAs) for lumbar spine radiography improves radiographic contrast but increases patient dose.

3. True/False: Placing a lead blocker mat behind the patient for lateral lumbar spine positions improves image quality.

4. True/False: Gonadal shielding should always be used for male and female patients for studies of the lumbar spine, sacrum, and coccyx.

5. True/False: The anteroposterior (AP) projection of the lumbar spine opens the intervertebral joint spaces better than the posteroanterior (PA) projection.

6. True/False: The knees and hips should be extended for an AP projection of the lumbar spine.

7. True/False: An increased source image receptor distance (SID) of 44 or 46 inches (112 to 117 cm) reduces distortion of spine anatomy.

8. True/False: The lead blocker mat and close collimation must not be used when performing digital imaging of the lumbar spine.

9. Select the imaging modality that best demonstrates each of the following pathologic features or conditions. (Answers may be used more than once.)

   _____ A. Osteoporosis

   _____ B. Soft tissues of lumbar spine

   _____ C. Structures within subarachnoid space

   _____ D. Inflammatory conditions such as Paget's disease

   _____ E. Compression fractures of the lumbar spine

   1. Magnetic resonance imaging (MRI)

   2. Computed tomography (CT)

   3. Myelography

   4. Bone densitometry

   5. Nuclear medicine

10. Match each of the following clinical indications to the correct definition or statement. (Use each choice only once.)

    _____ A. Lateral curvature of the vertebral column

    _____ B. Fracture of the vertebral body caused by hyperflexion force

    _____ C. Congenital defect in which the posterior elements of the vertebrae fail to unite

    _____ D. Most common at the L4-L5 level and may result in sciatica

    _____ E. Forward displacement of one vertebra onto another vertebra

    _____ F. Inflammatory condition that is most common in males in their thirties

    _____ G. Dissolution and separation of the pars interarticularis

    _____ H. A type of fracture that rarely causes neurologic deficits

    1. Spina bifida

    2. Herniated nucleus pulposus (HNP)

    3. Chance fracture

    4. Spondylolisthesis

    5. Compression fracture

    6. Spondylolysis

    7. Ankylosing spondylitis

    8. Scoliosis

11. With a 35- × 43-cm (14- × 17-inch) IR, the central ray is centered at the level of the

    _____ for AP and lateral lumbar spine projections.

12. Which two structures can be evaluated to determine whether rotation is present on a radiograph of an AP projection of the lumbar spine?

    A. _____   B. _____

13. How much rotation is required to properly visualize the zygapophyseal joints at the L5-S1 level?

    _____

14. Which specific set of zygapophyseal joints is demonstrated with an LAO position?

    _____

15. The _____, which is the eye of the "Scottie dog," should be near the center of the vertebral body on a correctly obliqued lumbar spine.

16. Which positioning error has been committed if the structures described in the previous question are projected too far posterior with a 45° oblique position of the lumbar spine? _____

17. Which position or projection of the lumbar spine series best demonstrates a possible compression fracture?

    _____

18. A patient with a wide pelvis and narrow thorax may require a central ray angle of

    _____° _____ (caudad or cephalad) for a lateral position of the lumbar spine.

19. How should the spine of a patient with scoliosis be positioned for a lateral position of the lumbar spine?

    _____

20. Why should the knees and hips be flexed for an AP lumbar spine projection? _____

21. True/False: The female ovarian dose used for a PA lumbar spine projection is approximately 30% less than the dose used for an AP projection.

22. Where is the central ray centered for a lateral L5-S1 projection of the lumbar spine?

    _____

23. What amount and direction of central ray angulation is required for an AP axial L5-S1 projection on a male

    patient? _____

24. True/False: A PA or AP projection for a scoliosis series frequently includes one erect and one recumbent position for comparison.

25. True/False: The lower margin of the cassette must include the symphysis pubis for a scoliosis series.

26. True/False: A PA projection for a scoliosis series produces only about ¹⁄₁₀ the dose to the breasts as compared with the AP projection, even if proper collimation is used.

27. Which one of the following techniques or devices produces a more uniform density along the vertebral column for an AP/PA scoliosis projection?

    A. Use of a 35- × 90-cm (14- × 36-inch) cassette

    B. Lower kV

    C. Higher mAs

    D. Compensating filter

28. Which side of the spine should be elevated for the second exposure for the AP/PA projection (Ferguson method) scoliosis series (by having the patient stand on a block with one foot)? _____

29. During the AP (PA) right and left bending projections of the lumbar spine, the

_____ must remain stationary during positioning.

30. Which projections should be taken to evaluate flexibility following spinal fusion surgery?

_____

31. How much central ray angulation is required for an AP projection of the sacrum for a typical male patient?

_____

32. If a patient cannot lie on his back for the AP sacrum because it is too painful, what alternate projection can be taken to achieve a similar view of the sacrum? _____

33. Where is the central ray centered for an AP projection of the coccyx? _____

34. True/False: The AP projections of the sacrum and coccyx can be taken as one single projection to decrease gonadal dose.

35. Patients should be asked to empty the urinary bladder before performing which projection(s) of the vertebral

column? _____

36. In addition to good collimation, what should be done to minimize overall "fogging" on a lateral lumbar spine or

lateral sacrum and coccyx radiograph? _____

37. Which sacroiliac (SI) joint is visualized with an RPO position? _____

38. How much rotation of the body is required for oblique positions of the SI joints?

_____

39. What type of CR angle is recommended for the AP axial projection of the SI joints on a female patient?
    A. 20° cephalad   C. 30° caudad
    B. 30° cephalad   D. 35° cephalad

40. Where is the CR centered for an oblique projection of the SI joints? _____

REVIEW EXERCISE C: Problem Solving for Technical and Positioning Errors

1. A radiograph of an AP projection of the lumbar spine reveals that the spinous processes are not midline to the vertebral column and distortion of the vertebral bodies is present. Which specific positioning error is present on this radiograph?

_____

2. A radiograph of an LPO projection of the lumbar spine reveals that the downside pedicles and zygapophyseal joints are projected over the anterior portion of the vertebral bodies. Which specific positioning error is present on this radiograph?

_____

3. A radiograph of a lateral projection of a female lumbar spine reveals that the mid- to lower intervertebral joint spaces are not open. The technologist supported the midsection of the spine with sponges to straighten the spine.

What else can be done to open the joint spaces during the repeat exposure?

_____

4. A radiograph of a lateral L5-S1 projection reveals that the joint space is not open. The technologist did support the middle aspect of the spine with a sponge. What else can the technologist do to open up the joint space during the repeat exposure?

_____

5. A radiograph of an AP axial projection of the coccyx reveals that the distal tip is superimposed over the symphysis pubis. What must the technologist do to eliminate this problem during the repeat exposure?

_____

6. A radiograph of an oblique position of the lumbar spine reveals that the downside pedicle and zygapophyseal joint are posterior in relation to the vertebral body. What modification of the position must be made during the repeat exposure to produce a more diagnostic image?

_____

7. **Situation:** A patient comes to the radiology department for a follow-up study for a compression fracture of L3. The radiologist requests that collimated projections be taken of L3. Which specific projections and centering would provide a quality study of L3 and the intervertebral joint spaces?

_____

8. **Situation:** A young female patient comes to the radiology department for a scoliosis series. She has had repeated radiation exposure over a period of time and is understandably concerned about the radiation. What three things can the technologist do to minimize the dose delivered to the patient's breasts?

A. _____

B. _____

C. _____

9. **Situation:** A patient with an injury to the coccyx enters the emergency room. When attempting the AP projection, the patient complains that it is too uncomfortable to lie on his back. He is unable to stand. What other options are available to complete the study?

_____

10. **Situation:** A patient with a clinical history of spondylolisthesis at the L5-S1 level comes to the radiology department. Which specific lumbar spine position is most diagnostic in demonstrating the extent of this condition?

_____

11. **Situation:** A positioning series for sacroiliac (SI) joints is performed on a patient. The resultant radiographs do not demonstrate the inferior portion of the joints. What can be done during the repeat exposure to demonstrate this aspect of the SI joints?

_____

12. **Situation:** A patient comes to the radiology department for a lumbar spine series. He has a clinical history of advanced spondylolysis. Which specific projection(s) of the lumbar spine series will best demonstrate this condition?

_____

13. **Situation:** A patient comes to the radiology department with a clinical history of HNP. Which of the following imaging modalities provide the most diagnostic study for this condition?

    A. Sonography   C. Nuclear medicine

    B. MRI   D. Radiography

14. **Situation:** A patient comes to the radiology department for a lumbar spine study following spinal fusion surgery. Her surgeon wants a study to assess mobility of the spine at the fusion site. Which radiographic positions provide this information?

_____

15. **Situation:** A patient comes to the radiology department for a lumbar spine series. She has a clinical history of severe kyphosis. How should the lumbar spine series be modified for this patient?

_____

REVIEW EXERCISE D: Critique Radiographs of the Lumbar Spine, Sacrum, and Coccyx (see textbook p. 351)

The following questions relate to the radiographs found at the end of Chapter 9 of the textbook. Evaluate these radiographs for the radiographic criteria categories (1 through 5) that follow. Describe the corrections needed to improve the overall image. The major, or "repeatable," errors are specific errors that indicate the need for a repeat exposure, regardless of the nature of the other errors.

A. Lateral lumbar spine (Fig. C9-83)

    1. Anatomy demonstrated: _____

    2. Part positioning: _____

    3. Collimation and central ray: _____

    4. Exposure: _____

    5. Anatomic side markers: _____

Repeatable error(s): _____

B. Lateral lumbar spine (Fig. C9-84)

    1. Anatomy demonstrated: _____

    2. Part positioning: _____

    3. Collimation and central ray: _____

    4. Exposure: _____

    5. Anatomic side markers: _____

Repeatable error(s): _____

C. Lateral L5-S1 (Fig. C9-85)

1. Anatomy demonstrated: _____

2. Part positioning: _____

3. Collimation and central ray: _____

4. Exposure: _____

5. Anatomic side markers: _____

Repeatable error(s): _____

D. RPO lumbar spine (Fig. C9-86)

1. Anatomy demonstrated: _____

2. Part positioning: _____

3. Collimation and central ray: _____

4. Exposure: _____

5. Anatomic side markers: _____

Repeatable error(s): _____

E. AP lumbar spine (Fig. C9-87)

1. Anatomy demonstrated: _____

2. Part positioning: _____

3. Collimation and central ray: _____

4. Exposure: _____

5. Anatomic side markers: _____

Repeatable error(s): _____

F. LPO lumbar spine (Fig. C9-88)

1. Anatomy demonstrated: _____

2. Part positioning: _____

3. Collimation and central ray: _____

4. Exposure: _____

5. Anatomic side markers: _____

Repeatable error(s): _____

G. AP lumbar spine (Fig. C9-89)

1. Anatomy demonstrated: _____

2. Part positioning: _____

3. Collimation and central ray: _____

4. Exposure: _____

5. Anatomic side markers: _____

Repeatable error(s): _____

PART III: LABORATORY EXERCISES

You must gain experience in positioning each part of the lumbar spine, sacrum, and coccyx before performing the following exams on actual patients. You can get experience in positioning and radiographic evaluation of these projections by performing exercises using radiographic phantoms and practicing positioning on other students (although you will not be taking actual exposures).

The following suggested activities assume that your teaching institution has an energized lab and radiographic phantoms. If not, perform Laboratory Exercises B and C, the radiographic evaluation and the physical positioning exercises. (Check off each step and projection as you complete it.)

Laboratory Exercise A: Energized Laboratory

1. Using the abdomen/lumbosacral radiographic phantom, produce radiographs of the following basic routines:

_____ AP lumbar spine   _____ AP sacrum   _____ Posterior oblique lumbar spine

_____ Lateral lumbar spine   _____ AP coccyx   _____ Anterior oblique lumbar spine

_____ Lateral L5-S1   _____ Lateral sacrum and coccyx   _____ AP axial L5-S1

_____ Oblique SI joints   _____ AP axial SI joints

Laboratory Exercise B: Radiographic Evaluation

1. Evaluate and critique the radiographs produced during the previous experiments, additional radiographs provided by your instructor, or both. Evaluate each radiograph for the following points.

_____ Evaluate the completeness of the study. (Are all of the pertinent anatomic structures included on the radiograph?)

_____ Evaluate for positioning or centering errors (e.g., rotation, off centering).

_____ Evaluate for correct exposure factors and possible motion. (Are the density and contrast of the images acceptable?)

_____ Determine whether anatomic side markers and an acceptable degree of collimation and/or area shielding are visible on the images.

Laboratory Exercise C: Physical Positioning

On another person, simulate performing all basic and special projections of the lumbar spine, sacrum, and coccyx as follows. (Check off each when completed satisfactorily.) Include the following six steps as described in the textbook.

Step 1. Appropriate size and type of image receptor with correct markers

Step 2. Correct central ray placement and centering of part to central ray and/or IR

Step 3. Accurate collimation

Step 4. Area shielding of patient where advisable

Step 5. Use of proper immobilizing devices when needed

Step 6. Approximate correct exposure factors, breathing instructions where applicable, and initiating exposure

Projections	Step 1	Step 2	Step 3	Step 4	Step 5	Step 6
● AP lumbar spine	_____	_____	_____	_____	_____	_____
● Lateral lumbar spine	_____	_____	_____	_____	_____	_____
● Lateral L5-S1	_____	_____	_____	_____	_____	_____
● AP sacrum	_____	_____	_____	_____	_____	_____
● AP coccyx	_____	_____	_____	_____	_____	_____
● Lateral sacrum and coccyx	_____	_____	_____	_____	_____	_____
● Posterior oblique lumbar spine	_____	_____	_____	_____	_____	_____
● Anterior oblique lumbar spine	_____	_____	_____	_____	_____	_____
● AP axial L5-S1	_____	_____	_____	_____	_____	_____

Spinal fusion series

● AP (PA) R and L bending	_____	_____	_____	_____	_____	_____
● Lateral hyperextension and hyperflexion	_____	_____	_____	_____	_____	_____

Scoliosis series

● PA (AP) and lateral erect	_____	_____	_____	_____	_____	_____

SI joint series

● AP axial SI joints	_____	_____	_____	_____	_____	_____
● RPO and LPO SI joints	_____	_____	_____	_____	_____	_____

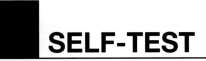 **SELF-TEST**

MY SCORE = _____%

This self-test should be taken only after completing all of the readings, review exercises, and laboratory activities for a particular section. The purpose of this test is not only to provide a good learning exercise but also to serve as a strong indicator of what your final evaluation exam for this chapter will cover. It is strongly suggested that if you do not get at least a 90% to 95% grade on each self-test, you should review those areas in which you missed questions before going to your instructor for the final evaluation exam.

1. Compared with the spinous processes of the cervical and thoracic spine, the lumbar spinous processes are:

   A. Smaller   C. Larger and more blunt

   B. Pointed downward more   D. Absent

2. The anterior/superior ridge of the upper sacrum is called the:

   A. Median sacral crest   C. Promontory

   B. Cornua   D. Sacral horns

3. Each sacroiliac joint opens obliquely _____° posteriorly

   A. 20   C. 45

   B. 30   D. 50

4. The angle of the midlumbar spine zygapophyseal joints in relation to the midsagittal plane is

   _____.

5. Where is the pars interarticularis found?

   A. Superior and inferior aspect of the pedicle   C. Between the superior and inferior articular processes

   B. Between the intervertebral disk and vertebra   D. Between the lamina and body spinous processes

Chapter **9 Lumbar Spine, Sacrum, and Coccyx: Self-Test**

6. Identify the labeled parts of the sacrum and coccyx on the following drawings (Figs. 9-6 and 9-7).

A. _____

B. _____

C. _____

D. _____

E. _____

F. _____

G. _____

H. _____

I. _____

J. _____

K. _____

L. _____

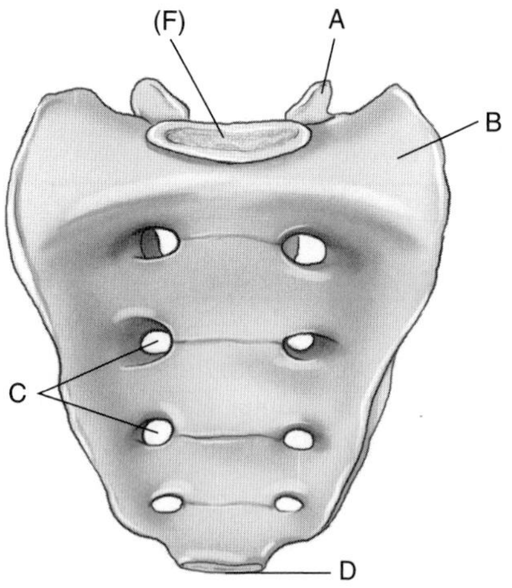

Fig. 9-6. Sacrum.

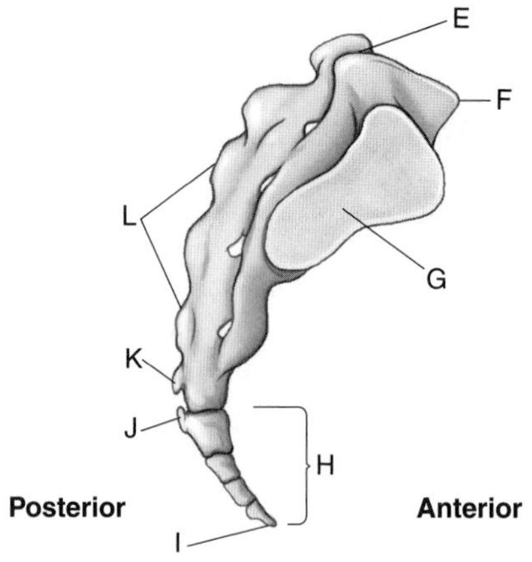

Fig. 9-7. Sacrum and coccyx.

7. Identify the labeled parts on these radiographs of individual vertebrae (Figs. 9-8 and 9-9).

A. _____

B. _____

C. _____

D. _____

E. _____

F. _____

G. _____

H. _____

I. _____

J. _____

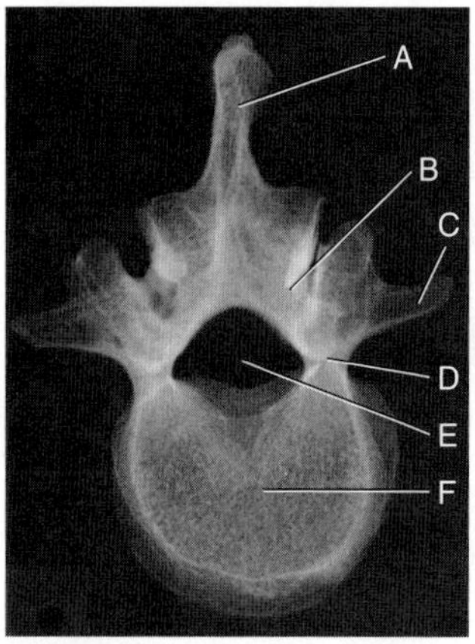

Fig. 9-8. Individual vertebra, A-F.

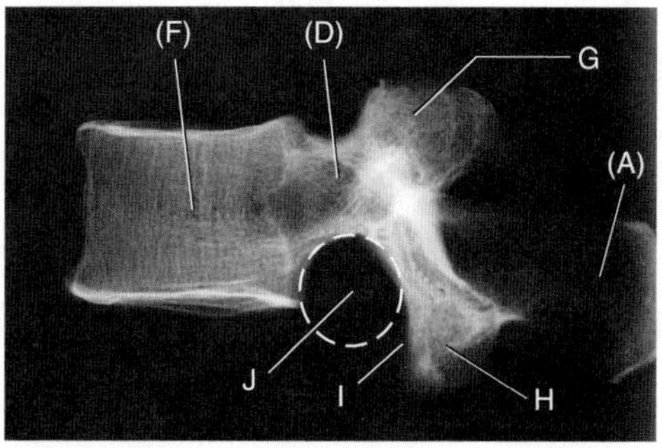

Fig. 9-9. Individual vertebra, G-J.

8. What are the characteristics of the vertebra in Fig. 9-9 that identify it as a lumbar vertebra rather than a thoracic?

_____

9. The zygapophyseal joints of the lumbar spine are classified as _____ joints with

_____ type of joint movement.

10. List the correct terms of the lumbar vertebra that correspond to the following labeled parts of the "Scottie dog" as seen on an oblique radiograph of the lumbar spine (Fig. 9-10).

A. _____

B. _____

C. _____

D. _____

E. _____

F. _____ joint

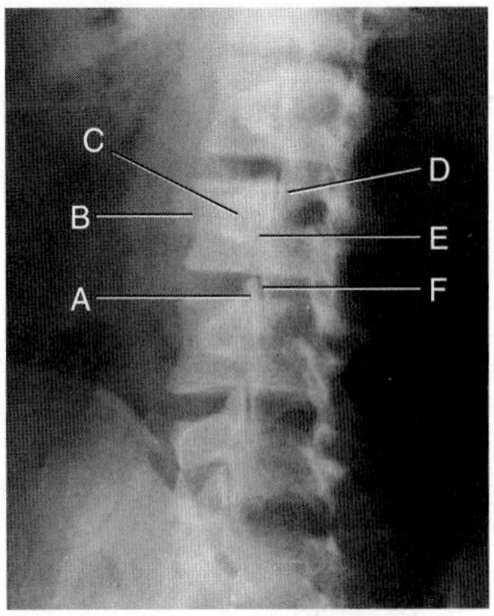

Fig. 9-10. Oblique lumbar spine.

11. The ear and front leg of the "Scottie dog" make up the _____ joint, best seen in the oblique position.

12. Which one of the following topographic landmarks corresponds to the L2-L3 level?

A. Xiphoid process   C. Iliac crest

B. Lower costal margin   D. ASIS

13. True/False: It is possible to shield females for an AP projection of the sacrum or coccyx if the gonadal shields are correctly placed.

14. True/False: The female gonadal dose is approximately equal for either AP or PA projections of the lumbar spine.

15. Why should the knees and hips be flexed for an AP projection of the lumbar spine?

_____

16. True/False: A lead blocker mat for lateral positions of the lumbar spine should not be used with digital imaging.

17. True/False: The efficiency of CT and MRI of the spine is reducing the number of myelograms being performed.

18. Anterior wedging and loss of vertebral body height are characteristic of:

A. Chance fracture   C. Compression fracture

B. Spina bifida   D. Spondylolysis

19. Which one of the following conditions is often diagnosed by prenatal ultrasound?

A. Scoliosis   C. Spondylolisthesis

B. Spina bifida   D. Ankylosing spondylitis

20. True/False. Ankylosing spondylitis usually requires an increase in manual exposure factors?

21. Where is the central ray centered for an AP projection of the lumbar spine with a 30- × 35-cm (11- × 14-inch) IR?

_____

22. Which set of zygapophyseal joints of the lumbar spine is best demonstrated with an LAO position?

_____

23. How much rotation of the spine is required to demonstrate the zygapophyseal joint space between L1-L2?

_____

24. Describe the body build that may require central ray angulation to open the intervertebral joint spaces with a lateral projection of the lumbar spine, even if the patient has some support under the waist.

_____

25. What type of central ray angulation should be used for the lateral L5-S1 projection if the waist is not supported?

A. Central ray perpendicular to IR   C. 10° to 15° cephalad

B. 5° to 8° caudad   D. 3° to 5° cephalad

26. For the lateral L5-S1 projection, the CR is parallel to the _____ plane.

A. Midsagittal   C. Midsagittal

B. Midcoronal   D. Interiliac

27. Where is the central ray centered for an AP axial projection for L5-S1?

_____

28. True/False: A kV range of 90 to 100 kV can be used for a lateral L5-S1 projection when using a digital imaging system.

29. Which projection or method is designed to demonstrate the degree of scoliosis deformity between the primary and compensatory curves as part of a scoliosis study?

_____

30. Which projections are designed to measure mobility of the vertebral column at the site of a spinal fusion?

_____

31. Where is the central ray centered for an AP projection of the sacrum?

_____

32. What two things can be done to reduce the high amounts of scatter reaching the IR during a lateral projection of the sacrum and coccyx?

A. _____   B. _____

33. Why should a single lateral projection of the sacrum and coccyx be performed rather than separate laterals of the sacrum and coccyx?

_____

34. True/False: The pelvis must remain as stationary as possible when positioning for the hyperextension and hyperflexion projections.

35. A radiograph of an AP projection of the lumbar spine reveals that the sacroiliac (SI) joints are not equidistant from the spine. The right ala of the sacrum appears wider, and the left SI joint is more open than the left. Which specific positioning error is evident on this radiograph?

_____

36. A radiograph of an LPO projection of the lumbar spine reveals that the downside pedicles are projected toward the posterior aspect of the vertebral bodies. What must be done to correct this error during the repeat exposure?

_____

37. An AP projection of the sacrum reveals that the sacrum is foreshortened and the foramina are not open. What positioning error may have led to this radiographic outcome?

_____

38. **Situation:** A patient with a possible compression fracture of L3 enters the emergency room. Which projection(s) of the lumbar spine best demonstrate(s) the extent of this injury?

_____

39. **Situation:** A patient with a clinical history of spondylolisthesis of the L5-S1 region comes to the radiology department. What basic (i.e., routine) and special (i.e., optional) projections should be included in this study? (Hint: If the oblique positions are included, how much spine rotation should be used?)

_____

40. **Situation:** A study of the sacroiliac joints demonstrates that the joints are not open and the upper iliac wings are nearly superimposing the joints. The technologist performed 35° RPO and LPO positions with a perpendicular CR. What can be done during the repeat exposure to open the joints?

_____

10 Bony Thorax—Sternum and Ribs

CHAPTER OBJECTIVES

After you have successfully completed the activities in this chapter, you will be able to:

_____ 1. Using drawings and radiographs, identify specific anatomic structures of the sternum and ribs.

_____ 2. Classify ribs as either true, false, or floating ribs.

_____ 3. Classify specific joints in the bony thorax according to their structural classification, mobility classification, and movement type.

_____ 4. Define specific types of clinical indications of the bony thorax as described in the textbook.

_____ 5. Identify basic and special projections of the ribs and sternum, including the correct size and type of image receptor (IR), and the location, direction, and angulation of the central ray for each position.

_____ 6. Identify which structures are best seen with specific projections of the ribs and sternum.

_____ 7. Identify the technical considerations important in radiography of the ribs and sternum, including breathing instructions, general body position, kV range, and other imaging options.

_____ 8. Given various hypothetic situations, identify the correct modification of a position and/or exposure factors to improve the radiographic image.

_____ 9. Given radiographs of specific bony thorax projections or positions, identify specific positioning and exposure factor errors.

POSITIONING AND RADIOGRAPHIC CRITIQUE

_____ 1. Using a peer, position for basic and special projections of the bony thorax.

_____ 2. Using a chest radiographic phantom, produce satisfactory radiographs of specific positions (if equipment is available).

_____ 3. Critique and evaluate cranial radiographs based on the five divisions of radiographic criteria: (1) anatomy demonstrated, (2) position, (3) collimation and central ray, (4) exposure, and (5) anatomic markers.

_____ 4. Distinguish between acceptable and unacceptable bony thorax radiographs based on exposure factors, motion, collimation, positioning, or other errors.

LEARNING EXERCISES

Complete the following review exercises after reading the associated pages in the textbook as indicated by each exercise. Answers to each review exercise are given at the end of the review exercises.

PART I: RADIOGRAPHIC ANATOMY

REVIEW EXERCISE A: Radiographic Anatomy of the Bony Thorax, Sternum, and Ribs (see textbook pp. 354-356)

1. List the three structures that make up the bony thorax.

   A. ________________ B. ________________ C. ________________

2. Identify the parts of the sternum and ribs labeled in Fig. 10-1.

   A. ________________

   B. ________________

   C. ________________

   D. ________________

   E. ________________

   F. ________________

   G. ________________

   H. ________________

   I. ________________

   J. ________________

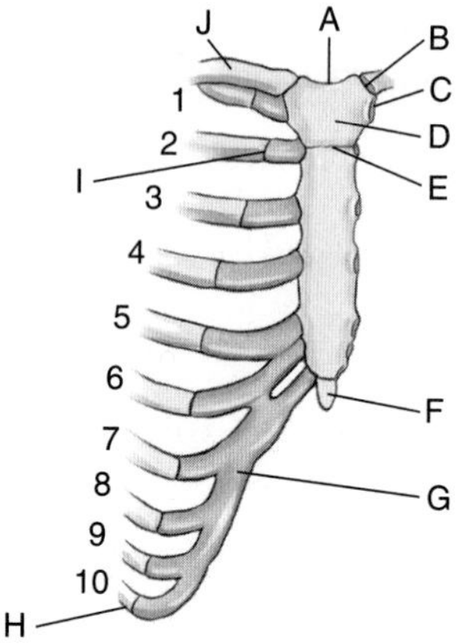

Fig. 10-1. Sternum and ribs.

3. What is the term for the long, middle aspect of the sternum? ________________________________

4. The most distal aspect of the sternum does not ossify until a person is approximately

   ________________________________ years of age.

5. The total sternum length on an average adult is about ________________ inches (________________ cm).

6. A. The xiphoid process of the sternum is at the approximate level of the ________________________________ vertebra.

   B. The sternal angle is at the level of ________________________________.

   C. What is another term for the sternal angle? ________________________________.

7. What is the name of the joint that connects the upper limb to the bony thorax (the only bony connection between the bony thorax and upper limbs)? ________________________________

8. What is the name of the section of cartilage that connects the anterior end of the rib to the sternum?

   ____

9. What distinguishes a true rib from a false rib? ________________________________

10. True/False: The eleventh and twelfth ribs are classified as false and floating ribs.

11. True/False: The anterior end of the ribs is called the vertebral end.

12. Which aspect of the ribs articulates with the transverse process of the thoracic vertebrae?

A. Head   C. Neck

B. Costal angle   D. Tubercle

13. List the three structures found within the costal groove of each rib.

A. _____   B. _____   C. _____

14. Answer the following questions as you study Fig. 10-2.

A. Which end of the ribs is most superior—the posterior vertebral ends or the anterior sternal ends?

_____

B. Approximately how much difference in height is there between these two ends of the ribs?

_____

C. Which ribs articulate with the upper lateral aspect of the manubrium of the sternum?

_____

D. The bony thorax is widest at the lateral margins

of which ribs? _____

E. How many posterior ribs are shown above the diaphragm? (Hint: Recall from Chapter 2 that a minimum of 10 posterior ribs must be seen on an average inspiration posteroanterior [PA] chest projection.)

_____

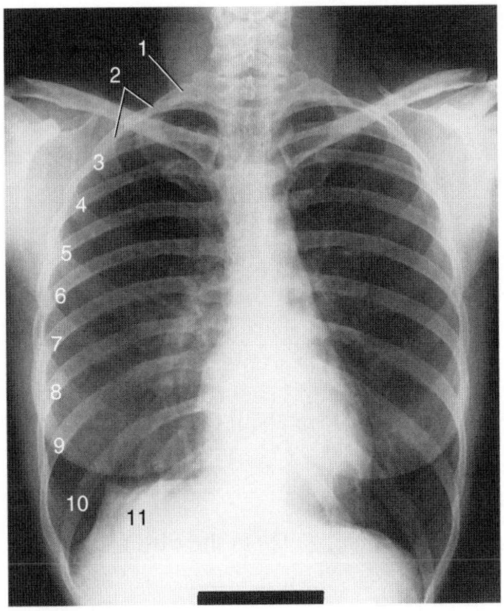

Fig. 10-2. Rib radiograph.

15. Match each of the following joints with the correct movement type.

A. Movable—diarthrodial (plane or gliding)

B. Immovable—synarthrodial

C. Fibrous—syndesmosis

_____ 1. First sternocostal

_____ 2. First through twelfth costovertebral joints

_____ 3. First through tenth costochondral unions (between costicartilage and ribs)

_____ 4. First through tenth costotransverse joints (between ribs and transverse processes of T vertebrae)

_____ 5. Second through seventh sternocostal joints (between second and seventh ribs and sternum)

_____ 6. Sixth through ninth interchondral joints (between anterior sixth and ninth costal cartilage)

_____ 7. Ninth and tenth interchondral joints between the cartilages

16. The joints from the previous question that have diarthrodial movement are classified as

_____.

17. Classify the following groups of ribs (labeled on the diagram as *A, B,* and *C)* and identify the number of the ribs in each category (Fig. 10-3).

A. _____

B. _____

C. _____

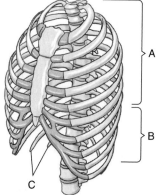

Fig. 10-3. Rib groups.

18. What is unique about the ribs in category A in the previous question?

_____

19. What is unique about the ribs in category C in the previous question?

_____

20. Identify the labeled parts of this posterior view of a typical rib (Fig. 10-4).

A. _____

B. _____

C. _____

D. _____

E. _____

F. _____

G. _____

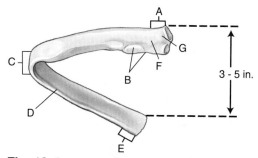

Fig. 10-4. Posterior view of a typical rib.

PART II: RADIOGRAPHIC POSITIONING
REVIEW EXERCISE B: Positioning of the Ribs and Sternum (see textbook pp. 357-370)

1. True/False: It is virtually impossible to visualize the sternum with a direct PA or anteroposterior (AP) projection.

2. True/False: A large, "deep-chested" (hypersthenic) patient requires more obliquity for a frontal view of the sternum as compared with a "thin-chested" (asthenic) patient.

3. How much rotation should be used for the oblique position of the sternum for a large, "deep-chested" patient?

_____

4. List the recommended ranges for the following **analog** exposure factors as they apply to an oblique position of the sternum (orthostatic-breathing technique).

A. kV range: _____

B. mA (low or high): _____

C. Exposure time (short or long): _____

5. What is the advantage of performing an orthostatic (breathing) technique for radiography of the sternum?

_____

6. What is the primary reason that a source image receptor distance (SID) of less than 40 inches (102 cm) should not

be used for sternum radiography? _____

7. What other imaging option is available to study the sternum if routine RAO and lateral radiographs do not provide

sufficient information? _____

8. Identify the preferred positioning factors to demonstrate an injury to the ribs found **below** the diaphragm:

A. General body position (erect or recumbent): _____

B. Breathing instructions (inspiration or expiration): _____

C. Recommended kV range (analog and digital): _____

9. An injury to the region of the eighth or ninth rib requires the _____ (above or below) diaphragm technique.

10. To properly elongate and visualize the axillary aspect of the ribs, the patient's spine should be rotated

_____ (toward or away from) the area of interest.

11. Which projections (AP or PA and anterior or posterior oblique) should be performed for an injury to the anterior

aspect of the ribs? _____

12. Which two rib projections should be performed for an injury to the right posterior ribs?

_____

13. How can the site of injury be marked for a rib series? _____

14. If the physician suspects a pneumothorax or hemothorax has occurred as a result of a rib fracture, which additional radiographic projection(s) should be performed in addition to the routine rib projections?

_____

15. A flail chest is defined as a(n):

   A. Asthenic body habitus

   B. Pulmonary injury caused by blunt trauma to two or more ribs

   C. Chronic obstructive pulmonary disease (COPD; e.g., emphysema)

   D. Cardiac injury caused by blunt trauma

16. Osteolytic metastases of the ribs produce which of the following radiographic appearances?

   A. Irregular bony margins   C. Sharp lucent lines through the ribs

   B. Increased bony density of the ribs   D. Smooth lucent "holes" in the rib

17. Which of the following definitions applies to pectus excavatum?

   A. Multiple fractures of the sternum with fragments in the pericardium

   B. Abnormally prominent lower aspect of sternum

   C. Depressed sternum caused by congenital defect

   D. Separation between ribs and sternum resulting from trauma

18. A proliferative bony lesion of increased density is generally termed:

   A. Osteoblastic   C. Osteolytic

   B. Osteoporotic   D. Osteostenotic

19. True/False: MRI provides a more diagnostic image of rib metastases as compared with a nuclear medicine scan.

20. True/False: Patients can develop osteomyelitis as a postoperative complication following open heart surgery.

21. Which is preferred for a study of the sternum: RAO or LAO? _____

   Why? _____

22. Where is the central ray centered for the oblique and lateral projections of the sternum?

   _____

23. What other position can be performed if the patient cannot assume a prone position for the RAO sternum?

   _____

24. What is the recommended SID for a lateral projection of the sternum? _____

   Why?_____

25. Which of the following criteria apply to a radiograph for an evaluation of the oblique sternum?

   A. The entire sternum should be adjacent to the spine and adjacent to the heart shadow.

   B. The entire sternum should lie over the heart shadow and be adjacent to the spine.

   C. The left sternoclavicular joint should be adjacent to the spinal column.

   D. The second rib should lie directly over the manubrium of the sternum.

26. Where is the central ray centered for a PA projection of the sternoclavicular joints?

   A. Level of T7   C. At the vertebra prominens

   B. Level of T2-T3   D. Level of xiphoid process

27. What type of breathing instructions should be given to the patient for a PA projection of the sternoclavicular joints?

    A. Suspend respiration on inspiration.

    B. Use an orthostatic-breathing technique.

    C. Suspended breathing is not necessary.

28. How much rotation of the thorax is recommended for an anterior oblique of the sternoclavicular joints?

    _____

29. Which specific oblique position best demonstrates the left sternoclavicular joint adjacent to the spine?

    _____

30. What are the three points that must be included in the patient's clinical history before a rib series?

    A. _____

    B. _____

    C. _____

31. Where is the central ray centered for an AP projection of the ribs for an injury located above the diaphragm?

    _____

32. Which two specific oblique positions can be used to elongate the left axillary portion of the ribs?

    _____

33. Which two basic projections or positions should be performed for an injury to the right anterior ribs?

    _____

34. How many degrees of rotation are required for an oblique projection of the axillary ribs?

    _____

35. What is the recommended SID for a bilateral lower rib study on an adult?

    _____

36. True/False: The recommended kV range for a digital study of the unilateral, lower anterior ribs is 80 to 90 kV.

37. Which region of the ribs is best demonstrated with an RAO projection?

    _____

38. True/False: An RAO of the SC joints projects the left joint closest to the spine.

39. To minimize patient dose for a RAO projection of the sternum, the patient's skin should be at least

    _____ below the collimator.

    A. 40 inches (102 cm)   C. 38 inches (97 cm)

    B. 72 inches (183 cm)   D. 2 inches (5 cm)

40. Which one of the following conditions may require a chest routine be included along with a study of the ribs?

    A. Pectus carinatum   C. Pectus excavatum

    B. Hemothorax   D. Osteomyelitis

REVIEW EXERCISE C: Problem Solving for Technical and Positioning Errors

1. A radiograph of an RAO sternum reveals that part of the sternum is superimposed over the thoracic spine. Which specific positioning error is visible on this radiograph?

_____

2. A radiograph of an RAO sternum reveals that the sternum is difficult to visualize because of excessive density. The following analog exposure factors were used for this image: 80 kV, 25 mA, 3-second exposure, 40-inch (102-cm) SID, Bucky, and 100-speed screens. Which one of these factors should be modified during the repeat exposure to produce a more diagnostic image?

_____

3. A radiograph of an RAO sternum reveals that the sternum is poorly visualized because of excessive lung markings superimposed over the sternum. The following analog exposure factors were used for this image: 65 kV, 200 mA, 1-second exposure, 40-inch (102-cm) SID, Bucky, and 100-speed screens. Which of these factors can be altered to increase the visibility of the sternum?

_____

4. A radiograph of a lateral projection of the sternum reveals that the patient's breasts are obscuring the sternum. What can be done to minimize the breast artifact over the sternum?

_____

5. Repeat PA projections of the sternoclavicular joints do not clearly demonstrate them. What other imaging modality may produce a more diagnostic image of these joints?

_____

6. **Situation:** A patient with trauma to the sternum and the left sternoclavicular joint region enters the emergency room. In addition to the sternum routine, the ER physician asks for a specific projection to better demonstrate the left sternoclavicular joint. Describe the positioning routine, including the breathing instructions that you would use. (Hint: Three projections are required.)

_____

_____

7. A radiograph of the upper ribs demonstrates that the diaphragm is superimposed over the seventh to eighth ribs, which is in the area of interest. The following analog exposure factors were used for the initial exposure: 65 kV, 400 mA, ¹⁄₄₀ second, 400-speed screens, grid, suspended respiration on expiration, erect position, 40-inch (102-cm) SID. Which one of these factors can be modified to increase the visibility of the area of interest?

_____

8. **Situation:** A patient enters the emergency room on a backboard after being involved in a motor vehicle accident. Because of the condition of the patient, the physician orders a portable study of the sternum in the ER. Which two projections of the sternum would be most diagnostic yet minimize movement of the patient? (See Chapter 15 in the textbook for a demonstration.)

_____

9. **Situation:** A patient with trauma to the right upper anterior ribs enters the ER. He is able to sit in an erect position. Which positioning routine of the ribs should be performed? (Include general body position, breathing instructions, and specific projections or positions performed.)

_____

10. **Situation:** A patient with trauma to the left lower anterior ribs enters the ER. Which positioning routine of the ribs should be performed? (Include general body position, breathing instructions, and specific positions performed.)

_____

11. **Situation:** An elderly patient comes to the radiology department for a complete rib series with an emphasis on the posterior ribs. She has advanced osteoporosis and has difficulty moving and lying down. Her physician wants both upper and lower ribs examined. What type of positions should be performed? How would you adjust technical factors for this patient?

_____

12. **Situation:** A patient enters the ER with blunt trauma to the chest. He is restricted on a backboard. The ER physician suspects a flail chest. Beyond the initial chest projections, what positioning routine would confirm the diagnosis of flail chest?

_____

REVIEW EXERCISE D: Critique Radiographs of the Bony Thorax (see textbook p. 371)

The following questions relate to the radiographs found at the end of Chapter 10 of the textbook. Evaluate these radiographs for the radiographic criteria categories (1 through 5) that follow. Describe the corrections needed to improve the overall image. The major, or "repeatable," errors are specific errors that indicate the need for a repeat exposure, regardless of the nature of the other errors.

A. Bilateral ribs above diaphragm (Fig. C10-46)

1. Anatomy demonstrated: _____

2. Part positioning: _____

3. Collimation and central ray: _____

4. Exposure: _____

5. Anatomic side markers: _____

Repeatable error(s): _____

B. Oblique sternum (Fig. C10-47)

1. Anatomy demonstrated: _____

2. Part positioning: _____

3. Collimation and central ray: _____

4. Exposure: _____

5. Anatomic side markers: _____

Repeatable error(s): _____

C. AP ribs below diaphragm (Fig. C10-48)

1. Anatomy demonstrated: _____

2. Part positioning: _____

3. Collimation and central ray: _____

4. Exposure: _____

5. Anatomic side markers: _____

Repeatable error(s): _____

D. Lateral sternum (Fig. C10-49)

1. Anatomy demonstrated: _____

2. Part positioning: _____

3. Collimation and central ray: _____

4. Exposure: _____

5. Anatomic side markers: _____

Repeatable error(s): _____

PART III: LABORATORY EXERCISES

You must gain experience in positioning each part of the sternum and ribs before performing the following exams on actual patients. You can get experience in positioning and radiographic evaluation of these projections by performing exercises using radiographic phantoms and practicing positioning on other students (although you will not be taking actual exposures).

The following suggested activities assume that your teaching institution has an energized lab and radiographic phantoms. If not, perform Laboratory Exercises B and C, the radiographic evaluation, and the physical positioning exercises. (Check off each step and projection as you complete it.)

Laboratory Exercise A: Energized Laboratory

1. Using the chest radiographic phantom, produce radiographs of the following basic routines:

_____ RAO sternum

_____ PA sternoclavicular joints

_____ AP (PA) ribs

_____ AP (PA) ribs, above and below diaphragm

_____ Lateral sternum

_____ RAO (LAO) sternoclavicular joints

_____ Posterior and anterior oblique ribs, above the diaphragm

_____ Horizontal beam lateral sternum

Laboratory Exercise B: Radiographic Evaluation

1. Evaluate and critique the radiographs produced in the preceding, additional radiographs provided by your instructor, or both. Evaluate each radiograph for the following points.

_____ Evaluate the completeness of the study. (Are all of the pertinent anatomic structures included on the radiograph?)

_____ Evaluate for positioning or centering errors (e.g., rotation, off centering).

_____ Evaluate for correct exposure factors and possible motion. (Are the density and contrast of the images acceptable?)

_____ Determine whether markers and an acceptable degree of collimation and/or area shielding are visible on the images.

Laboratory Exercise C: Physical Positioning

On another person, simulate performing all basic and special projections of the sternum and ribs as follows. Include the six steps listed in the following and described in the textbook. (Check off each step when completed satisfactorily.)

Step 1. Appropriate size and type of image receptor with correct markers

Step 2. Correct central ray placement and centering of part to central ray and/or image receptor

Step 3. Accurate collimation

Step 4. Area shielding of patient where advisable

Step 5. Use of proper immobilizing devices when needed

Step 6. Approximate correct exposure factors, breathing instructions where applicable, and initiating exposure

Projections	Step 1	Step 2	Step 3	Step 4	Step 5	Step 6
● RAO sternum	_____	_____	_____	_____	_____	_____
● Erect lateral sternum	_____	_____	_____	_____	_____	_____
● Recumbent left posterior oblique (LPO) sternum	_____	_____	_____	_____	_____	_____
● Horizontal beam lateral sternum	_____	_____	_____	_____	_____	_____
● PA sternoclavicular joints	_____	_____	_____	_____	_____	_____
● Oblique sternoclavicular joints	_____	_____	_____	_____	_____	_____
● Rib routine for injury to right upper anterior ribs	_____	_____	_____	_____	_____	_____
● Rib routine for injury to left lower posterior ribs	_____	_____	_____	_____	_____	_____

Optional exercise if the school or medical center has a linear tomography unit

● Linear tomogram of the sternum	_____	_____	_____	_____	_____	_____

SELF-TEST

MY SCORE = _____%

This self-test should be taken only after completing all of the readings, review exercises, and laboratory activities for a particular section. The purpose of this test is not only to provide a good learning exercise but also to serve as a strong indicator of what your final evaluation exam for this chapter will cover. It is strongly suggested that if you do not get at least a 90% to 95% grade on each self-test, you should review those areas in which you missed questions before going to your instructor for the final evaluation exam.

1. List the three parts of the sternum.

   A. _____

   B. _____

   C. _____

2. What is the most distal aspect of the sternum? _____

3. What is the name of the palpable junction between the upper and midportion of the sternum?

   _____

4. Which aspect of the sternum possesses the jugular notch?

   A. Body   C. Xiphoid process

   B. Sternal angle   D. Manubrium

5. What distinguishes a true rib from a false rib?

   A. A true rib attaches directly to the sternum with its own costicartilage.

   B. A true rib possesses a costovertebral and a costotransverse joint.

   C. A false rib does not possess a head.

   D. A false rib is composed primarily of cartilage.

6. What distinguishes a floating rib from a false rib?

   A. A floating rib is found only at the T1, T10, and T11 levels.

   B. A floating rib does not possess a head.

   C. A floating rib has no costal groove.

   D. A floating rib does not possess costicartilage.

7. The fifth rib is an example of a _____ (true rib or false rib).

8. Which part of the sternum do the second ribs articulate?

   A. Midbody   C. Middle manubrium

   B. Upper manubrium   D. Sternal angle

9. Which of the following structures is (are) found in the costal groove of each rib?

A. Nerve   C. Vein

B. Artery   D. All of the above

10. Match each of the following joints with the correct type of movement.

_____ 1. Sternoclavicular   A. Plane (gliding)—diarthrodial

_____ 2. Costovertebral joint   B. Immovable—synarthrodial

_____ 3. First sternocostal joint

_____ 4. Eighth interchondral joint

_____ 5. Third costochondral union

11. Identify the structures labeled on the following radiographs of the sternum (Figs. 10-5 and 10-6).

Fig. 10-5

A. _____

B. _____ (joint)

C. _____

D. _____

E. _____

F. _____

G. _____

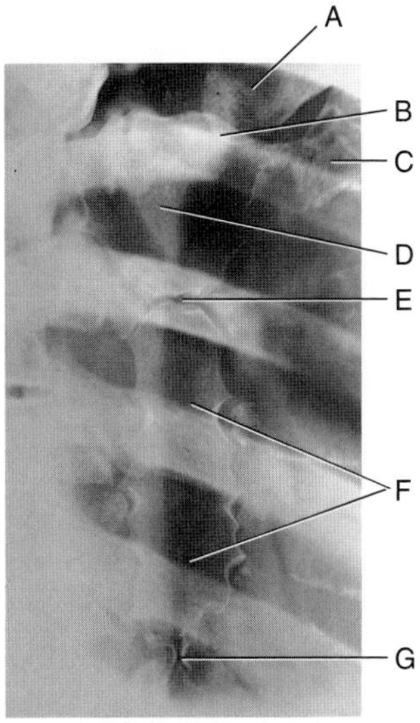

Fig. 10-5. The sternum, A-G.

Fig. 10-6

H. _____

I. _____

J. _____

K. _____

L. _____

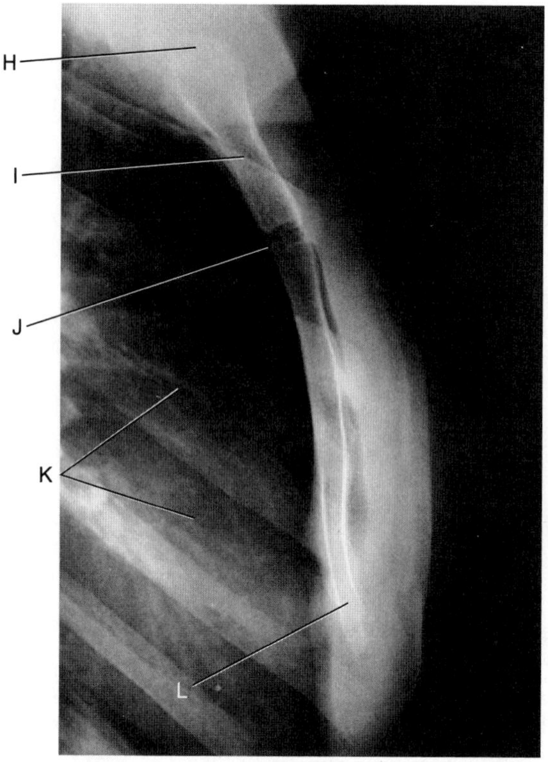

Fig. 10-6. The sternum, H-L.

12. List the correct positioning considerations for a study of the ribs above the diaphragm.

    A. Breathing instructions: _____

    B. kV range: _____

    C. General body position: _____

13. What is the minimum SID for radiography of the sternum? (Note: This is a radiation safety concern.)

_____

14. Which one of the following breathing instructions should be employed for an RAO position of the sternum to maximize visibility of it?

    A. Suspended inspiration   C. Suspended expiration

    B. Orthostatic-breathing technique   D. Valsalva maneuver

15. List the two factors to be considered when determining which specific projections to include in the rib routine.

    A. _____

    B. _____

16. List three chest pathologic conditions that may result from a rib injury and may require a PA and lateral chest projections be included with the rib routine.

    A. _____

    B. _____

    C. _____

17. A. What is the range of body rotation for an RAO position of the sternum?

    _____

    B. Does an asthenic patient require a little more or a little less obliquity than a hypersthenic patient?

    _____

18. For which of the following conditions of the bony thorax are nuclear medicine bone scans not normally performed?

    A. Possible fractures   C. History of multiple myeloma

    B. Osteoporosis   D. Osteomyelitis

19. Pathology of the sternum is most commonly caused by:

    A. Metastases   C. Infection

    B. Osteoporosis   D. Blunt trauma

20. The most common cause of osteomyelitis is _____.

21. What other position can be used for the sternum if the patient cannot assume the recumbent RAO position?

    A. LAO   C. LPO

    B. RPO   D. Left lateral decubitus

22. How should the arms be positioned for an erect lateral projection of the sternum?

    A. Raised over the head   C. Depressed by holding 5 to 10 lb in each hand

    B. Drawn back   D. Extended in front of the thorax

23. Which radiographic sign can be evaluated to determine whether rotation is present on a PA projection of the

    sternoclavicular joints? _____

24. How much rotation of the thorax is required for the anterior oblique projection of the sternoclavicular joints?

    _____

25. Where is the central ray centered for an AP projection of the ribs below the diaphragm?

    _____

26. What range of kV for analog imaging should be used for ribs above the diaphragm?

    A. 55 to 65 kV   C. 80 to 90 kV

    B. 65 to 70 kV   D. 90 to 100 kV

27. Which one of the following positions or projections will best demonstrate the right axillary ribs?

    A. LAO   C. RAO

    B. LPO   D. PA

28. A radiograph of an RAO projection of the sternum reveals that the width of the sternum is foreshortened and the sternum is shifted away from the spine and out of the heart shadow. The patient has a large "barrel" chest. The technologist performed the RAO with 20° to 25° of rotation and used a breathing technique. Which positioning error led to this radiographic outcome?

_____

29. A radiograph of a lateral sternum reveals that anterior ribs are superimposed over the sternum. Which specific

positioning error led to this radiographic outcome? _____

30. **Situation:** A patient with an injury to the right lower posterior ribs comes to the emergency room. She is unable to stand. List the positioning routine that would be performed for this patient. Include breathing instructions.

    A. Positions performed: _____

    B. Breathing instructions: _____

31. **Situation:** A patient with an injury to the left upper anterior ribs comes to the ER. He is unable to stand but can lie on his abdomen. List the positioning routine that would be used for this patient. Include breathing instructions.

    A. Positions performed: _____

    B. Breathing instructions: _____

32. **Situation:** A routine chest study reveals a possible lesion near the right sternoclavicular joint. A PA projection of the sternoclavicular joints is taken, but the area of interest is superimposed over the spine. What specific position

can be used to better demonstrate this region? _____

33. **Situation:** A patient is brought into the ER with multiple injuries because of an MVA. The patient can move but cannot stand or lie prone because of his injuries. A sternum study is ordered. What positions should be performed

for this patient? _____

34. **Situation:** A patient comes to the ER with multiple rib fractures. The ER physician suspects a flail chest. The patient is able to stand and move. Beyond a rib series, what projections should be taken for this patient?

_____

35. True/False: The automatic exposure control (AEC) system is recommended for the RAO sternum projection if the center chamber is used.

36. True/False: An orthostatic-breathing technique is recommended for studies of the sternoclavicular joints.

37. **Situation:** A patient comes to the ER with a right, upper, anterior rib injury. A unilateral rib study is ordered. What are the basic projections taken for this patient?

_____

240

38. **Situation:** A patient comes to the ER with a left lower posterior rib injury. A unilateral rib study is ordered. The patient is unable to stand because of multiple injuries. What are the basic projections taken for this patient?

_____

39. **Situation:** A patient comes to radiology with a clinical history of pectus excavatum. What positioning routine would best demonstrate the condition?

_____

40. **Situation:** A patient comes to radiology with widespread metastases involving the bony thorax. Beyond radiographic studies, what other imaging modality demonstrates the extent of this condition?

_____

11 Skull and Cranial Bones

CHAPTER OBJECTIVES
Cranium

After you have successfully completed the activities in this chapter, you will be able to:

_____ 1. List the eight cranial bones and describe their features, related structures, location, and function.

_____ 2. Using drawings and/or radiographs, identify specific structures of the eight cranial bones.

_____ 3. Define specific terminology, reference points, positioning lines, and topographic landmarks of the cranium.

_____ 4. Identify specific radiographic and topographic landmarks of the cranium.

_____ 5. List the location, joint classification, and related terminology for the sutures and joints of the cranium.

_____ 6. List the differences among the three shape and size (morphology) classifications of the skull and their implications for radiography of the cranium.

_____ 7. Identify alternative imaging modalities that best demonstrate specific conditions or disease processes of the cranium and brain.

_____ 8. Match specific clinical indications of the cranium to the correct definition or statements.

_____ 9. List the three main portions of the temporal bones.

_____ 10. Identify specific structures of the external, middle, and internal ear.

_____ 11. Using drawings, identify the three divisions of the ear and the structures found in each division.

_____ 12. List the specific features, characteristics, location, and functions of the 14 facial bones.

_____ 13. List the seven cranial and facial bones that make up the bony orbit.

_____ 14. Using drawings and/or radiographs, identify specific structures of the facial bone region.

_____ 15. Match specific clinical indications of the temporal bone to the correct definition.

_____ 16. Using radiographs, identify specific structures of the temporal bone.

_____ 17. List the location, function, and characteristics of the four groups of paranasal sinuses.

_____ 18. Using drawings and radiographs, identify specific paranasal sinuses.

_____ 19. Match specific clinical indications of the paranasal sinuses to the correct definition.

_____ 20. Identify the correct size and type of image receptor and central ray location, direction, and angle for routine and special projections of the cranium.

_____ 21. Identify which structures are best seen with specific projections of the cranium.

_____ 22. Given various hypothetic situations, identify the correct modification of a position and/or exposure factors to improve the radiographic image.

Facial Bones and Paranasal Sinuses

After you have successfully completed the activities in this chapter, you will be able to:

_____ 1. Explain the technical and positioning considerations for facial bone routines.

_____ 2. Identify alternative imaging modalities that best demonstrate specific facial bone and paranasal sinus pathology.

_____ 3. Identify specific types of fractures of the facial bone region.

_____ 4. Identify routine and special projections of the facial bones and list the correct size of the image receptor, as well as the location, direction, and angulation of the central ray for each projection.

_____ 5. List which structures are best seen with basic and special projections of the facial bones.

_____ 6. List technical and positioning considerations when performing a mandible study using the orthopanto-mography (panoramic tomography) imaging system.

_____ 7. Identify routine and special projections of the paranasal sinuses and list the correct size and type of image receptor, as well as the location, direction, and angulation of the central ray for each position.

_____ 8. Given various hypothetic situations, identify the correct modification of a position and/or exposure factors to improve the radiographic image.

_____ 9. Given radiographs of specific facial and paranasal sinus projections/positions, identify specific errors in positioning and exposure factors.

POSITIONING AND RADIOGRAPHIC CRITIQUE

_____ 1. Using a peer, position for routine and special projections of the cranium, facial bones, and sinuses.

_____ 2. Using a cranial radiographic phantom, produce satisfactory radiographs of specific positions (if equipment is available).

_____ 3. Critique and evaluate cranial radiographs based on the five divisions of radiographic criteria: (1) anatomy demonstrated, (2) position, (3) collimation and central ray, (4) exposure, and (5) anatomic side markers.

_____ 4. Distinguish between acceptable and unacceptable cranial radiographs based on exposure factors, motion, collimation, positioning, or other errors.

LEARNING EXERCISES

Complete the following review exercises after reading the associated pages in the textbook as indicated by each exercise. Answers to each review exercise are given at the end of the review exercises.

PART I: RADIOGRAPHIC ANATOMY

REVIEW EXERCISE A: Radiographic Anatomy of the Cranium (see textbook pp. 375-382)

1. Fill in the total number of bones.

   A. Cranium ________________ B. Facial bones ________________

2. List the four cranial bones that form the calvaria (skull cap).

   A. ________________ C. ________________

   B. ________________ D. ________________

3. List the four cranial bones that form the floor of the cranium.

   A. ________________ C. ________________

   B. ________________ D. ________________

4. Identify the cranial bones labeled on Figs. 11-1 and 11-2. (Note: All eight cranial bones, including each paired bone, are visible in at least one of the following drawings.)

   A. ________________

   B. ________________

   C. ________________

   D. ________________

   E. ________________

   F. ________________

   G. ________________

   H. ________________

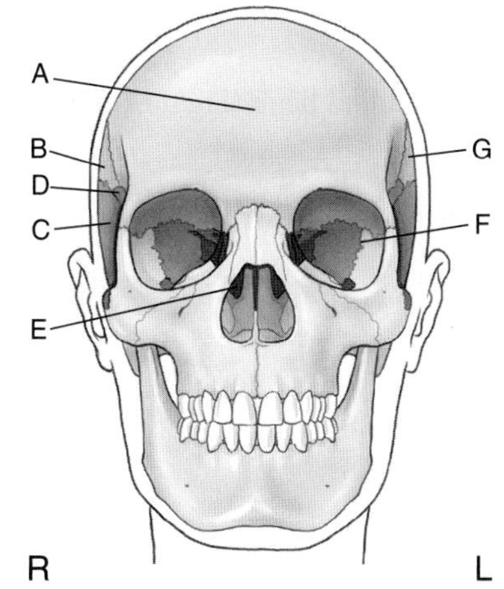

Fig. 11-1. Frontal view.

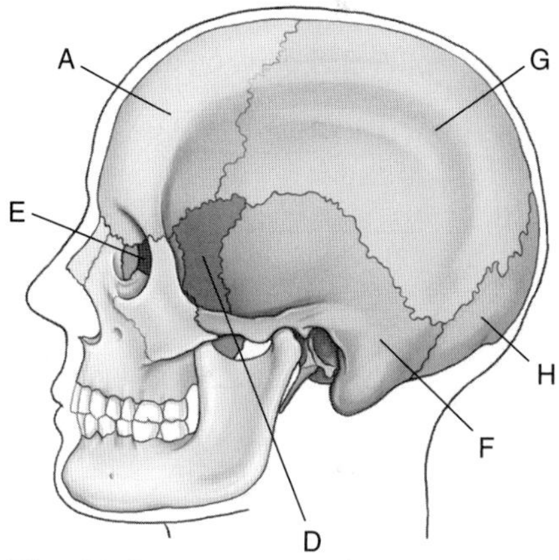

Fig. 11-2. Lateral view.

5. Identify all eight cranial bones on the two superior-view drawings (Figs. 11-3 and 11-4).

A. _____

B. _____

C. _____

D. _____

E. _____

F. _____

G. _____

H. _____

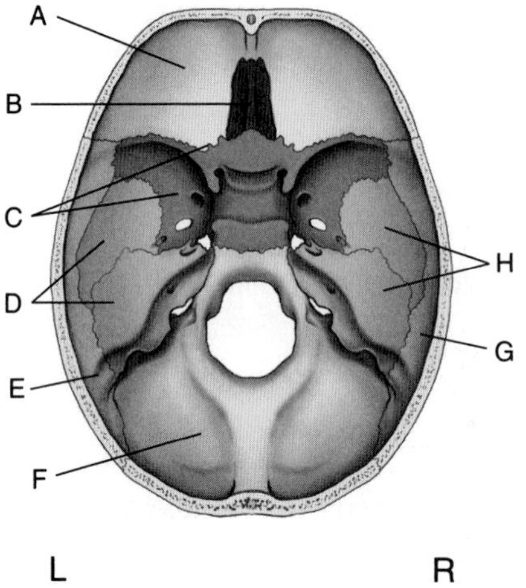

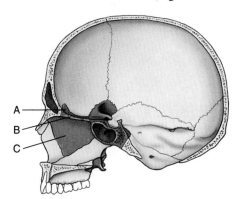

Fig. 11-3. Superior, cut-away view.

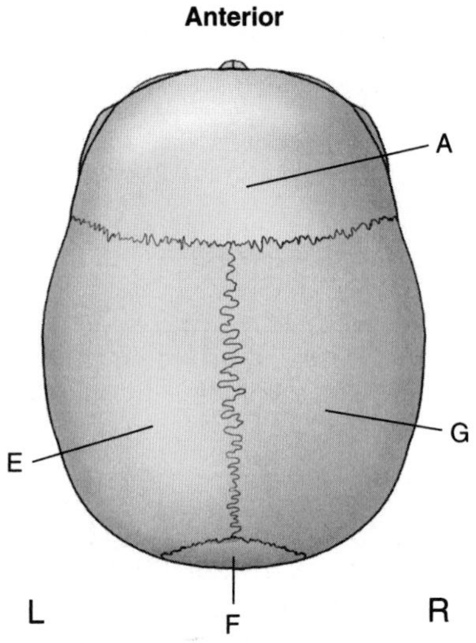

Fig. 11-4. Superior view.

Identify the labeled parts on the three views of the ethmoid bone (Figs. 11-5 and 11-6).

A. _____

B. _____

C. _____

D. _____

E. _____

Fig. 11-5. Medial sectional view.

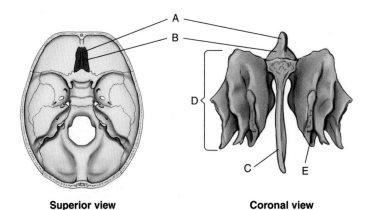

Superior view

Coronal view

Fig. 11-6. Superior (left) and coronal sectional (right) views.

6. The small horizontal plate of the ethmoid seen in the preceding drawings is called the

   _____.

7. The vertical plate of the ethmoid bone forming the upper portion of the bony nasal septum is the

   _____.

8. Identify the labeled parts on the four views of the sphenoid in Figs. 11-7 through 11-10. (Note: Most of the parts are identified on more than one drawing.)

A. _____

B. _____

C. _____

D. _____

E. _____

F. _____

G. _____

Foramina (H-L)

H. _____

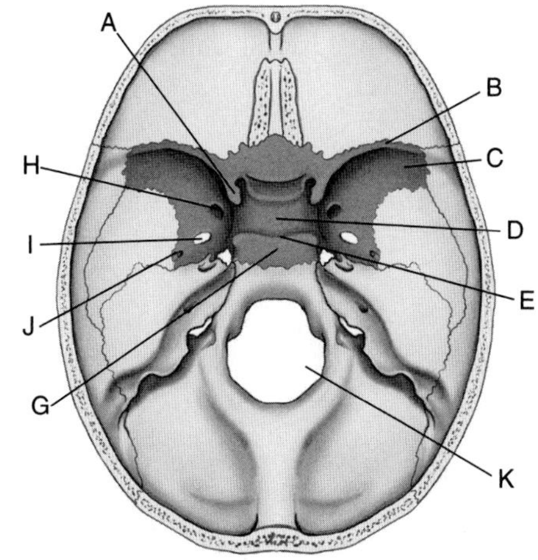

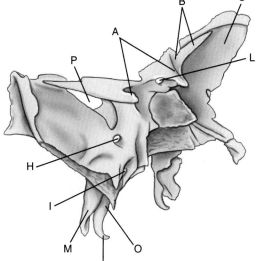

Fig. 11-7. Sphenoid, superior view.

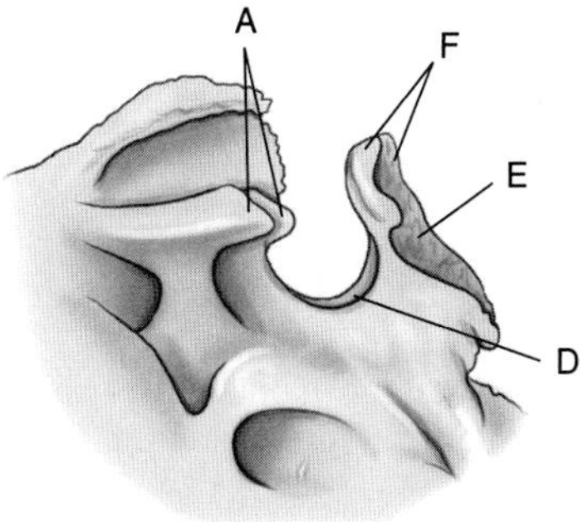

I. _____

J. _____

K. _____

L. _____

M. _____

N. _____

O. _____

P. _____

Q. _____

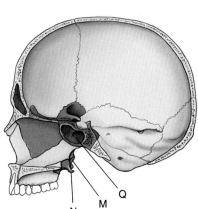

Fig. 11-8. Sphenoid, lateral view.

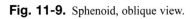

Fig. 11-9. Sphenoid, oblique view.

Fig. 11-10. Sphenoid, medial sectional view.

9. A structure found in the middle of the sphenoid bone that surrounds the pituitary gland is the

    _____.

10. The posterior aspect of the sella turcica is called the _____.

11. Which structure of the sphenoid bone allows for the passage of the optic nerve and is the actual opening into the

    orbit? _____.

12. Which structures of the sphenoid bone help form part of the lateral walls of the nasal cavities?

    _____

13. Which radiographic projection best demonstrates the sella turcica and dorsum sellae?

    _____

14. Which aspect of the frontal bone forms the superior aspect of the orbit? _____

15. Identify the four major sutures and the six associated asterions and fontanels labeled on these drawings of an adult
    cranium and an infant cranium (Figs. 11-11 to 11-14).

Sutures

    A. _____

    B. _____

    C. _____

    D. _____

Asterions

    E. _____

    F. _____

    G. Right and left _____

    H. Right and left _____

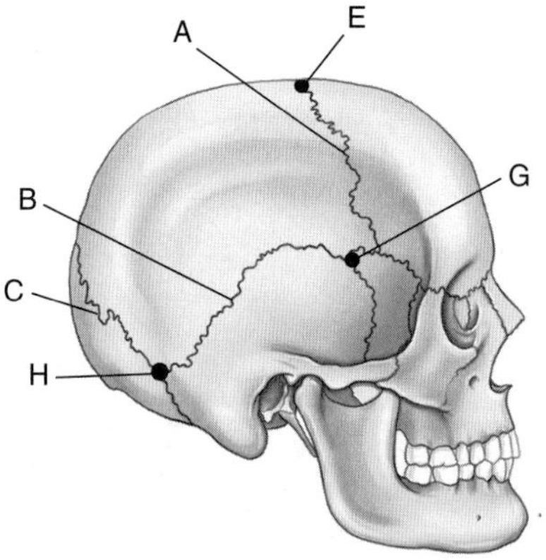

Fig. 11-11. Adult cranium, lateral view.

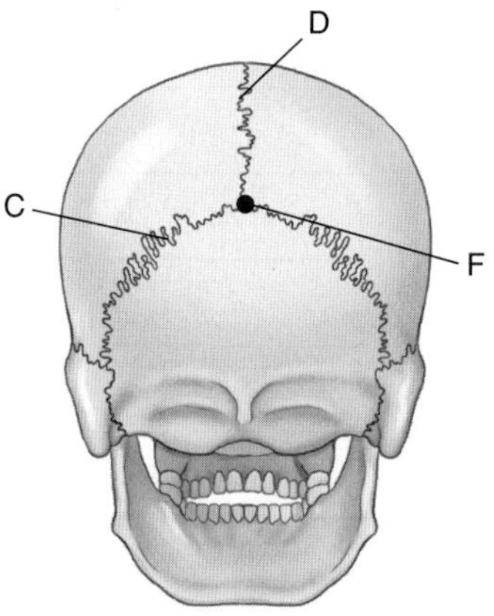

Posterior view
Fig. 11-12. Posterior view.

Fontanels: associated adult asterion

    I. _____ (_____)

    J. _____ (_____)

    K. Right and left _____ (_____)

    L. Right and left _____ (_____)

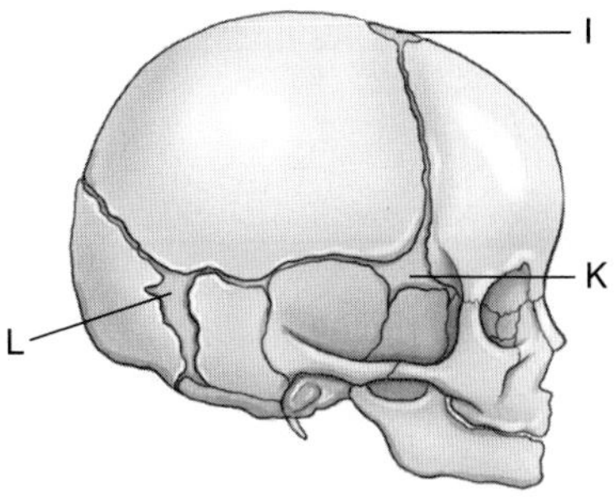

16. Cranial sutures are classified as being

    _____ joints.

Fig. 11-13. Infant cranium, lateral view.

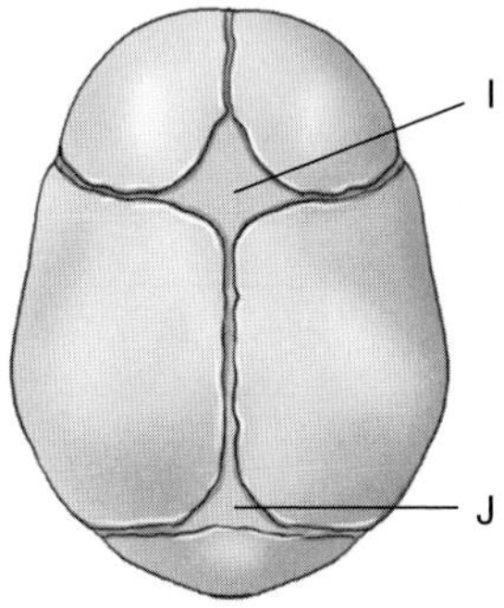

17. Small, irregular bones that sometimes develop in adult skull sutures are

    called _____ or

    _____ bones and are most frequently found in

    the _____ suture.

18. Which term describes the superior rim of the orbit? (Include the abbreviation

    also.) _____

Fig. 11-14. Infant cranium, superior view.

19. What is the name of the notch that separates the orbital plates from each

    other? _____

20. Which cranial bones form the upper lateral walls of the calvarium? _____

21. Which cranial bone contains the foramen magnum? _____

22. A small prominence located on the squamous portion of the occipital bone is called the

    _____.

23. What is the name of the oval processes found on the occipital bone that helps form the **occipitoatlantal** joint?

    _____

24. List the three aspects of the temporal bones.

    A. _____   B. _____   C. _____

25. True/False: The mastoid portion of the temporal bone is the densest of the three aspects of the temporal bone.

26. Which external landmark corresponds with the level of the petrous ridge? _____

27. Which opening in the temporal bone serves as a passageway for nerves of hearing and equilibrium?

    _____

28. Identify the following cranial structures labeled on Figs. 11-15 and 11-16.

Fig. 11-15

    A. _____

    B. _____

    C. _____ (suture)

    D. _____ (suture)

    E. _____

Fig. 11-16

    A. _____

    B. _____

    C. _____

    D. _____ (suture)

    E. _____

    F. _____

    G. _____

    H. _____

    I. _____

    J. _____ (suture)

    K. _____

    L. _____

    M. _____

    N. _____

    O. _____

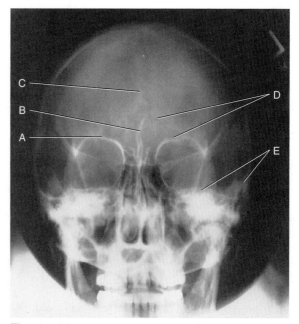

Fig. 11-15. Cranial structures, PA axial (Caldwell) projection.

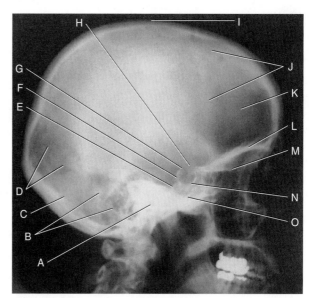

Fig. 11-16. Cranial structures, lateral projection.

REVIEW EXERCISE B: Specific Anatomy and Pathology of the Temporal Bone (see textbook pp. 383-386)

1. List the three aspects of the temporal bone.

   A. _____   B. _____   C. _____

2. Which aspect of the temporal bone is considered the densest? _____

3. Which structure makes up the cartilaginous external ear? _____

4. How long is the average external acoustic meatus (EAM)? _____

5. Which small membrane marks the beginning of the middle ear? _____

6. What is the collective term for the small bones of the middle ear? _____

7. Which structure allows for communication between the nasopharynx and middle ear?

   _____

8. What is the major function of the structure described in question 7? _____

9. Which structure serves as an opening between the mastoid portion of the temporal bone and the middle ear?

   _____

10. What is the name of the thin plate of bone that separates the mastoid air cells from the brain?

    _____

11. Which one of the auditory ossicles picks up sound vibrations from the tympanic membrane?

    _____

12. Which one of the auditory ossicles is considered to be the smallest? _____

13. Which one of the auditory ossicles resembles a premolar tooth? _____

14. What is the name of the small membrane that connects the middle to the inner ear?

    _____

15. Which two sensory functions occur within the inner ear?

    A. _____   B. _____

16. What is the name of the small membrane that will move outward to transmit impulses to the auditory nerve, thus

    creating the sense of hearing? _____

17. True/False: The cochlea is a closed system relating to the sense of hearing.

18. Identify the structures labeled on Fig. 11-17.

A. _____

B. _____

C. _____

D. _____

E. _____

F. _____

G. _____

H. _____

I. _____

J. _____

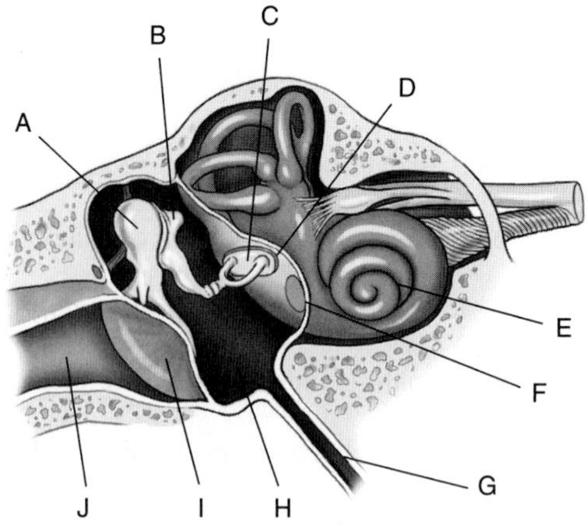

Fig. 11-17. Structures of the middle and internal ear.

19. Match each of the following clinical indications for the temporal bone to the correct definition or description. (Use each choice only once. Pathology of temporal bone found on p. 402.)

_____ A. Neoplasia   1. Bacterial infection of the mastoid process

_____ B. Otosclerosis   2. Growth arising from a mucous membrane

_____ C. Mastoiditis   3. Hereditary disease involving excessive bone formation of middle and inner ear

_____ D. Acoustic neuroma 4. Benign, cystlike mass or tumor of the middle ear

_____ E. Polyp   5. New and abnormal growth

_____ F. Cholesteatoma   6. Benign tumor of the auditory nerve sheath

20. Which one of the following radiographic appearances pertains to an acoustic neuroma?

A. Expansion of the internal acoustic canal   C. Increased density in the sinus

B. Bone destruction within the middle ear   D. Sinus mucosal thickening

21. Which one of the following imaging modalities best demonstrates otosclerosis?

A. Nuclear medicine   C. Conventional radiography

B. CT   D. Sonography

1. Which of the following bones is not a facial bone?

   A. Middle nasal conchae   C. Lacrimal bone

   B. Vomer   D. Mandible

2. What is the largest immovable bone of the face? _____

3. List the four processes of the maxilla.

   A. _____   C. _____

   B. _____   D. _____

4. Which one of the mentioned processes is considered most superior? _____

5. Which soft tissue landmark is found at the base of the anterior nasal spine? _____

6. Which facial bones form the posterior aspect of the hard palate? _____

7. Which two cranial bones articulate with the maxilla? _____

8. Which facial bones are sometimes called the "cheek bones"? _____

9. Which of the following bones does not articulate with the zygomatic bone?

   A. Temporal   C. Frontal

   B. Maxilla   D. Sphenoid

10. Which facial bone is associated with the tear ducts? _____

11. The purpose of the _____, or _____, is to divide the nasal cavity into compartments and circulate air coming into the nasal cavities. (Include both terms for these bones.)

12. True/False: The majority of the nose is formed by the right and left nasal bones.

13. A deviated nasal septum is most likely to occur at the junction between _____ and

    _____.

14. Match each of the following mandibular terms to the correct definition or description. (Use each choice only once.)

    A. Gonion   1. Vertical portion of mandible

    B. Mandibular notch   2. The chin

    C. Body   3. Mandibular angle

    D. Condyloid process   4. The point of union between both halves of the mandible

    E. Coronoid process   5. Bony process located anterior to mandibular notch

    F. Ramus   6. Horizontal portion of mandible

    G. Mentum   7. Posterior process of upper ramus

    H. Symphysis menti   8. U-shaped notch

Identify the labeled facial bones visible on Figs. 11-18 and 11-19.

Paired Bones

A. _____

B. _____

C. _____

D. _____

E. _____

Single Bone

F. _____

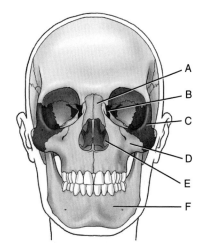

Fig. 11-18. Frontal view.

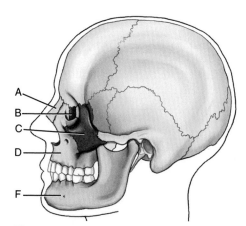

Fig. 11-19. Side view.

15. The one single facial bone and the one pair of facial bones not visible from the exterior and not demonstrated on

Figs. 11-18 and 11-19 are the _____ and _____, respectively. (These are demonstrated on special view drawings in the following questions.)

Identify the labeled structures (and the facial bones of which they are a part) on this inferior surface view of the maxillae (Fig. 11-20).

Structure   **Bone(s)**

A. _____   (_____)

B. _____   (_____)

C. _____   (_____)

D. _____   (_____)

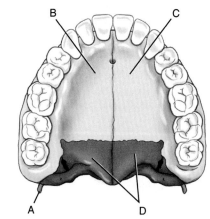

Fig. 11-20. Inferior surface view of the maxillae.

List the three structures that form the nasal septum as shown on Fig. 11-21.

A. _____

B. _____

C. _____

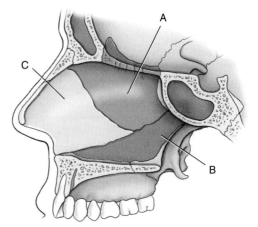

Fig. 11-21. Nasal septum.

Identify the parts of the mandible and skull as labeled on Figs. 11-22 and 11-23.

A. _____

B. _____

C. _____

D. _____

E. _____

F. _____

G. _____

H. _____

I. _____

J. _____

K. (Cranial bone) _____

L. (Joint) _____

M. (Key landmark) _____

N. (Landmark) _____

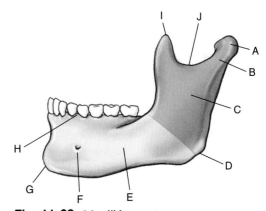

Fig. 11-22. Mandible.

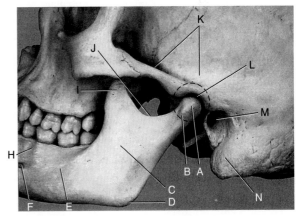

Fig. 11-23. Lateral skull and mandible.

16. Identify the seven bones that form the orbit and indicate whether they are cranial or facial bones (Fig. 11-24). (See pp. 396-397.)

Bone   **Cranial or Facial?**

A. _____   (_____)

B. _____   (_____)

C. _____   (_____)

D. _____   (_____)

E. _____   (_____)

F. _____   (_____)

G. _____   (_____)

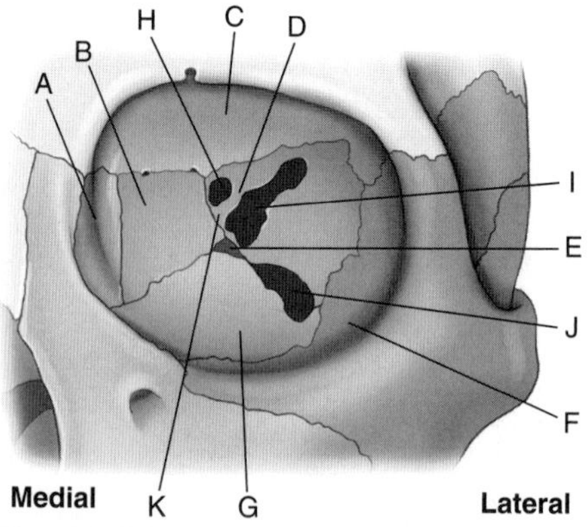

Fig. 11-24. Slightly oblique frontal view of orbit, A-K.

17. Identify the three foramina found within the orbits as labeled on Fig. 11-24.

H. _____

I. _____

J. _____

Small section of bone:

K. _____

18. From anterior to posterior, the cone-shaped orbits project upward at an angle of _____ °

and toward the midsagittal plane at an angle of _____ °.

19. Which facial bone opening has the maxillary branch of the fifth cranial nerve passing through it?

_____

20. Which one of the facial bone openings is formed by a cleft between the greater and lesser wings of the sphenoid bone?

A. Superior orbital fissure   C. Inferior orbital fissure

B. Optic foramen   D. Optic canal

21. What is another term for the second cranial nerve?

A. Olfactory nerve   C. Maxillary nerve

B. Optic nerve   D. Trigeminal nerve

REVIEW EXERCISE D: Radiographic Anatomy of the Paranasal Sinuses (see textbook pp. 393-395)

1. What is the older term for the maxillary sinuses? _____

2. An infection of the teeth may travel upward and involve the _____ sinus.

3. Specifically, where are the frontal sinuses located? _____

4. The frontal sinuses rarely become aerated before the age of _____.

5. Which specific aspect of the ethmoid bone contains the ethmoid sinuses? _____

6. The drainage pathway for the paranasal sinuses is called the:

   A. Uncinate process   C. Paranasal meatus

   B. Ostiomeatal complex   D. Lateral masses

7. Which sinus is projected through the open mouth with a PA axial transoral projection?

   _____

Identify the sinuses, structures, or bones labeled on Fig. 11-25.

A. _____

B. _____

C. _____

D. _____

E. _____

F. _____

G. _____

H. _____

I. _____

J. _____

K. _____

L. _____

M. _____

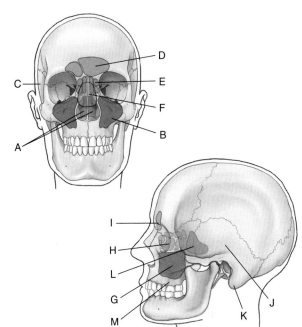

Fig. 11-25. Frontal and lateral views.

8. Identify the following paranasal sinuses labeled on Figs. 11-26 and 11-27.

Fig. 11-26

A. _____

B. _____

C. _____

D. _____

Fig. 11-27

E. _____

F. _____

G. _____

H. _____

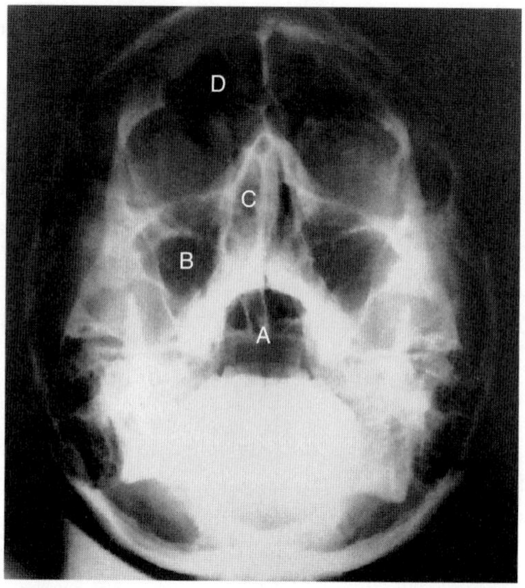

Fig. 11-26. Paranasal sinuses. PA axial transoral projection.

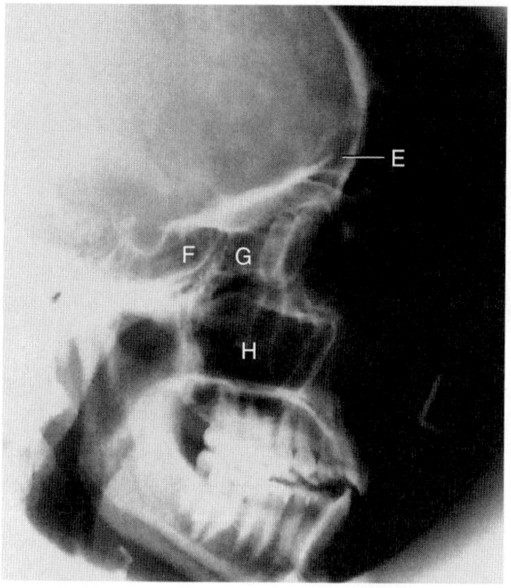

9. What is the name of the passageway between the maxillary sinuses and the middle nasal meatus?

_____

10. True/False: Most CT studies of the sinuses do not require the use of contrast media.

11. Which position is most often used when performing a CT study of the sinuses?

A. Supine   C. Erect

B. Prone   D. Supine with 20° oblique of skull from AP position

Fig. 11-27. Paranasal sinuses. Lateral projection.

PART II: RADIOGRAPHIC POSITIONING OF CRANIUM
REVIEW EXERCISE A: Skull Morphology, Topography, Pathology, and Positioning of the Cranium (see textbook pp. 403-407 and 410-416)

1. List the three classifications of the skull; then match them with the correct shape description listed on the right.

Classification	*Shape Description*
A. _____	a. Width less than 75% of length
B. _____	b. Width 80% or more than length
C. _____	c. Width between 75% and 80% of length

2. Central ray angles and degree of rotation stated for basic skull positions are based on the

_____ (average) skull, which has an approximate angle of

_____ between the midsagittal plane and the long axis of the petrous bone.

3. The long, narrow-shaped skull has an angle of approximately _____° between the midsagittal plane and the long axis of the petrous bone.

4. True/False: Two older terms for the orbitomeatal line (OML) are Reid's base line and the anthropologic base line.

5. There is a _____° difference between the orbitomeatal and infraorbitomeatal lines,

and _____° between the orbitomeatal and glabellomeatal lines.

6. Match each of the following cranial landmarks and positioning lines with the correct definition. (Use each choice only once.)

_____ 1. Lateral junction of the eyelid

_____ 2. Posterior angle of the jaw

_____ 3. A line between the infraorbital margin and EAM

_____ 4. Corresponds to the highest "nuchal" line of the occipital bone

_____ 5. A line between the glabella and alveolar process of the maxilla

_____ 6. A line between the mental point and EAM

_____ 7. Located at the junction of the two nasal bones and the frontal bone

_____ 8. The small cartilaginous flap covering the ear opening

_____ 9. Corresponds to the highest level of the facial bone mass

_____ 10. A line between the midlateral orbital margin and the EAM

_____ 11. The center point of the EAM

_____ 12. A positioning line that is primarily used for the modified Waters projection

_____ 13. A line used in positioning to ensure that the skull is in a true lateral position

_____ 14. Corresponds to the level of the petrous ridge

_____ 15. A smooth, slightly depressed area between the eyebrows

A. TEA

B. Supraorbital groove

C. Interpupillary line

D. Nasion

E. Gonion

F. Tragus

G. Outer canthus

H. Glabelloalveolar line

I. OML

J. Infraorbitomeatal line (IOML)

K. Mentomeatal line

L. Lips-meatal line

M. Glabella

N. Inion

O. Auricular point

7. What is the average kV range for analog skull radiography? kV range for digital imaging?

_____

8. List the five most common errors made during skull radiography.

A. _____   C. _____   E. _____

B. _____   D. _____

9. Of the five causes listed in the previous question, which two are the most common?

A. _____   B. _____

10. Bilateral horizontal fractures of the maxillae describes a _____ fracture.

A. LeFort   C. Tripod

B. Blowout   D. Contrecoup

11. Which one of the following imaging modalities is the most common neuroimaging procedure performed for the cranium?

A. Computed tomography (CT)   C. Magnetic resonance imaging (MRI)

B. Ultrasound   D. Nuclear medicine

12. Which of the following imaging modalities is commonly performed on neonates with a possible intracranial hemorrhage?

A. CT   C. MRI

B. Ultrasound   D. Nuclear medicine

13. Which of the following imaging modalities is most commonly performed to evaluate patients for Alzheimer's disease?

A. CT   C. MRI

B. Ultrasound   D. Nuclear medicine

14. Match each of the following clinical indications to the correct definition or statement. (Use each choice only once.)

A. Fracture that may produce an air-fluid level in the sphenoid sinus   1. Osteoblastic neoplasm

B. Destructive lesion with irregular margins   2. Pituitary adenoma

C. Also called a "ping-pong" fracture   3. Basal skull fracture

D. Proliferative bony lesion of increased density   4. Paget's disease

E. A tumor that may produce erosion of the sella turcica   5. Osteolytic neoplasm

F. Also known as osteitis deformans   6. Depressed skull fracture

G. A bone tumor that originates in the bone marrow   7. Multiple myeloma

15. Which one of the following clinical indications may require an increase in manual exposure factors?

A. Advanced Paget's disease   C. Multiple myeloma

B. Metastatic neoplasm   D. Basal skull fracture

16. Which cranial bone is best demonstrated with an AP axial (Towne method) projection of the skull?

_____

17. When using a 30° caudad angle for the AP axial (Towne method) projection of the skull, which positioning line should be perpendicular to the image receptor?

    A. OML   C. GAL

    B. IOML   D. AML

18. A properly positioned AP axial (Towne method) projection should place the dorsum sellae into the middle aspect of the:

    A. Orbits   C. Foramen magnum

    B. Clivus   D. Anterior arch of C1

19. A lack of symmetry of the petrous ridges indicates which of the following problems with a radiograph of an AP axial projection?

    A. Tilt   C. Flexion or extension

    B. Central ray angle   D. Rotation

20. If the patient cannot flex the head adequately for the AP axial (Towne method) projection, the technologist could

    place the _____ perpendicular to the image receptor and angle the central ray

    _____° caudad.

21. What evidence on an AP axial (Towne method) radiograph indicates whether the correct central ray angle and

    correct head flexion were used? _____

22. What central ray angle should be used for the PA axial (Haas method) projection for the cranium?

    _____

23. Where is the central ray centered for a lateral projection of the skull? _____

24. Which specific positioning error is present if the mandibular rami are not superimposed on a lateral skull radiograph?

    A. Tilt   C. Overflexion of head and neck

    B. Rotation   D. Incorrect central ray angle

25. Where will the petrous ridges be projected with a 15° PA axial (Caldwell) projection of the cranium?

    _____

26. Which specific positioning error is present if the petrous ridges are projected higher in the orbits than expected for

    a 15° PA axial projection? _____

27. Which projection of the cranium produces an image of the frontal bone with little or no distortion?

    _____

28. With a possible trauma patient, what must be determined before performing the SMV projection of the skull?

    _____

29. What positioning error has been committed if the EAMs are not superimposed with one of them more superior than the other on a lateral projection of the cranium? _____

30. Which skull positioning line is placed parallel to the plane of the IR for the SMV projection?
    A. OML   C. AML
    B. IOML   D. GML

31. Which one of the following projections best demonstrates the sella turcica in profile?
    A. AP axial   C. 15° PA axial
    B. SMV   D. Lateral

32. Which one of the following projections best demonstrates the foramen rotundum?
    A. SMV   C. 25° to 30° PA axial
    B. 25° to 30° AP axial   D. Lateral

33. Which one of the following projections best demonstrates the clivus in profile?
    A. AP axial   C. Lateral
    B. 15° PA   D. SMV

34. Where does the CR exit for a PA axial (Haas method) projection of the skull?
    A. 1½ inches (4 cm) superior to the nasion
    B. ¾ inch (2 cm) anterior to EAM
    C. 2½ inches (6.5 cm) above the glabella
    D. Level of nasion

35. Which imaging modality is best to differentiate between an epidural and subdural hemorrhage?
    A. CT
    B. MRI
    C. Nuclear medicine
    D. PET

REVIEW EXERCISE B: Problem Solving for Technical and Positioning Errors of the Cranium

1. A radiograph of an AP axial (Towne method) projection of the cranium reveals that the right petrous ridge is wider than the left side. Which specific positioning error is present on this radiograph?

   _____

2. A radiograph of a 15° PA axial (Caldwell) projection of the cranium demonstrates that the petrous ridges are projected at the inferior orbital margin. Which positioning error(s) led to this radiographic outcome?

   _____

3. A radiograph of a 15° PA axial (Caldwell) projection demonstrates that the distance between the right midlateral orbital borders and lateral margin of the skull cortex is greater than the left side. Which positioning error led to this radiographic outcome?

   _____

4. A radiograph of an SMV projection of the skull reveals that the mandibular condyles are within the petrous bone. Which specific positioning error led to this problem?

_____

5. A radiograph of a lateral projection of the skull reveals that the orbital plates are not superimposed. (One orbital plate is slightly superior to the other.) Which specific positioning error led to this radiographic outcome?

_____

6. A lateral skull radiograph demonstrates one mandibular ramus about 0.5 cm more anterior than the other. Which positioning error occurred?

_____

7. An AP axial (Towne method) radiograph for cranium demonstrates the dorsum sellae projected above or superior to, the foramen magnum. The foramen magnum is distorted. Which positioning error(s) occurred?

_____

8. **Situation:** A patient comes to the radiology department with a possible tumor of the pituitary gland. Which radiographic projection of the cranium best demonstrates any bony involvement of the sella turcica?

_____

9. **Situation:** A patient with a possible linear fracture of the right parietal bone enters the emergency room. Which single radiographic projection of the skull best demonstrates this fracture?

_____

10. **Situation:** A patient comes to the radiology department for a skull series, but the patient cannot assume the correct position for either version of the AP axial (Towne method) projection because of a very short neck and severe spinal kyphosis. What can the technologist do to demonstrate the occipital bone?

_____

11. **Situation:** A patient with a possible basal skull fracture enters the emergency room. No CT scanner is available. Which specific position may provide radiographic evidence of this fracture?

_____

12. **Situation:** A neonate has a clinical history of craniosynostosis. Because of the age of the patient, the physician does not order a radiographic procedure of the cranium. What other imaging modality can be performed to evaluate the patient for this condition?

_____

13. **Situation:** A patient with a clinical history of acoustic neuroma comes to the radiology department. Which imaging modality(-ies) can be performed for this type of pathology?

_____

14. A radiograph of an AP axial (Towne method) projection for cranium reveals that the posterior arch of C1 is projected within the foramen magnum. The dorsum sellae is superimposed on the posterior arch as well. What is the positioning error(s)?

_____

15. A radiograph of an AP axial (Towne method) projection for cranium reveals that the mid to lower mandible is cut off and not demonstrated. What should the technologist do?

_____

PART III: RADIOGRAPHIC POSITIONING OF FACIAL BONES, MANDIBLE, AND PARANASAL SINUSES
REVIEW EXERCISE A: Positioning of the Facial Bones (see textbook pp. 408-409 and 418-427)

1. True/False: Facial bone studies should always be performed recumbent whenever possible.

2. True/False: The common basic PA axial projection for facial bones requires a 15° caudad angle of the central ray, which projects the dense petrous ridges into the lower one-third of the orbits.

3. True/False: An increase in kV of 25% to 30% (using manual techniques) is often required for the geriatric patient with advanced osteoporosis.

4. True/False: CT is ideal for facial bone studies because it allows for visualization of bony structures as well as related soft tissues of the facial bones.

5. True/False: Nuclear medicine is not helpful in diagnosing occult facial bone fractures.

6. True/False: MRI is an excellent imaging modality for the detection of small metal foreign bodies in the eye.

7. What is the name of the fracture that results from a direct blow to the orbit leading to a disruption of the inferior

   orbital margin? _____

8. A "free-floating" zygomatic bone is the frequent result of a _____ fracture.

9. What is the major disadvantage of performing a straight PA projection for facial bones, with no CR angulation or neck extension, as compared with other PA facial bone projections?

_____

10. Where is the CR centered for a lateral position for facial bones?
    A. Outer canthus   C. Zygoma
    B. Acanthion   D. Nasion

11. What is the proper method name for the parietoacanthial projection of the facial bones?

_____

12. Which facial bone structures are best seen with a parietoacanthial projection?

_____

13. What CR angle must be used to project the petrous ridges just below the orbital floor with the PA axial (Caldwell method) projection?
    A. None. CR is perpendicular.   C. 20°
    B. 30°   D. 45°

14. Which structures specifically are visualized better on the modified parietoacanthial (Waters) projection as compared with the basic Waters projection?

_____

15. Give two reasons why projections of the facial bones are performed PA rather than AP when possible.

    A. _____   B. _____

16. What are two positioning differences between the lateral projection of the cranium and the lateral projection for the facial bones?

    A. _____

    B. _____

17. The parietoacanthial (Waters) projection for the facial bones has the _____ line perpendicular to the image receptor, which places the orbitomeatal line (OML) at a _____ ° angle to the tabletop and image receptor.

18. Where does the CR exit for a parietoacanthial (Waters) projection of the facial bones?

    _____

19. Where does the CR exit for a 15° PA axial (Caldwell) projection for facial bones?

    _____

20. The modified parietoacanthial (modified Waters) projection requires that the _____ line is perpendicular to the image receptor, which places the OML at a _____° angle to the tabletop and image receptor.

21. True/False: Lateral projections for nasal bones generally are taken bilaterally for comparison.

22. True/False: The tangential projection for a unilateral zygomatic arch requires that the skull be rotated and tilted 15° *away from* the affected side.

23. True/False: Both oblique inferosuperior (tangential) projections for the zygomatic arch are generally taken for comparison.

24. For a parietoacanthial (PA Waters) projection, the petrous ridges should be projected directly below the

    _____ and projected into the lower half of the maxillary sinuses or below the

    _____ for a modified Waters projection.

25. For the superoinferior projection of the nasal bones, the image receptor is placed perpendicular to the

    _____ line. (Include the full term and abbreviation.)

26. Which specific facial bone structures (other than the mandible) are best demonstrated with the submentovertex (SMV) projection if the correct exposure factors are used (soft tissue technique)?

    _____

27. Where is the CR centered for an AP axial projection for the zygomatic arches?

    _____

28. List the proper method name and the common descriptive name for the parieto-orbital oblique projection for the optic foramen.

A. _____   B. _____

29. The three aspects of the face that should be in contact with the head unit or tabletop when beginning positioning for

the parieto-orbital oblique projection are the (A) _____, _____,

and _____. The final angle between the midsagittal plane and the IR should be

(B) _____, with the (C) _____ line perpendicular to

the IR. This places the optic foramen in the (D) _____ quadrant of the orbit.

30. Match each of the following structures to the facial bone projection that best demonstrates the structure(s). (Use each choice only once.)

_____ 1. Floor of orbits (blowout fractures)   A. Lateral (nasal bones)

_____ 2. Optic foramen   B. Parietoacanthial projection

_____ 3. View of single zygomatic arch   C. Parieto-orbital oblique projection

_____ 4. Profile image of nasal bones and nasal septum   D. Submentovertex (SMV) projection

_____ 5. Bilateral zygomatic arches   E. Modified Waters method

_____ 6. Inferior orbital rim, maxillae, nasal septum, nasal   F. Oblique inferosuperior projection
           spine, zygomatic bone and arches

REVIEW EXERCISE B: Positioning of the Mandible and Temporomandibular Joints (TMJ) (see textbook pp. 428-435)

1. True/False: The PA axial projection of the mandible produces an elongated view of the condyloid processes.

_____

2. Which projection of the mandible projects the opposite half of the mandible away from the side of interest?

_____

3. What must be done to prevent the ramus of the mandible from being superimposed over the cervical spine with an axiolateral oblique projection of the mandible?

_____

4. How much skull rotation (from the lateral skull position) toward the image receptor is required with an axiolateral oblique projection for demonstrating each of the following?

A. Body of the mandible: _____

B. Mentum region: _____

C. Ramus region: _____

D. General survey of the mandible: _____

E. What is the maximum CR angle needed for all of these projections? _____

Chapter 11 Skull and Cranial Bones

5. What specific positioning error has been committed if both sides of the mandible are superimposed with an axiolateral oblique projection?

_____

6. Where should the CR exit for a PA axial projection of the mandible?

_____

7. Which cranial positioning line is placed perpendicular to the image receptor for a PA or PA axial projection of the

   mandible? _____

8. True/False: For a true PA projection of the mandibular body (if this is the area of interest), the AML should be perpendicular to the image receptor.

9. True/False: The CR should be angled 20° to 25° caudad for the PA axial projection of the mandible.

10. Which aspect of the mandible is best visualized with an AP axial projection?

_____

11. A. What CR angle is required for the AP axial projection of the mandible if the OML is placed perpendicular to

      the image receptor? _____

    B. If the infraorbitomeatal line (IOML) is perpendicular to IR, what CR angle is needed?

       _____

12. Where is the CR centered for an AP axial projection of the mandible?

_____

13. Which projection of the mandible will demonstrate the entire mandible, including the coronoid and condyloid processes?

_____

14. Which imaging system provides a single, frontal perspective of the entire mandible?

_____

15. What device provides inherent collimation during an orthopantomographic procedure?

_____

16. Which cranial line is placed parallel to the floor for orthopantomography of the mandible?

_____

17. What type of image receptor must be used with analog orthopantomography?

_____

18. True/False: The modified Law method provides a bilateral and functional study of the TMJ.

19. True/False: The mandibular condyles move anteriorly as the mouth is opened.

20. Which projection/method of the TMJ requires that the skull be kept in a true lateral position?

    A. Modified Law   C. Axiolateral oblique projection

    B. Schuller   D. Modified Towne

21. The axiolateral (Schuller method) projection for the TMJ requires a CR angle of _____° (caudad or cephalad).

22. The axiolateral oblique projection of the TMJ is commonly referred to as the

    (A) _____ method, which requires a (B) _____°

    head rotation from lateral and a (C) _____° caudad CR angle.

23. If the area of interest is the temporomandibular fossae, angle the CR _____ to the OML for the AP axial (modified Towne) projection to reduce superimposition of the TM fossae and mastoid portions of the temporal bone.

24. Aligning the _____ plane perpendicular to the IR prevents rotation of either a PA or AP axial mandible.

REVIEW EXERCISE C: Positioning of the Paranasal Sinuses (see textbook pp. 436-440)

1. What analog kV range should be used for sinus radiography? _____ Digital kV

    range? _____

2. To demonstrate any possible air or fluid levels within the sinuses, it is important to:

    A. _____

    B. _____

3. True/False: Ultrasound exams of the maxillary sinuses to rule out sinusitis are possible.

4. True/False: Magnetic resonance imaging is the preferred modality to study soft tissue changes and masses within the sinuses.

5. True/False: Secondary osteomyelitis is often caused by tumor invasion.

6. List the four most commonly performed routine projections for paranasal sinuses.

    A. _____   C. _____

    B. _____   D. _____

7. Which single projection for a paranasal sinus routine provides an image of all four sinus groups?

    _____

8. If the patient cannot stand for the lateral projection of the paranasal sinuses, it should be taken with:

    _____

9. Which paranasal sinuses are best demonstrated with a PA (Caldwell) projection?

    _____

10. To avoid angling the CR for the erect PA Caldwell sinus projection, the head should be adjusted so that the OML is

_____° from horizontal.

11. A. Which group of paranasal sinuses is best demonstrated with a parietoacanthial (Waters) projection?

_____

B. The OML forms a _____° angle with the image receptor with this projection.

12. Which positioning line is placed perpendicular to the image receptor for a parietoacanthial projection?

_____

13. Where are the petrous ridges located on a well-positioned parietoacanthial projection?

_____

14. Which paranasal sinuses are demonstrated with an SMV projection of the paranasal sinuses?

_____

15. Where should the CR exit for both the PA parietoacanthial (Waters) and the PA transoral (open-mouth Waters)

projection? _____

16. What is the one major difference in positioning between the parietoacanthial and PA axial transoral projections?

_____

17. Which sinuses are projected through the oral cavity with the PA axial transoral projection?

_____

18. Match each of the following sinus projections with the anatomy best seen. (Use each choice only once.)

_____ 1. Lateral   A. Sphenoid sinus in oral cavity

_____ 2. Parietoacanthial   B. Inferosuperior view of sphenoid and ethmoid sinus

_____ 3. PA Caldwell   C. All four paranasal sinuses demonstrated

_____ 4. PA transoral   D. Best view of maxillary sinuses

_____ 5. SMV for sinuses   E. Best view of frontal and ethmoid sinuses

REVIEW EXERCISE D: Problem Solving for Technical and Positioning Errors for Facial Bones, Mandible, and Paranasal Sinuses

1. **Situation:** A radiograph of a lateral projection of the facial bones reveals that the mandibular rami are not superimposed. What positioning error led to this radiographic outcome?

_____

2. **Situation:** A radiograph of a parietoacanthial (Waters) projection reveals that the petrous ridges are projected within the maxillary sinuses. Is this an acceptable image? If not, what must be done to improve the image during

the repeat exposure? _____

3. **Situation:** A radiograph of a parietoacanthial (Waters) projection reveals that the distance between the lateral margins of the orbits and the lateral aspect of the cranial cortex is not equal. What type of positioning error led to this radiographic outcome?

_____

4. **Situation:** A radiograph of a 30° PA axial projection of the facial bones reveals that the petrous ridges are projected at the level of the inferior orbital margins. Is this an acceptable image for this projection? If not, what must be done to improve the quality of the image during the repeat exposure?

_____

5. **Situation:** A radiograph of a superoinferior projection of the nasal bones reveals that the glabella are superimposed over the nasal bones. What positioning error led to this radiographic outcome, and how can it be corrected during the repeat exposure?

_____

_____

6. **Situation:** A lateral radiograph of the facial bones demonstrates that the bodies of the mandible are not superimposed; one is about 1 cm superior to the other. How would this be corrected on a repeat exposure?

_____

7. **Situation:** A radiograph of a parieto-orbital oblique (Rhese) projection reveals that the optic foramen is located in the upper outer quadrant of the orbit. Is this an acceptable image for this projection? If not, what must be done to correct this problem during the repeat exposure?

_____

8. **Situation:** A radiograph of an axiolateral oblique projection of the mandible reveals that the body of the mandible is severely foreshortened. The body of the mandible is the area of interest. What positioning error led to this radiographic outcome?

_____

9. **Situation:** A patient with a possible fracture of the nasal bones enters the emergency room. The physician is concerned about deviation of the bony nasal septum along with possible nasal bones fracture. What radiographic routine would be best for this situation?

_____

_____

10. **Situation:** A patient with a possible blowout fracture of the right orbit enters the emergency room. In addition to the basic facial bone routine, what single projection would best demonstrate this type of injury?

_____

11. **Situation:** A patient with a possible fracture of the left zygomatic arch enters the emergency room. Neither the AP axial nor the SMV projection demonstrates the left side well. The radiologist is indecisive as to whether this zygomatic arch is fractured. What other projections can the technologist provide to better define this area?

_____

12. **Situation:** As part of a study of the zygomatic arches, the technologist attempts to perform the SMV position. Because of the size of the patient's shoulders, he is unable to flex his neck adequately to place the IOML parallel to the image receptor. What other options does the technologist have to produce an acceptable SMV projection?

_____

13. **Situation:** A radiograph of a PA (Caldwell) projection for sinuses reveals that the petrous ridges are projected into the lower half of the orbits and are obscuring the ethmoid sinuses. The technologist used a horizontal x-ray beam for the projection. The skull was positioned to place the OML at a 15° angle from the horizontal plane. What positioning modification is needed to correct this problem during the repeat exposure?

_____

14. **Situation:** A radiograph of a parietoacanthial projection reveals that the distance between the midsagittal plane and the outer orbital margin is not equal. What positioning error is present on this radiograph?

_____

15. **Situation:** A radiograph of an SMV projection for sinuses reveals that the distance between the mandibular condyles and lateral border of the skull is not equal. What specific positioning error is present on this radiograph?

_____

16. **Situation:** A radiograph of a PA transoral projection reveals that the sphenoid sinus is superimposed over the upper teeth and the nasal cavity. How must the position be modified to avoid this problem during the repeat exposure?

_____

17. **Situation:** A radiograph of a parietoacanthial projection (Waters method) reveals that the petrous ridges are projected just below the maxillary sinuses. What positioning error (if any) is present?

_____

18. **Situation:** A patient with a clinical history of sinusitis comes to the radiology department for a sinus study. The patient is quadriplegic and cannot be placed erect. Which single projection demonstrates any possible air-fluid levels in the sinuses?

_____

19. **Situation:** A patient comes to the radiology department to rule out a possible polyp within the sphenoid sinus. What routine and/or special projection provides the best overall assessment of the sinuses for this patient?

_____

20. **Situation:** A patient comes to the radiology department with a clinical history of a deviated bony nasal septum. Which facial bone projections best demonstrate the degree of deviation? (More than one correct answer is possible.)

_____

_____

The following review exercises should be completed only after careful study of the associated pages in the textbook as indicated by each exercise. Answers to each review exercise are given at the end of the review exercises.

REVIEW EXERCISE A: Critique Radiographs of the Cranium (see textbook p. 441)

The following questions relate to the radiographs found at the end of Chapter 11 of the textbook. Evaluate these radiographs for the radiographic criteria categories (1 through 5) that follow. Describe the corrections needed to improve the overall image. The major, or "repeatable," errors are specific errors that indicate the need for a repeat exposure, regardless of the nature of the other errors.

A. Lateral skull: 4-year-old (Fig. C11-198)

1. Anatomy demonstrated: _____

2. Part positioning: _____

3. Collimation and central ray: _____

4. Exposure: _____

5. Anatomic side markers: _____

Repeatable error(s): _____

B. Lateral skull: 54-year-old, post-traumatic injury (Fig. C11-199)

1. Anatomy demonstrated: _____

2. Part positioning: _____

3. Collimation and central ray: _____

4. Exposure: _____

5. Anatomic side markers: _____

Repeatable error(s): _____

C. AP axial skull (Towne) (Fig. C11-200)

1. Anatomy demonstrated: _____

2. Part positioning: _____

3. Collimation and central ray: _____

4. Exposure: _____

5. Anatomic side markers: _____

Repeatable error(s): _____

D. AP or PA skull (Fig. C11-201)

How can you determine whether this was a PA or an AP projection? _____

1. Anatomy demonstrated: _____

2. Part positioning: _____

3. Collimation and central ray: _____

4. Exposure: _____

5. Anatomic side markers: _____

Repeatable error(s): _____

E. AP or PA skull (Fig. C11-202)

Is this an AP or a PA skull? (Compare with Fig. C11-201, looking at the size of the orbits.) _____

1. Anatomy demonstrated: _____

2. Part positioning: _____

3. Collimation and central ray: _____

4. Exposure: _____

5. Anatomic side markers: _____

Repeatable error(s): _____

REVIEW EXERCISE B: Critique Radiographs of the Facial Bones (see textbook p. 442)

The following questions relate to the radiographs found at the end of Chapter 11 of the textbook. Evaluate these radiographs for the radiographic criteria categories (1 through 5) that follow. Describe the corrections needed to improve the overall image. The major, or "repeatable," error(s) are specific errors that indicate the need for a repeat exposure, regardless of the nature or degree of the other errors.

A. Parietoacanthial (Waters method) projection (Fig. C11-203)

Description of possible error:

1. Anatomy demonstrated: _____

2. Part positioning: _____

3. Collimation and central ray: _____

4. Exposure: _____

5. Anatomic side markers: _____

Repeatable error(s): _____

B. SMV mandible (Fig. C11-204)

Description of possible error:

    1. Anatomy demonstrated: _____

    2. Part positioning: _____

    3. Collimation and central ray: _____

    4. Exposure: _____

    5. Anatomic side markers: _____

Repeatable error(s): _____

C. Optic foramina, parieto-orbital oblique Rhese method (Fig. C11-205)

Description of possible error:

    1. Anatomy demonstrated: _____

    2. Part positioning: _____

    3. Collimation and central ray: _____

    4. Exposure: _____

    5. Anatomic side markers: _____

Repeatable error(s): _____

D. Optic foramina, parieto-orbital oblique Rhese method (Fig. C11-206)

Description of possible error:

    1. Anatomy demonstrated: _____

    2. Part positioning: _____

    3. Collimation and central ray: _____

    4. Exposure: _____

    5. Anatomic side markers: _____

Repeatable error(s): _____

E. Lateral facial bones (Fig. C11-207)

Description of possible error:

1. Anatomy demonstrated: _____

2. Part positioning: _____

3. Collimation and central ray: _____

4. Exposure: _____

5. Anatomic side markers: _____

Repeatable error(s): _____

REVIEW EXERCISE C: Critique Radiographs of the Paranasal Sinuses (see textbook p. 443)

The following questions relate to the radiographs found at the end of Chapter 11 of the textbook. Evaluate these radiographs for positioning accuracy as well as exposure factors, collimation, and correct use of anatomic markers. Describe the corrections needed to improve the overall image. The major, or "repeatable," error(s) imply that these specific errors require a repeat exposure be taken regardless of the nature or degree of the other errors. Answers to each critique are given at the end of the laboratory activities.

A. Parietoacanthial transoral (open-mouth Waters method) (Fig. C11-208)

Description of possible error:

1. Anatomy demonstrated: _____

2. Part positioning: _____

3. Collimation and central ray: _____

4. Exposure: _____

5. Anatomic side markers: _____

Repeatable error(s): _____

B. Parietoacanthial (Waters) (Fig. C11-209)

Description of possible error:

1. Anatomy demonstrated: _____

2. Part positioning: _____

3. Collimation and central ray: _____

4. Exposure: _____

5. Anatomic side markers: _____

Repeatable error(s): _____

C. Submentovertex (SMV) (Fig. C11-210)

Description of possible error:

1. Anatomy demonstrated: _____

2. Part positioning: _____

3. Collimation and central ray: _____

4. Exposure: _____

5. Anatomic side markers: _____

Repeatable error(s): _____

D. Lateral projection (Fig. C11-211)

Description of possible error:

1. Anatomy demonstrated: _____

2. Part positioning: _____

3. Collimation and central ray: _____

4. Exposure: _____

5. Anatomic side markers: _____

Repeatable error(s): _____

PART V: LABORATORY EXERCISES OF CRANIUM

You must gain experience in positioning each part of the cranium before performing the following exams on actual patients. You can get experience in positioning and radiographic evaluation of these projections by performing exercises using radiographic phantoms and practicing on other students (although you will not be taking actual exposures).

The following suggested activities assume that your teaching institution has an energized lab and radiographic phantoms. If not, perform the laboratory exercises, the radiographic evaluation, and the physical positioning exercises. (Check off each step and projection as you complete it.)

Laboratory Exercise A: Energized Laboratory

1. Using the skull radiographic phantom, produce radiographs of the following basic routines:

_____ 15° PA axial (Caldwell) skull   _____ PA axial (Haas)

_____ Lateral skull   _____ SMV

_____ AP axial skull

Laboratory Exercise B: Radiographic Evaluation

1. Evaluate and critique the radiographs produced in the preceding, additional radiographs provided by your instructor, or both. Evaluate each radiograph for the following points.

_____ Evaluate the completeness of the study. (Are all of the pertinent anatomic structures included on the radiograph?)

_____ Evaluate for positioning or centering errors (e.g., rotation, off centering).

_____ Evaluate for correct exposure factors and possible motion. (Are the density and contrast of the images acceptable?)

_____ Determine whether anatomic side markers and an acceptable degree of collimation and/or area shielding are visible on the images.

Laboratory Exercise C: Physical Positioning

On another person, simulate performing all basic and special projections of the sternum and ribs as follows. Include the six steps listed in the following and described in the textbook. (Check off each step when completed satisfactorily.)

Step 1. Appropriate size and type of image receptor with correct markers

Step 2. Correct central ray placement and centering of part to central ray and/or image receptor

Step 3. Accurate collimation

Step 4. Area shielding of patient where advisable

Step 5. Use of proper immobilizing devices when needed

Step 6. Approximate correct exposure factors, breathing instructions where applicable, and initiating exposure

Projections	*Step 1*	*Step 2*	*Step 3*	*Step 4*	*Step 5*	*Step 6*
Skull series: routine						
● AP axial (Towne)	_____	_____	_____	_____	_____	_____
● Lateral skull	_____	_____	_____	_____	_____	_____
● PA 15° axial (Caldwell)	_____	_____	_____	_____	_____	_____
Skull series: special						
● PA axial (Haas)	_____	_____	_____	_____	_____	_____
● SMV	_____	_____	_____	_____	_____	_____

PART VI: LABORATORY EXERCISES FOR FACIAL BONES, MANDIBLE, AND PARANASAL SINUSES

You must gain experience in positioning each part of the facial bones before performing the following exams on actual patients. You can get experience in positioning and radiographic evaluation of these projections by performing exercises using radiographic phantoms and practicing on other students (although you will not be taking actual exposures).

The following suggested activities assume that your teaching institution has an energized lab and radiographic phantoms. If not, perform the laboratory exercises, the radiographic evaluation, and the physical positioning activities. (Check off each step and projection as you complete it.)

Laboratory Exercise A: Energized Laboratory

1. Using the skull radiographic phantom, produce radiographs of the following routine facial bone studies:

Facial bones

_____ Parietoacanthial (Waters)

_____ Modified Waters

_____ Lateral

_____ 15° PA axial (Caldwell)

Temporomandibular joints

_____ Submentovertex (SMV)

_____ Oblique tangential

_____ AP axial

Zygomatic arches

_____ Modified Law

_____ Schuller method

_____ AP axial

Nasal bones

_____ Lateral

_____ Superoinferior (tangential)

_____ SMV

Mandible

_____ Axiolateral oblique

_____ PA

_____ AP axial

Optic foramina

_____ Parieto-orbital oblique (Rhese)

2. Using the skull radiographic phantom, produce radiographs of the following basic routines:

Sinuses

_____ Parietoacanthial (Waters)

_____ Lateral

_____ PA

_____ Submentovertex (SMV)

Laboratory Exercise B: Radiographic Evaluation

1. Evaluate and critique the radiographs produced during the previous experiments, additional radiographs provided by your instructor, or both. Evaluate each radiograph for the following points.

_____ Evaluate the completeness of the study. (Are all pertinent anatomic structures included on the radiograph?)

_____ Evaluate for positioning or centering errors (e.g., rotation, off-centering).

_____ Evaluate for correct exposure factors and possible motion. (Are the density and contrast of the images acceptable?)

_____ Determine whether anatomic side markers and an acceptable degree of collimation and/or area shielding are visible on the images.

Laboratory Exercise C: Physical Positioning

On another person, simulate performing all basic and special projections of the facial bones as follows. Include the six steps listed in the following and described in the textbook. (Check off each step when completed satisfactorily.)

Step 1. Appropriate size and type of image receptor (IR) with correct markers

Step 2. Correct CR placement and centering of part to CR and/or IR

Step 3. Accurate collimation

Step 4. Area shielding of patient where advisable

Step 5. Use of proper immobilizing devices when needed

Step 6. Approximate correct exposure factors, breathing instructions where applicable, and initiating exposure

Projections	Step 1	Step 2	Step 3	Step 4	Step 5	Step 6
Facial bones						
• Parietoacanthial (Waters)	_____	_____	_____	_____	_____	_____
• Modified parietoacanthial	_____	_____	_____	_____	_____	_____
• Lateral facial bones	_____	_____	_____	_____	_____	_____
• 15° PA axial (Caldwell)	_____	_____	_____	_____	_____	_____
Nasal bones						
• Laterals	_____	_____	_____	_____	_____	_____
• Superoinferior nasal bones	_____	_____	_____	_____	_____	_____
Zygomatic arches						
• Submentovertex (SMV)	_____	_____	_____	_____	_____	_____
• Oblique tangential	_____	_____	_____	_____	_____	_____
• AP axial	_____	_____	_____	_____	_____	_____
Optic foramina						
• Parieto-orbital oblique (Rhese)	_____	_____	_____	_____	_____	_____
Mandible						
• PA	_____	_____	_____	_____	_____	_____
• AP axial	_____	_____	_____	_____	_____	_____
• Axiolateral oblique (general survey)	_____	_____	_____	_____	_____	_____
Temporomandibular joints						
• Modified law	_____	_____	_____	_____	_____	_____
• Schuller method	_____	_____	_____	_____	_____	_____
• AP axial	_____	_____	_____	_____	_____	_____
Paranasal sinus projections						
• Parietoacanthial (Waters)	_____	_____	_____	_____	_____	_____
• Lateral	_____	_____	_____	_____	_____	_____
• PA	_____	_____	_____	_____	_____	_____
• Submentovertex (SMV)	_____	_____	_____	_____	_____	_____
• Parietoacanthial transoral (open-mouth Waters)	_____	_____	_____	_____	_____	_____

This self-test should be taken only after completing all of the readings, review exercises, and laboratory activities for a particular section. The purpose of this test is not only to provide a good learning exercise but also to serve as a strong indicator of what your final evaluation exam for this chapter will cover. It is strongly suggested that if you do not get at least a 90% to 95% grade on each self-test, you should review those areas in which you missed questions before going to your instructor for the final evaluation exam. The self-test is divided into two regions of study: cranium and facial bones/paranasal sinuses.

ANATOMY AND POSITIONING OF CRANIUM

1. Which one of the following bones is not part of the floor of the cranium?

   A. Temporal   B. Ethmoid   C. Occipital   D. Sphenoid

2. Which aspect of the frontal bone is thin-walled and forms the forehead?

   A. Orbital   B. Horizontal   C. Squamous   D. Superciliary margin

3. Which four cranial bones articulate with the frontal bone?

   A. _____   C. _____

   B. _____   D. _____

4. Which structures are found at the widest aspect of the skull? _____

5. What is the name of a prominent landmark (or "bump") found on the external surface of the occipital bone?

   _____

6. List the number of individual bones that articulate with the following cranial bones.

   A. Parietal bone: _____

   B. Occipital bone: _____

   C. Temporal bone: _____

   D. Sphenoid: _____

   E. Ethmoid: _____

7. What is the thickest and densest structure in the cranium? _____

8. True/False: The hypophysis is another term for the pituitary gland.

9. True/False: The sphenoid bone articulates with all the other cranial bones.

10. The shallow depression just posterior to the base of the dorsum sellae and anterior to the foramen magnum is the

   _____.

11. What is the name of the paired collections of bone found inferior to the cribriform plate that contain numerous air cells and help form the lateral walls of the nasal cavity?

   _____

12. Which small section of bone is located superior to the cribriform plate?

   _____

13. What is the formal term for the left sphenoid fontanel in the adult?

   _____

14. What is the name of the cranial suture formed by the inferior junction of the parietals to the temporal bones?

   _____

15. What are the two terms for the small, irregular bones found in the adult skull sutures?

   _____

16. Match each of the following structures to its related cranial bone.

   _____   1. Pterygoid hamulus   A. Occipital

   _____   2. Anterior clinoid processes   B. Frontal

   _____   3. Glabella   C. Sphenoid

   _____   4. Foramen ovale   D. Ethmoid

   _____   5. Perpendicular plate   E. Temporal

   _____   6. Superior nasal conchae   F. Parietal

   _____   7. Foramen magnum

   _____   8. Cribriform plate

   _____   9. Zygomatic process

   _____   10. Lateral condylar portions

   _____   11. Superciliary arch

   _____   12. EAM

   _____   13. Inion

   _____   14. Sella turcica

   _____   15. Petrous ridge

Identify the cranial structures, sutures, and regions labeled on the following radiographs (Figs. 11-28 and 11-29):

Structure	*Bone(s)*
A. _____	_____
B. _____	_____
C. _____	_____
D. _____ (suture)	_____
E. _____	_____
F. _____	_____
G. _____	_____
H. _____	_____
I. _____	_____
J. _____	_____
K. _____	_____
L. _____	_____
M. _____	_____

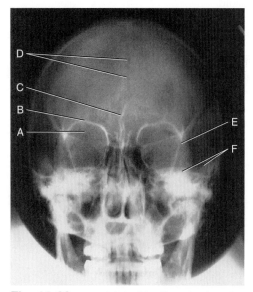

Fig. 11-28. PA axial (Caldwell) projection of cranium.

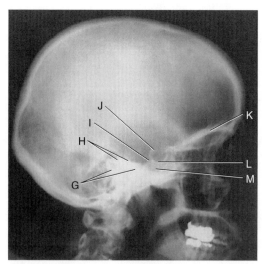

Fig. 11-29. Lateral cranium.

17. Which one of the following skull classifications applies to a skull with an angle of 54° between the midsagittal plane and the long axis of the pars petrosa?

    A. Mesocephalic   C. Brachycephalic

    B. Dolichocephalic   D. None of these

18. Which of the preceding classifications is considered the average-shaped skull? _____

Identify the labeled landmarks and positioning lines used in skull and facial bone positioning, as shown in Fig. 11-30 (including abbreviations).

    A. _____

    B. _____

    C. _____

    D. _____

    E. _____

    F. _____

    G. _____

    H. _____

    I. _____

    J. _____

    K. _____

    L. _____

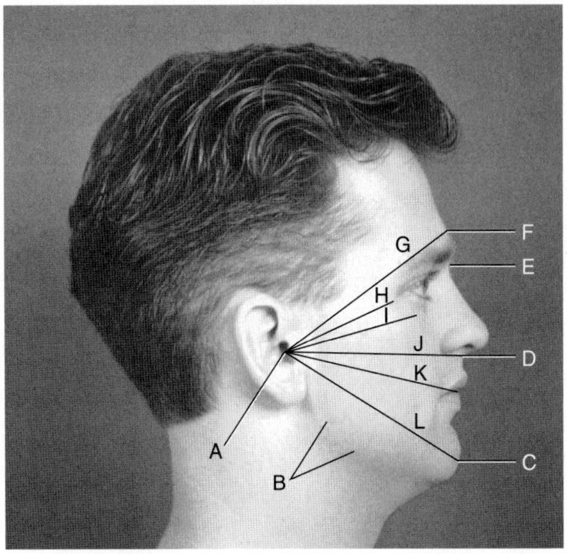

Fig. 11-30. Skull and facial bone landmarks and positioning lines.

19. Which of the following landmarks corresponds to the highest level of the petrous ridge?

    A. EAM   C. Outer canthus

    B. TEA   D. Acanthion

20. Which one of the following terms is defined as the large cartilaginous aspect of the external ear?

    A. Pinna   C. Glabella

    B. Tragus   D. Acanthion

21. Reid's base line is an older term for:

    A. GML   C. OML

    B. IOML   D. GAL

22. How much of a difference in degrees is there between the OML and IOML?

    A. 10°   C. 3°

    B. 7° to 8°   D. None (They represent the same positioning line.)

23. Which one of the following positioning errors frequently results in a repeat exposure of a cranial position?

    A. Rotation   C. Slight flexion

    B. Incorrect central ray placement   D. Slight extension

24. Match each of the following pathologic indications to the correct definition or description. (Use each choice only once.)

    _____ A. Bone tumor originating in the bone marrow   1. Linear fracture

    _____ B. Fracture evident by sphenoid sinus effusion   2. Paget's disease

    _____ C. Condition that begins with bony destruction followed by bony repair   3. Depressed fracture

    _____ D. Destructive lesion with irregular margins   4. Osteolytic neoplasm

    _____ E. Fracture of the skull with jagged or irregular lucent line that lies at a   5. Multiple myeloma
            right angle to the axis of the bone.

                                                                  6. Basal fracture

    _____ F. Tangential view may be helpful to determine extent or degree of
            this fracture

25. Which one of the following clinical indications may require a decrease in manual exposure factors?

    A. Pituitary adenoma   C. Paget's disease

    B. Linear skull fracture   D. Multiple myeloma

26. Which one of the following imaging modalities may be used to examine a possible cranial bleed caused by trauma?

    A. CT   C. Ultrasound

    B. MRI   D. Nuclear medicine

27. Which one of the following imaging modalities provides an excellent distinction between normal and abnormal brain tissue?

    A. CT   C. Ultrasound

    B. MRI   D. Nuclear medicine

28. Which aspect of the temporal bone is considered to be thinnest?

    _____

29. Which aspect of the temporal bone contains the organs of hearing and balance?

    _____

30. The correct term for the eardrum is the _____.

31. Which one of the following middle ear structures is considered to be most lateral?

    A. Malleus   C. Stapes

    B. Incus   D. Oval window

32. Which structure helps equalize atmospheric pressure in the middle ear? _____

33. What passes through the internal acoustic meatus? _____

34. The aditus is an opening between the _____ and the

    _____ portion of the temporal bone.

35. An infection of the mastoid air cells, if untreated, can lead to a serious infection of the brain called

    _____.

36. Which auditory ossicle attaches to the oval window?

    A. Malleus   C. Stapes

    B. Incus   D. None

37. The internal ear is divided into the osseous or bony labyrinth and the _____
    labyrinth.

38. List the three divisions of the bony labyrinth of the inner ear.

    A. _____   B. _____   C. _____

39. Identify the structures labeled on Fig. 11-31.

    A. _____

    B. _____

    C. _____

    D. _____

    E. _____

    F. _____

    G. _____

    H. _____

    I. _____

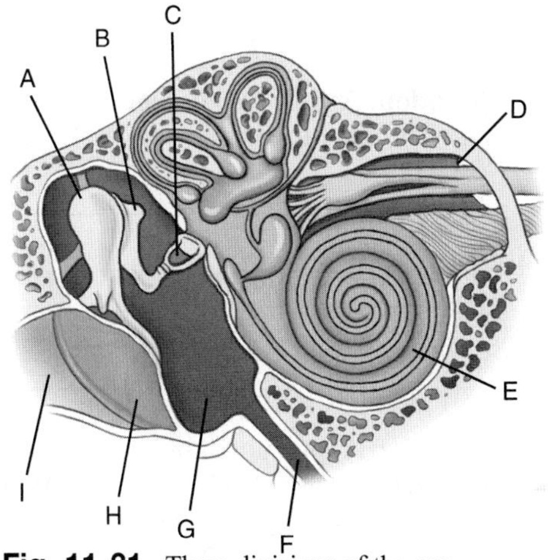

Fig. 11-31. Three divisions of the ear.

40. A benign, cystlike mass of the middle ear is a(n):

    A. Acoustic neuroma   C. Cholesteatoma

    B. Osteomyelitis   D. Acoustic sarcoma

41. True/False: Otosclerosis is a hereditary disease.

42. Which two projections of the cranium project the dorsum sellae within the foramen magnum?

    A. _____

    B. _____

43. A. How much central ray angle is required for the AP axial projection (Towne method) for skull with the IOML perpendicular to the image receptor?

_____

B. What is the central ray angle for this same projection with a perpendicular OML?

_____

44. Where is the central ray centered for a lateral projection of the cranium?

_____

45. To prevent tilting of the skull for the lateral projection of the cranium, the _____ line is placed perpendicular to the image receptor.

46. Where should the petrous ridges be located (on the image) for a well-positioned, 25° caudad PA axial (Haas method) projection? _____

47. Where is the central ray centered for an SMV projection of the skull?

_____

48. Which positioning line is parallel to the IR for the SMV projection of the skull?

_____

49. **Situation:** A radiograph of an AP axial projection for the cranium reveals that the dorsum sellae is projected superior to the foramen magnum. What must be modified during the repeat exposure to correct this problem?

_____

50. **Situation:** A radiograph of a lateral projection of the cranium reveals that the greater wings of sphenoid are not superimposed. What type of positioning error is present on this radiograph?

_____

51. **Situation:** A radiograph of a 15° caudad PA axial projection of the cranium reveals that the petrous ridges are at the level of the supraorbital margin. Without changing the central ray angle, how must the head position be modified during the repeat exposure to produce a more acceptable image?

_____

52. **Situation:** A patient with a possible basilar skull fracture enters the emergency room. The physician wants a projection to demonstrate a possible sphenoid sinus effusion. Which projection of the cranium is best for this situation?

_____

53. **Situation:** The same patient in the previous situation also requires a frontal projection of the skull. The physician wants the projection to demonstrate the frontal bone and place the petrous ridges in the lower one-third of the orbits, but it has not been determined whether the patient's cervical spine has been fractured, so the patient cannot be moved from a supine position. What should the technologist do to obtain this image?

_____

54. **Situation:** A patient comes to the radiology department for a skull series. Because of the size of the patient's shoulders, he is unable to flex his neck sufficiently to place the OML perpendicular to the IR for the AP axial projection. His head cannot be raised because of possible cervical trauma. What other options does the technologist have to obtain an acceptable AP axial projection?

_____

55. **Situation:** A radiograph of an AP axial (Towne method) projection for cranium reveals that the posterior arch of C1 and dorsum sellae are superimposed. Both are projected into the foramen magnum. What modification is needed to correct this error present on the initial radiograph?

_____

56. **Situation:** A radiograph of a lateral skull demonstrates that the orbital plates (roof) of the frontal bone are not superimposed. What is the positioning error present on this radiograph?

_____

57. **Situation:** A radiograph of an AP axial (Towne method) for cranium reveals that the left petrous portion of the temporal bone is wider than the right. What is the specific positioning error present on this radiograph?

_____

58. **Situation:** A radiograph of a SMV projection of the cranium demonstrates that mandibular condyles are projected into the petrous portion (pyramids) of the temporal bone. How must the position be altered during the repeat exposure to correct this error?

_____

ANATOMY AND POSITIONING OF FACIAL BONES, MANDIBLE, AND PARANASAL SINUSES

1. The majority of the hard palate is formed by:

   A. Maxilla   C. Zygomatic bone

   B. Palatine bones   D. Mandible

2. Which of the following is _not_ an aspect of the maxilla?

   A. Frontal process   C. Zygomatic process

   B. Body   D. Ramus

3. Match each of the following definitions or characteristics to the correct facial bone. (Use each choice only once.)

   _____ A. Mandible   1. Contains four processes

   _____ B. Lacrimal bones   2. Forms lower, outer aspect of orbit

   _____ C. Palatine bones   3. Lie just anterior and medial to the frontal process of maxilla

   _____ D. Inferior nasal conchae   4. Unpaired bone in the adult

   _____ E. Nasal bones   5. Located anteriorly in medial aspect of orbit

   _____ F. Maxilla   6. Help to mix air drawn into nasal cavity

   _____ G. Zygomatic bone   7. Possesses a vertical and horizontal portion

Identify the seven (cranial and facial) bones that form the bony orbit (Fig. 11-32).

A. _____

B. _____

C. _____

D. _____

E. _____

F. _____

G. _____

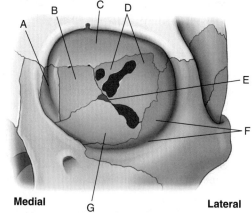

Fig. 11-32. Slightly oblique frontal view of orbit, A-G.

4. On average, how many separate cavities make up the frontal sinus? _____

5. True/False: All of the paranasal sinuses are contained within cranial bones, except the maxillary sinuses.

6. True/False: All of the paranasal sinuses except the sphenoid communicate with the nasal cavity.

7. True/False: In general, all the paranasal sinuses are fully developed by the age of 6 or 7 years.

8. True/False: The frontal sinuses are usually larger in men than in women.

9. Identify the labeled structures on these radiographs of the paranasal sinuses (Figs. 11-33, 11-34, and 11-35).

A. _____   H. _____

B. _____   I. _____

C. _____   J. _____

D. _____   K. _____

E. _____   L. _____

F. _____   M. _____

G. _____

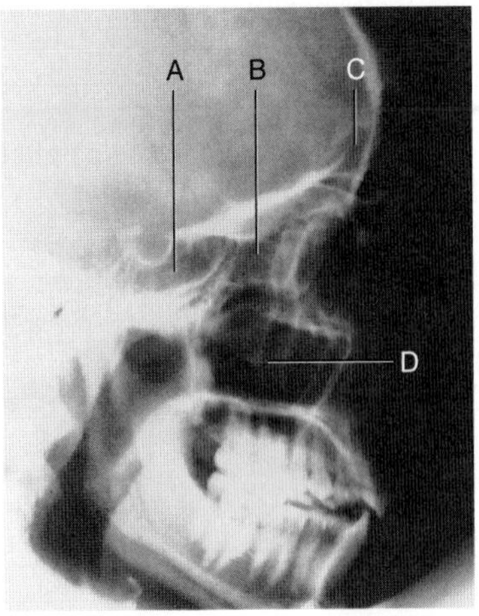

Fig. 11-33. Paranasal sinuses, A-D.

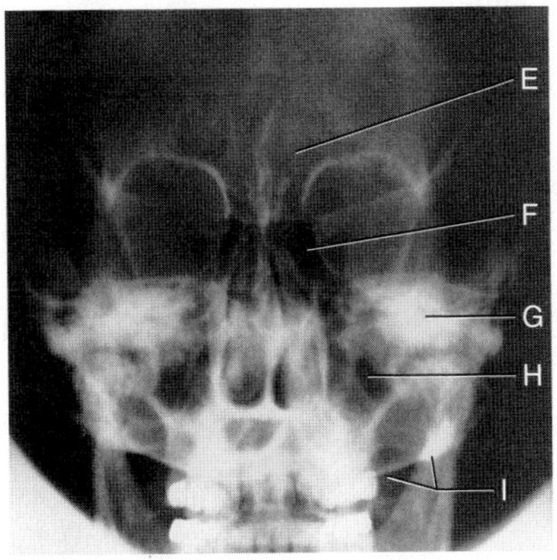

Fig. 11-34. Paranasal sinuses, E-I.

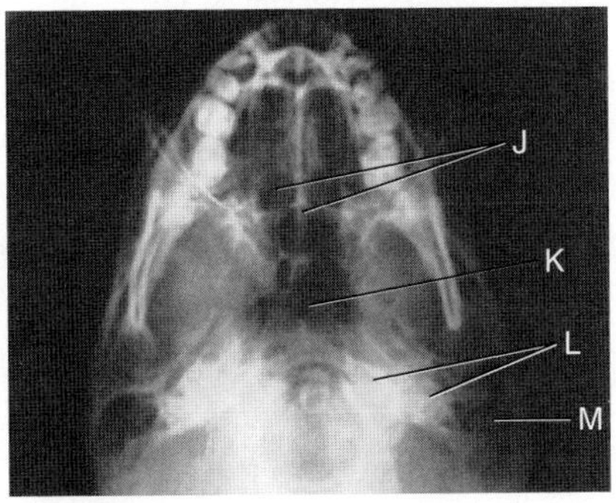

Fig. 11-35. Paranasal sinuses, J-M.

10. Which aspect of the ethmoid bone contains the ethmoid air cells?

_____

11. The sphenoid sinus lies directly inferior to the _____.

12. True/False: Ultrasound of the sphenoid sinus can be performed to rule out sinusitis.

13. Which one of the following imaging modalities best demonstrates bony erosion of the maxillary sinus resulting from acute sinusitis?

A. CT   C. Ultrasound

B. MRI   D. Conventional radiography

14. True/False: Facial bone studies should be performed erect whenever possible.

15. True/False: A Le Fort fracture produces a "free-floating" zygomatic bone.

16. Which frontal projection of the facial bones best visualizes the region of the maxilla and orbits?

_____

17. Which single projection of the facial bones best demonstrates any possible air-fluid levels in the sinuses if the patient cannot stand or sit erect?

_____

18. Which plane is placed parallel to the IR with a true lateral projection of the facial bones?

_____

19. A. What is the angle between the OML and plane of image receptor with a parietoacanthial (Waters method)

projection? _____

   B. This places the _____ positioning line perpendicular to the IR.

20. The CR is centered to exit at the level of the _____ for a well-positioned parietoacanthial projection.

   A. Nasion   C. Inner canthus

   B. Glabella   D. Acanthion

21. The CR is centered to exit at the level of the _____ for a well-positioned 15° PA axial projection of the facial bones.

   A. Nasion   C. Midorbits

   B. Glabella   D. Acanthion

22. Where are the petrous ridges projected for a properly positioned modified parietoacanthial projection?

_____

23. True/False: The lateral projection of the nasal bones should be performed using a small focal spot, low-to-medium kV (analog), and close collimation.

24. True/False: The CR should be angled as needed to be parallel to the glabellomeatal line (GML) for the superoinferior tangential projection of the nasal bones.

25. Which positioning line is placed perpendicular to the image receptor for a modified parietoacanthial projection?

_____

26. Where is the CR centered for a lateral projection of the nasal bones?

_____

27. Which positioning line, if placed parallel to the image receptor, ensures adequate extension of the head for the submentovertex projection for zygomatic arches?

_____

28. How much skull tilt and rotation are required for the oblique inferosuperior (tangential) projection for zygomatic

arches? _____

29. How much CR angle is required for the AP axial projection of the zygomatic arches if the IOML is placed perpendicular to the IR? (Hint: This is the same as for an AP axial skull.)

_____

30. The proper method name for the "three-point landing" projection for the optic foramen is the

_____.

31. Where should the optic foramen be located with a well-positioned parieto-orbital oblique projection?

_____

32. What is the maximum amount of CR angulation that should be used for an axiolateral oblique projection of the

mandible?_____

33. Which one of the following factors prevents superimposition of the ramus on the cervical spine for the axiolateral oblique mandible projection?

    A. Angle CR 10° to 15° cephalad   C. Extend chin

    B. Have patient open mouth during exposure   D. Rotate head toward IR

34. How much skull rotation (from the lateral position) toward the image receptor is required for the axiolateral oblique projection specifically for the mentum?

    A. 10° to 15°   C. 45°

    B. 30°   D. None. Keep the skull in the true lateral position.

35. How much CR angulation should be used for a PA axial projection of the mandible?

    A. None   C. 20° to 25° cephalad

    B. 10° to 15° cephalad   D. 5° cephalad

36. What structures are better defined when the CR angulation is increased from 35° to 40° caudad for the AP axial projection of the mandible?

_____

37. Where is the CR centered for an SMV projection of the mandible?

_____

38. During an orthopantomographic procedure, it is important to keep the _____ positioning line parallel to the floor.

    A. OML   C. IOML

    B. AML   D. GAL

39. What CR angulation is used for the AP axial projection of the TMJ with the OML perpendicular to the image

receptor?_____

40. True/False: The modified Law method requires a tube angulation of 25° caudad.

41. True/False: The Schuller method requires that the skull be placed in a true lateral position.

42. True/False: A grid is not required for the lateral projection of the nasal bones.

43. Where is the CR centered for a lateral projection of the paranasal sinuses?

_____

44. Why should a patient remain in an erect position for at least 5 minutes before sinus radiography?

_____

45. Which routine projection is best for demonstrating the maxillary sinuses?

_____

46. Why should a horizontal CR be used for the erect PA (Caldwell) projection for sinuses rather than the usual

15° caudad angle? _____

47. A radiograph of a 15° PA projection of the facial bones reveals that the petrous ridges are projected at the level of the midorbital rims. What specific positioning or CR angling error led to this radiographic outcome?

_____

48. Which positioning line should be perpendicular to the image receptor for the parieto-orbital oblique (Rhese method) projections for optic foramina?

A. Acanthomeatal line (AML)   C. Infraorbitomeatal line (IOML)

B. Mentomeatal line (MML)   D. Glabellomeatal line (GML)

49. A radiograph of lateral position for sinuses reveals that the greater wings of the sphenoid bone are not superimposed. What specific positioning error is present?

_____

50. **Situation:** A patient with severe facial bone injuries comes into the emergency room. The patient is wearing a cervical collar and cannot be moved. What type of positioning routine should be performed for this situation?

_____

51. **Situation:** A superoinferior, tangential projection for the nasal bones was taken with the following analog exposure factors: 18- × 24-cm (8- × 10-inch) IR crosswise, 85 kV, 13 mAs, 40-inch (102-cm) SID. The resultant radiograph was unsatisfactory because of poor visibility of the nasal bones. Which technical factors should be changed for the repeat exposure?

_____

52. **Situation:** A patient with possible facial fractures, including a possible "blow-out" fracture to the right orbit, was brought from the emergency room to the radiology department. What special facial bone projection should be included with the basic facial bone routine of a lateral, parietoacanthial (Waters), and PA axial (Caldwell)?

_____

53. **Situation:** A patient with a clinical history of secondary osteomyelitis comes to the radiology department. Which imaging modalities or procedures can be performed to demonstrate the extent of damage to the sinuses?

_____

12 Biliary Tract and Upper Gastrointestinal System

Radiographic procedures involving the administration of some form of contrast media are described in the next four chapters. These include common procedures, which may make up 20% to 30% of the radiology department case load. You will likely be performing these examinations early in your clinical training. If you learn and understand the fundamentals provided in these next four chapters, combined with clinical experience, you will soon become a proficient technologist of these organ systems.

CHAPTER OBJECTIVES

After you have successfully completed the activities in this chapter, you will be able to:

_____ 1. Identify specific anatomy and functions of the liver, gallbladder, and biliary ductal system.

_____ 2. Describe the production, storage, and purpose of bile.

_____ 3. On drawings and radiographs, identify specific anatomy of the biliary system.

_____ 4. Describe the effect of body habitus on the location of the gallbladder.

_____ 5. Define specific terms related to conditions and procedures of the biliary system.

_____ 6. Define specific pathologies of the biliary system.

_____ 7. Match specific biliary pathologies to the correct radiographic appearances and signs.

_____ 8. List the major organs of the upper gastrointestinal system and specific accessory organs.

_____ 9. List the three primary functions of the digestive system.

_____ 10. List three divisions of the pharynx.

_____ 11. Identify the anatomic location, function, and features of the esophagus, stomach, and duodenum.

_____ 12. Identify the effect of body position on the distribution of air and contrast media in the stomach.

_____ 13. Describe the effect of body habitus on the position and shape of the stomach.

_____ 14. Using drawings and radiographs, identify specific anatomy of the upper gastrointestinal system.

_____ 15. Identify differences between mechanical digestion and chemical digestion.

_____ 16. Identify the contrast media, patient preparation, room preparation, and fluoroscopic procedure for an esophagram and an upper gastrointestinal series.

_____ 17. List and define the specific clinical indications and contraindications for an esophagogram and upper GI series.

_____ 18. Match specific types of pathology to the correct radiographic appearances and signs.

_____ 19. Describe specific breathing maneuvers and positioning techniques used to detect esophageal reflux.

_____ 20. List the routine and special positions or projections for the esophagogram and upper gastrointestinal (GI) series to include size and type of image receptor, central ray location, direction and angulation of the central ray, and anatomy best demonstrated.

_____ 21. Identify which anatomy is best demonstrated with specific projections of an esophagogram and upper GI series.

_____ 22. Given various hypothetic situations, identify the correct modification of a position and/or exposure factors to improve the radiographic image.

POSITIONING AND RADIOGRAPHIC TECHNIQUE

_____ 1. Using a peer, position for routine and special projections for the esophagogram and upper GI series.

_____ 2. Critique and evaluate esophagram and upper GI series radiographs based on the five divisions of radiographic criteria: (1) anatomy demonstrated, (2) position, (3) collimation and CR, (4) exposure, and (5) anatomic side markers.

_____ 3. Distinguish between acceptable and unacceptable esophagogram and upper GI series radiographs that result from exposure factors, motion, collimation, positioning, or other errors.

LEARNING EXERCISES

Complete the following review exercises after reading the associated pages in the textbook as indicated by each exercise. Answers to each review exercise are given at the end of the review exercises.

PART I: RADIOGRAPHIC ANATOMY
REVIEW EXERCISE A: Radiographic Anatomy and Clinical Indications of the Gallbladder and Biliary System (see textbook pp. 446-449)

1. What is the average weight of the adult human liver? _____

2. Which abdominal quadrant contains the gallbladder? _____

3. What is the name of the soft tissue structure that separates the right from the left lobe of the liver?

_____

4. Which lobe of the liver is larger, the right or the left? _____

5. List the other two lobes of the liver (in addition to right and left lobes):

   A. _____   B. _____

6. True/False: The liver performs more than 100 functions.

7. True/False: The average healthy adult liver produces 1 gallon, or 3000 to 4000 mL, of bile per day.

8. List the three primary functions of the gallbladder:

   A. _____

   B. _____

   C. _____

9. True/False: Concentrated levels of cholesterol in bile may lead to gallstones.

10. What is a common site for impaction, or lodging, of gallstones? _____

11. True/False: In about 40% of individuals, the end of the common bile duct and the end of the pancreatic duct are totally separated into two ducts rather than combining into one single passageway into the duodenum.

12. True/False: An older term for the main pancreatic duct is the duct of Vater.

13. The gallbladder is located more _____ (posteriorly or anteriorly) within the abdomen.

14. Match the following structures to their primary location within the abdomen.

_____ 1. Liver   A. Near midsagittal plane

_____ 2. Gallbladder on asthenic patient   B. To left of midsagittal plane

_____ 3. Gallbladder on hypersthenic patient   C. To right of midsagittal plane

_____ 4. Gallbladder on hyposthenic patient

15. Identify the major components of the gallbladder and biliary system labeled on Fig. 12-1.

A. _____

B. _____

C. _____

D. _____

E. _____

F. _____

G. _____

H. _____

I. _____

J. _____

K. _____

L. _____

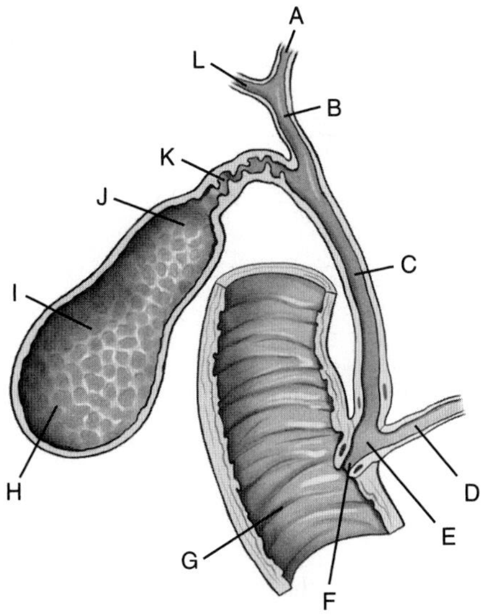

Fig. 12-1. Components of the gallbladder and biliary system.

16. List four advantages of a gallbladder ultrasound instead of the outdated OCG procedure:

A. _____

B. _____

C. _____

D. _____

17. Cholecystocholangiography is a radiographic examination of _____.

18. Which imaging modality produces cholescintigraphy?

A. CT   C. Radiography

B. MRI   D. Nuclear medicine

19. True/False: Acute cholecystitis may produce a thickened gallbladder wall.

20. Match each of the following clinical indications with its correct definition:

_____ 1. Cholelithiasis

_____ 2. Cholecystitis

_____ 3. Biliary stenosis

_____ 4. Cholecystectomy

_____ 5. Neoplasm

_____ 6. Choledocholithiasis

A. Surgical removal of the gallbladder

B. Enlargement or narrowing of the biliary ducts because of the presence of stones

C. Condition of having gallstones

D. Inflammation of the gallbladder

E. Benign or malignant tumors

F. Narrowing of the biliary ducts

REVIEW EXERCISE B: Specific Anatomy of the Upper Gastrointestinal System (see textbook pp. 450-456)

1. List the seven major components of the alimentary canal:

A. _____   E. _____

B. _____   F. _____

C. _____   G. _____

D. _____

2. List the four accessory organs of digestion:

A. _____   C. _____

B. _____   D. _____

3. What are the three primary functions of the digestive system?

A. _____

B. _____

C. _____

4. What two terms refer to a radiographic examination of the pharynx and esophagus?

_____ or _____

5. Which term describes the radiographic study of the distal esophagus, stomach, and duodenum?

_____

6. Which three pairs of salivary glands are accessory organs of digestion associated with the mouth?

    A. _____

    B. _____

    C. _____

7. The act of swallowing is called _____.

8. List the three divisions of the pharynx:

    A. _____   B. _____   C. _____

9. What structures create the two indentations seen along the lateral border of the esophagus?

    A. _____   B. _____

10. List the three structures that pass through the diaphragm.

    A. _____   B. _____   C. _____

11. What part of the upper GI tract is a common site for ulcer disease? _____

12. What term describes the junction between the duodenum and jejunum? _____
(This is a significant reference point in small bowel studies.)

13. The C-loop of the duodenum and pancreas are _____ (intraperitoneal or retroperitoneal) structures.

14. Name the following structures of the mouth and pharynx (Fig. 12-2):

    A. _____

    B. _____

    C. _____

    D. _____

    E. _____

    F. _____

    G. _____

    H. _____

    I. _____

    J. _____

    K. _____

    L. _____

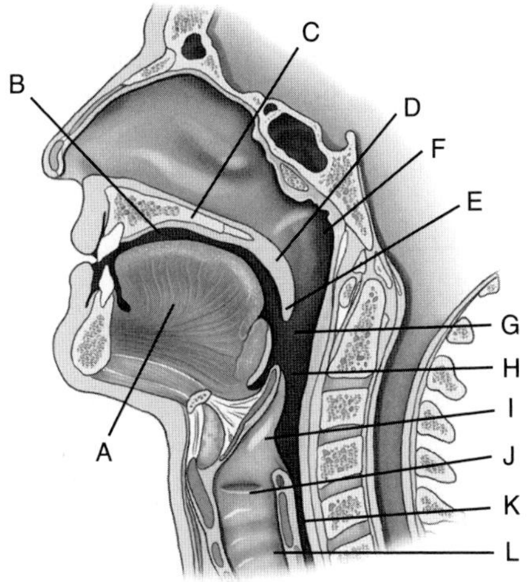

Fig. 12-2. Structures of the mouth and pharynx.

15. True/False: The body of the stomach curves inferiorly and posteriorly from the fundus.

16. Identify the parts labeled on Fig. 12-3:

A. _____

B. _____

C. _____

D. _____
(formed by rugae along lesser curvature)

E. _____

F. _____

G. _____

H. _____

I. _____

J. _____
(abdominal segment of esophagus)

K. _____

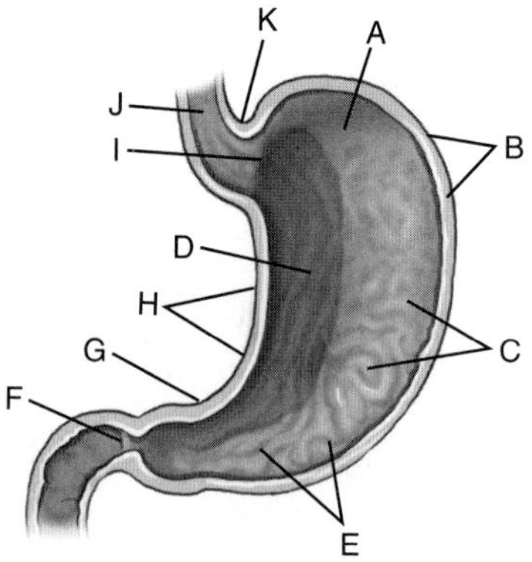

Fig. 12-3. Sectional anatomy of the stomach.

17. The three main subdivisions of the stomach are:

A. _____   B. _____   C. _____

18. The division of the stomach labeled *E* in Fig. 12-3 is divided into two parts: _____

and _____.

19. Another term for mucosal folds of the stomach is _____.

20. Identify the correct body position (erect, prone, or supine) for each of the preceding drawings of the stomach filled with air and barium (Fig. 12-4). (barium = white; air = black)

A. _____   B. _____   C. _____

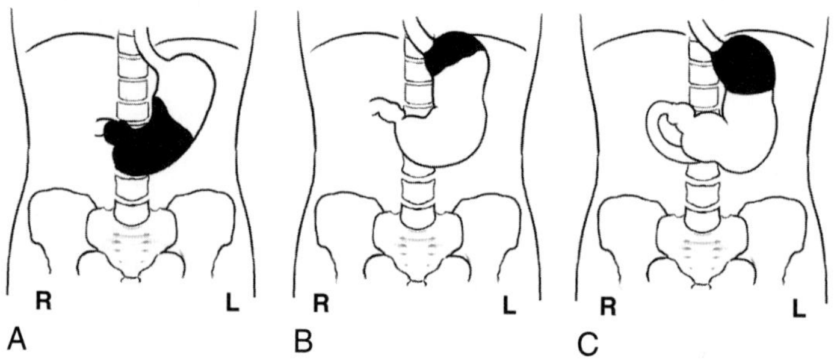

Fig. 12-4. Body position identification based on a stomach filled with air or barium.

21. Identify the parts labeled on Fig. 12-5:

A. _____

B. _____

C. _____

D. _____

E. _____

F. _____

G. _____

H. Region of _____

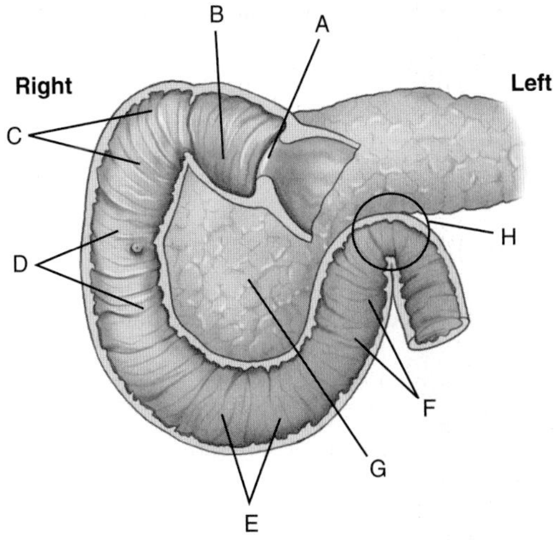

Fig. 12-5. Anatomy of the duodenum and pancreas.

22. Name the two anatomic structures implicated in the phrase "romance of the abdomen" illustrated in Fig. 12-5.

A. _____   B. _____

23. Identify the gastrointestinal structures labeled on Fig. 12-6.

A. _____

B. _____

C. _____

D. _____

E. _____

F. _____

G. _____

H. _____

I. _____

J. _____

K. _____

L. _____

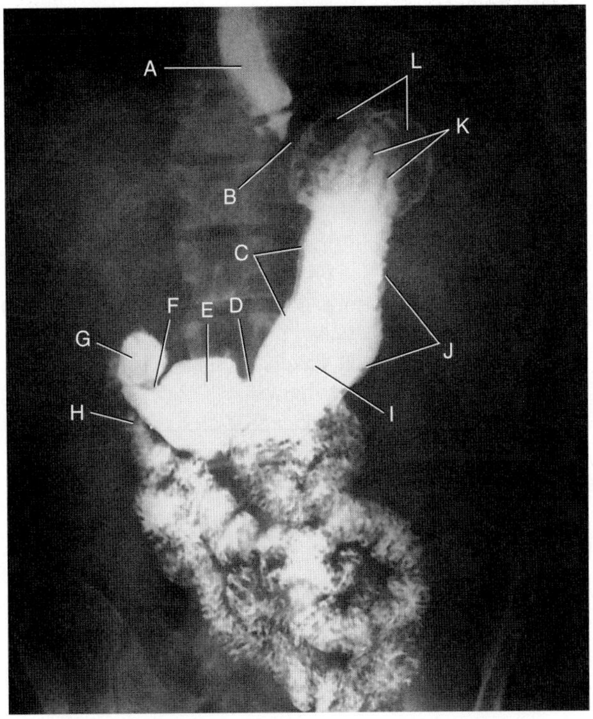

Fig. 12-6. Radiograph of gastrointestinal structures.

1. True/False: Mechanical digestion includes movements of the entire gastrointestinal tract.

2. Peristaltic activity is *not* found in which of the following structures?

   A. Pharynx   C. Stomach

   B. Esophagus   D. Small intestine

3. Stomach contents are churned into a semifluid mass called _____.

4. A churning or mixing activity present in the small bowel is called _____.

5. List the three classes of substances that are ingested and must be chemically digested.

   A. _____   B. _____   C. _____

6. Biologic catalysts that speed up the process of digestion are called _____.

7. List the end products of digestion for the following classes of food:

   A. Carbohydrates: _____

   B. Lipids: _____

   C. Proteins: _____

8. What is the name of the liquid substance that aids in digestion and is manufactured in the liver and stored in the

   gallbladder? _____

9. How does the material from question 8 assist in emulsification in fat?

10. Absorption of nutrients primarily takes place in the (A) _____, although some

    substances are absorbed through the lining of the (B) _____.

11. Of the three primary food substances listed in question 7, the digestion of which one begins in the mouth?

    _____

12. Any residues of digestion or unabsorbed digestive products are eliminated from the

    _____ as a component of feces.

13. Peristalsis is an example of which type of digestion? _____

14. Which term describes food once it is mixed with gastric secretions in the stomach?

    _____

15. A high and transverse stomach would be found in a(n) _____ patient.

    A. Hypersthenic   C. Hyposthenic

    B. Sthenic   D. Asthenic

16. A J-shaped stomach that is more vertical and lower in the abdomen with the duodenal bulb at the level of L3-L4

    would be found in a(n) _____ patient.

    A. Hypersthenic   C. Hyposthenic/asthenic

    B. Sthenic   D. None of the above

17. On the average, how much will abdominal organs drop in the erect position? _____

18. Name the two abdominal organs most dramatically affected, in relation to location, by body habitus:

    A. _____   B. _____

19. Would the fundus of the stomach be more superior or more inferior when one takes in a deep breath?

    _____ Why? _____

20. Match the types of mechanical digestion and/or movement that occur in each of the following anatomic sites.
    (Each anatomic site may have more than one type of digestion.)

    Anatomic Sites   **Types of Mechanical Digestion**

    _____ 1. Oral cavity   A. Mastication

    _____ 2. Pharynx   B. Deglutition

    _____ 3. Esophagus   C. Peristalsis

    _____ 4. Stomach   D. Mixing

    _____ 5. Small intestine   E. Rhythmic segmentation

PART II: RADIOGRAPHIC POSITIONING
REVIEW EXERCISE D: Contrast Media, Fluoroscopy, and Clinical Indications and Contraindications for Upper Gastrointestinal Studies (see textbook pp. 460-468)

1. True/False: With the use of digital fluoroscopy, the number of postfluoroscopy radiographs ordered has greatly diminished.

2. Another term for a negative contrast medium is _____.

3. What substance is most commonly ingested to produce carbon dioxide gas as a negative contrast medium for gastrointestinal studies?

   _____

4. What is the most common form of positive contrast medium used for studies of the gastrointestinal system?

   _____

5. Is a mixture of barium sulfate a suspension or a solution? _____

6. True/False: Barium sulfate never dissolves in water.

7. True/False: Certain salts of barium are poisonous to humans, so barium contrast studies require a pure sulfate salt of barium for human consumption during GI studies.

8. What is the ratio of water to barium for a thin mixture of barium sulfate?

_____

9. What is the chemical symbol for barium sulfate? _____

10. When is the use of barium sulfate contraindicated? _____

11. What patient condition prevents the use of a water-soluble contrast medium for an upper GI?

_____

12. What is the major advantage for using a double-contrast medium technique for esophagrams and upper GIs?

_____

13. The speed with which barium sulfate passes through the GI tract is called gastric

_____.

14. What is the purpose of the gas with a double-contrast media technique?

_____

15. Which of the following devices on a digital fluoroscopy system converts the analog into a digital signal?
    A. PACS   C. CCD
    B. Light converter   D. OTS

16. What device (found beneath the radiographic table when correctly positioned) greatly reduces exposure to the technologist from the fluoroscopic x-ray tube?

    A. Lead skirt   B. Lead drape   C. Bucky slot shield   D. Fluoroscopy tube shield

17. How is the device referred to in question 16 activated or placed in its correct position for fluoroscopy?

_____

18. What is the *minimum* level of protective apron worn during fluoroscopy?
    A. 0.25 mm Pb/Eq apron   C. 1.0 mm Pb/Eq apron
    B. 0.5 mm Pb/Eq apron   D. 1.5 mm Pb/Eq apron

19. What is the major benefit of using a compression paddle during an upper GI study?
    A. Reduces exposure to the patient   C. Reduces exposure to arms and hands of radiologist
    B. Reduces exposure to the eyes of radiologist D. Reduces exposure to the torso of radiologist

20. During an upper GI fluoroscopy procedure, if the technologist stands directly beside the radiologist next to the patient's head and shoulders (see textbook, p. 66 zone C in Fig. 1-188), how much radiation would the technologist receive to the lead apron at waist level during each fluoroscopic exam if the radiologist averaged 5 minutes of fluoroscopy exposure per patient? (Hint: Determine the exposure dose range in mR/min in zone C

    and multiply by 5 minutes.) _____

21. List the three cardinal principles of radiation protection:

    A. _____   B. _____   C. _____

22. Which one of the three cardinal principles is most effective in reducing exposure to the technologist during a

fluoroscopic procedure? _____

23. List the four advantages or unique features and capabilities of digital fluoroscopy over conventional fluoroscopic recording systems:

A. _____   C. _____

B. _____   D. _____

24. Which capability on most digital fluoroscopy systems demonstrates dynamic flow of contrast media through the

GI tract? _____

25. Match the following definitions or descriptions to the correct pathologic condition for the esophagram:

_____ A. Difficulty in swallowing

_____ B. Replacement of normal squamous epithelium with columnar epithelium

_____ C. May lead to esophagitis

_____ D. May be secondary to cirrhosis of the liver

_____ E. Large outpouching of the esophagus

_____ F. Also called cardiospasm

_____ G. Most common form is adenocarcinoma

1. Achalasia

2. Zenker's diverticulum

3. Esophageal varices

4. Carcinoma of esophagus

5. Barrett's esophagus

6. GERD

7. Dysphagia

26. Match the following definitions or descriptions to the correct pathology for the upper GI series:

_____ A. Blood in vomit

_____ B. Inflammation of lining of stomach

_____ C. Blind outpouching of the mucosal wall

_____ D. Undigested material trapped in stomach

_____ E. Synonymous with gastric or duodenal ulcer

_____ F. Portion of stomach protruding through the diaphragmatic opening

_____ G. Only 5% of ulcers lead to this condition

_____ H. Double-contrast upper GI is recommended for this type of tumor

1. Hiatal hernia

2. Gastric carcinoma

3. Bezoar

4. Hematemesis

5. Gastritis

6. Perforating ulcer

7. Peptic ulcer

8. Diverticula

27. Match the following pathologic conditions or diseases to the correct radiographic appearance:

_____ A. Its presence indicates a possible sliding hiatal hernia   1. Ulcers

_____ B. Speckled appearance of gastric mucus   2. Hiatal hernia

_____ C. "Wormlike" appearance of esophagus   3. Achalasia

_____ D. Stricture of esophagus   4. Zenker's diverticulum

_____ E. Gastric bubble above diaphragm   5. Schatzki's ring

_____ F. Irregular filling defect within stomach   6. Gastritis

_____ G. Enlarged recess in proximal esophagus   7. Esophageal varices

_____ H. "Lucent-halo" sign during upper GI   8. Gastric carcinoma

28. Which procedure is often performed to detect early signs of GERD? _____

29. Which specific structure of the gastrointestinal system is affected by HPS? _____

30. Which imaging modality is most effective in diagnosing HPS while reducing dose to the patient?

_____

REVIEW EXERCISE E: Patient Preparation and Positioning for Esophagogram and Upper Gastrointestinal Study (see textbook pp. 469-486)

1. What does the acronym *NPO* stand for, and what does it mean? _____

2. True/False: The patient must be NPO 4 to 6 hours before an esophagram.

3. True/False: The esophagogram usually begins with fluoroscopy with the patient in the erect position.

4. What materials may be used for swallowing to aid in the diagnosis of radiolucent foreign bodies in the esophagus?

_____

5. List the four radiographic tests that may be performed to detect signs of GERD (gastroesophageal reflux disease):

A. _____   C. _____

B. _____   D. _____

6. A breathing technique in which the patient takes in a deep breath and bears down is called the

_____.

7. What position is the patient usually placed in during the water test? _____

8. Which region of the GI tract is better visualized when the radiologist uses a compression paddle during an

esophagram? _____

9. What type of contrast medium should be used if the patient has a history of bowel perforation?

   _____.

10. What is the minimum amount of time that the patient should be NPO before an upper GI?

    _____.

11. Why should cigarette use and gum chewing be restricted before an upper GI?

    _____.

12. Why should the technologist review the patient's chart before the beginning of an upper GI?

    A. To identify any known allergies   C. To look for pertinent clinical history

    B. To ensure that the proper study has been ordered   D. All of the above

13. In which hand does the patient usually hold the barium cup during the start of an upper GI?

    _____

14. List the suggested dosages of barium sulfate during an upper GI for each of the following pediatric age groups:

    Newborn to 1 year: _____

    1 to 3 years: _____

    3 to 10 years: _____

    More than 10 years: _____

15. What type of fluoroscopy generator is recommended for pediatric procedures?

    _____

16. Which one of the following modalities is an alternative to an esophagram in detecting esophageal varices?

    A. Nuclear medicine   C. Sonography

    B. Computed tomography   D. Endoscopy

17. Gastric emptying studies are performed using:

    A. Intraesophageal sonography   C. Magnetic resonance imaging

    B. Radionuclides   D. Computed tomography

18. Why is the RAO preferred over the LAO for an esophagram? _____

19. How much rotation of the body should be used for the RAO projection of the esophagus?

    _____

20. Which optional position should be performed to demonstrate the upper esophagus located between the shoulders?

    _____

21. The three most common routine projections for an esophagram are:

    A. _____   B. _____   C. _____

22. Which aspect of the GI tract is best demonstrated with an RAO position during an upper GI?

    A. Fundus of stomach   C. Body of stomach

    B. Pylorus of stomach and C-loop   D. Fourth (ascending) portion of duodenum

23. How much rotation of the body is required for the RAO position during an upper GI on a sthenic patient?

    A. 30° to 35°   C. 40° to 70°

    B. 15° to 20°   D. 10° to 15°

24. What is the average kV range for an esophagram and upper GI when using barium sulfate (single-contrast study)?

_____

25. Which aspect of the upper GI tract will be filled with barium in the PA projection (prone position)?

_____

26. What is the purpose of the PA axial projection for the hypersthenic patient during an upper GI?

_____

27. What CR angle is required for the PA axial projection for a hypersthenic patient during an upper GI?

    A. 10° to 15° caudad   C. 35° to 45° cephalad

    B. 20° to 25° cephalad   D. 60° to 70° cephalad

28. Which projection taken during an upper GI will best demonstrate the retrogastric space?

    A. RAO   C. LPO

    B. Lateral   D. PA

29. What is the recommended kV range for a double-contrast upper GI projection?

_____

30. The upper GI series usually begins with the table and patient in the _____ position.

31. The five most common routine projections for an upper GI series are (not counting a possible AP scout projection):

    A. _____   C. _____   E. _____

    B. _____   D. _____

32. The major parts of the stomach on an average patient are usually confined to which abdominal quadrant?

_____

33. Most of the duodenum is usually found to the _____ (right or left) of the midline on a sthenic patient.

34. True/False: Respiration should be suspended during inspiration for upper GI radiographic projections.

1. **Situation:** A radiograph of an RAO projection taken during an esophagogram demonstrates incomplete filling of the esophagus with barium. What can the technologist do to ensure better filling of the esophagus during the repeat exposure?

   _____

   _____

2. **Situation:** A series of radiographs taken during an upper GI reveals that the stomach mucosa is not well visualized. The following factors were used during this positioning routine: high-speed screens, Bucky, 40-inch (102-cm) SID, 80 kV, 30 mAs, and 300 mL of barium sulfate ingested during the procedure. Which exposure factor should be changed to produce a more diagnostic study?

   _____

   _____

3. **Situation:** A radiograph taken during an upper GI (double-contrast study) reveals that the anatomic side marker is missing. The technologist is unsure whether it is a recumbent AP or PA projection. The fundus of the stomach is filled with barium. Which position does this radiograph represent?

   _____

   _____

4. **Situation:** A radiograph of an RAO projection taken during an upper GI reveals that the duodenal bulb is not well demonstrated and not profiled. The RAO was a 45° oblique performed on a hypersthenic type of patient. What positioning modification needs to be made to produce a better image of the duodenal bulb?

   _____

   _____

5. **Situation:** A radiograph of an upper GI was taken, but the student technologist is unsure of the position. The radiograph demonstrates that the fundus is filled with barium, but the duodenal bulb is air filled and seen in profile. Which position does this radiograph represent?

   _____

   _____

6. **Situation:** A patient with a clinical history of hiatal hernia comes to the radiology department. Which procedure should be performed on this patient to rule out this condition?

   _____

   _____

7. **Situation:** A patient with a possible lacerated duodenum enters the emergency room. The ER physician orders an upper GI to determine the extent of the injury. What type of contrast medium should be used for this examination?

   _____

   _____

8. **Situation:** A patient with a fish bone stuck in his esophagus enters the emergency room. What modification to a standard esophagogram may be needed to locate the foreign body?

_____

_____

9. **Situation:** An upper GI is being performed on a thin, asthenic-type patient. Because of room scheduling conflicts, this patient was brought into your room for the overhead follow-up images following fluoroscopy. Where would you center the CR and the 30- × 35-cm (11- × 14-inch) image receptor to ensure that you included the stomach and duodenal regions?

_____

_____

10. **Situation:** A patient with a clinical history of a possible bezoar comes to the radiology department. What is a bezoar, and what radiographic study should be performed to demonstrate this condition?

_____

_____

11. **Situation:** A radiograph of an RAO position taken during an esophagogram reveals that the esophagus is superimposed over the vertebral column. What positioning error led to this radiographic outcome? What must be altered to eliminate this problem during the repeat exposure?

_____

_____

12. **Situation:** A PA projection taken during an upper GI series performed on an infant reveals that the body and pylorus of the stomach are superimposed. What modification needs to be employed during the repeat exposure to separate these two regions?

_____

_____

13. **Situation:** A patient comes to radiology with a clinical history of possible gastric diverticulum in the posterior aspect of the fundus. Which projection taken during the upper GI series best demonstrates this defect?

_____

_____

14. **Situation:** A patient comes to radiology with a clinical history of Barrett's esophagus. In addition to an esophagogram, what other imaging modality is ideal in demonstrating this condition?

_____

_____

15. **Situation:** A patient has a clinical history of hemochromatosis. Which imaging modality is most effective in diagnosing this condition?

_____

_____

PART III: LABORATORY EXERCISES

You must gain experience in positioning each part of the esophagram and upper GI procedures before performing the following exams on actual patients. You can get experience in positioning and radiographic evaluation of these projections by performing exercises using radiographic phantoms and practicing on other students (although you will not be taking actual exposures).

Laboratory Exercise A: Radiographic Evaluation

1. Evaluate and critique the radiographs produced during the previous experiments, additional radiographs of esophagrams and upper GI procedures provided by your instructor, or both. Evaluate each position for the following points (check off when completed):

   _____ Evaluate the completeness of the study. (Are all the pertinent anatomic structures included on the radiograph?)

   _____ Evaluate for positioning or centering errors (e.g., rotation, off centering).

   _____ Evaluate for correct exposure factors and possible motion. (Are the density and contrast of the images acceptable?)

   _____ Determine whether anatomic side markers and an acceptable degree of collimation and/or area shielding are visible on the images.

Laboratory Exercise B: Physical Positioning

On another person, simulate performing all routine and special projections of the upper GI as follows. Include the six steps listed in the following and described in the textbook. (Check off each step when it is completed satisfactorily.)

Step 1. Appropriate size and type of image receptor holder with correct markers

Step 2. Correct CR placement and centering of part to CR and/or image receptor

Step 3. Accurate collimation

Step 4. Area shielding of patient where advisable

Step 5. Use of proper immobilizing devices when needed

Step 6. Approximate correct exposure factors, breathing instructions where applicable, and initiating exposure

Projections	Step 1	Step 2	Step 3	Step 4	Step 5	Step 6
● RAO esophagogram	_____	_____	_____	_____	_____	_____
● Left lateral esophagogram	_____	_____	_____	_____	_____	_____
● AP (PA) esophagogram	_____	_____	_____	_____	_____	_____
● LAO esophagogram	_____	_____	_____	_____	_____	_____
● Soft tissue lateral esophagogram	_____	_____	_____	_____	_____	_____
● RAO upper GI	_____	_____	_____	_____	_____	_____
● PA upper GI	_____	_____	_____	_____	_____	_____
● Right lateral upper GI	_____	_____	_____	_____	_____	_____
● LPO upper GI	_____	_____	_____	_____	_____	_____
● AP upper GI	_____	_____	_____	_____	_____	_____

This self-test should be taken only after completing all of the readings, review exercises, and laboratory activities for a particular section. The purpose of this test is not only to provide a good learning exercise but also to serve as a strong indicator of what your final evaluation exam for this chapter will cover. It is strongly suggested that if you do not get at least a 90% to 95% grade on each self-test, you should review those areas in which you missed questions before going to your instructor for the final evaluation exam.

1. The gallbladder is located in the _____ margin of the liver.

   A. Posterior inferior   C. Midaspect

   B. Posterior superior   D. Anterior superior

2. Which one of the following is not a recognized lobe of the liver?

   A. Caudate   C. Inferior

   B. Quadrate   D. Left

3. In which quadrant is the liver located in the sthenic patient?

   A. Right lower quadrant   C. Left upper quadrant

   B. Left lower quadrant   D. Right upper quadrant

4. What is the name of the soft tissue structure that divides the liver into left and right lobes?

   _____

5. What is the primary function of bile?

   _____

6. Which duct is formed by the union of the left and right hepatic ducts?

   _____

7. Which duct carries bile from the cystic duct to the duodenum?

   _____

8. What is the average capacity of the gallbladder?

   _____

9. Which process leads to concentration of bile within the gallbladder?

   _____

10. Which hormone leads to contraction of the gallbladder to release bile?

   _____

11. Match each of the following biliary structures to its correct description or definition:

_____ 1. Pancreatic duct

_____ 2. Fundus

_____ 3. Hepatopancreatic ampulla

_____ 4. Spiral valve

_____ 5. Hepatopancreatic sphincter

_____ 6. Duodenal papilla

_____ 7. Cystic duct

_____ 8. Neck

_____ 9. Body

A. Series of mucosal folds in cystic duct

B. A protrusion into the duodenum

C. Middle aspect of gallbladder

D. Duct connected directly to gallbladder

E. Narrowest portion of gallbladder

F. Broadest portion of gallbladder

G. Enlarged chamber in distal aspect of common bile duct

H. Duct of Wirsung

I. Circular muscle fibers adjacent to duodenal papilla

12. Identify the labeled parts and/or structures on the radiograph of an OCG (Fig. 12-7):

A. _____

B. _____

C. _____

D. _____

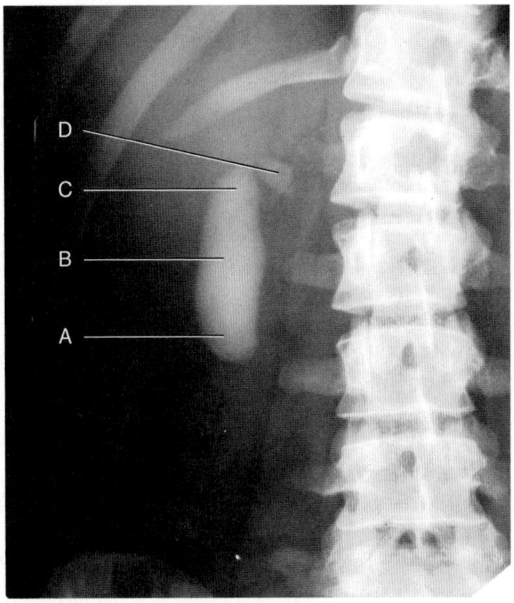

Fig. 12-7. Radiograph of an OCG and of biliary ducts.

13. Which of the following terms describes the condition of having gallstones?

A. Cholecystitis

B. Cholelithiasis

C. Cholecystectomy

D. Choleliths

14. Which one of the following is *not* a function of the gastrointestinal system?

A. Intake and digestion of food

B. Absorption of nutrients

C. Production of hormones

D. Elimination of waste products

15. What is another term for an esophagogram?

_____

16. Which one of the following is *not* a salivary gland?

   A. Parotid   C. Vallecula

   B. Sublingual   D. Submandibular

17. What is the name of the condition that results from a viral infection of the parotid gland?

_____

18. Which structure in the pharynx prevents aspiration of food and fluid into the larynx?

   A. Uvula   C. Soft palate

   B. Epiglottis   D. Laryngopharynx

19. The esophagus extends from C5-C6 to:

   A. T9   C. T10

   B. L1   D. T11

20. Which one of the following structures does not pass through the diaphragm?

   A. Trachea   C. Aorta

   B. Esophagus   D. Inferior vena cava

21. Wavelike involuntary contractions that help propel food down the esophagus are called

_____

22. The Greek term *gaster*, or *gastro*, means _____.

23. Which one of the following aspects of the stomach is defined as an indentation between the body and pylorus?

   A. Cardiac antrum   C. Cardiac notch (incisura cardiaca)

   B. Pyloric antrum   D. Angular notch (incisura angularis)

24. True/False: The numerous mucosal folds found in the small bowel are called rugae.

25. Which aspect of the stomach fills with air when the patient is prone?

   A. Fundus   C. Duodenal bulb

   B. Body   D. Pylorus

26. True/False: The lateral margin of the stomach is called the lesser curvature.

27. Which aspect of the stomach does barium gravitate to when the patient is in the supine position?

_____

28. Which two structures create the "romance of the abdomen"?

_____

29. Match each of the following aspects of the upper gastrointestinal system with the correct definition.

_____ 1. Pyloric orifice

_____ 2. Cardiac notch

_____ 3. Fundus

_____ 4. Fourth portion of duodenum

_____ 5. Mucosal folds

_____ 6. Body

_____ 7. Esophagogastric junction

_____ 8. Angular notch

_____ 9. Third portion of duodenum

A. Middle aspect of stomach

B. Horizontal portion of duodenum

C. Rugae

D. Opening between esophagus and stomach

E. Opening leaving the stomach

F. Found along superior aspect of fundus

G. Indentation found along lesser curvature

H. Ascending portion of duodenum

I. Most posterior aspect of stomach

30. Identify the structures labeled on Fig. 12-8:

A. _____

B. _____

C. _____

D. _____

E. _____

F. _____

G. _____

H. _____

I. _____

J. _____

K. _____

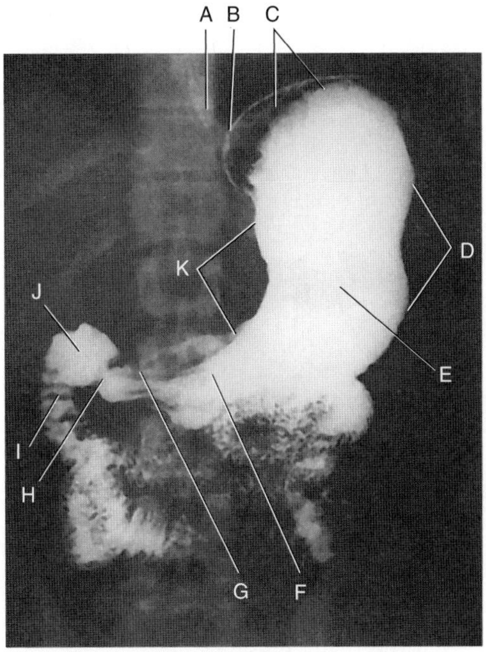

Fig. 12-8. Radiograph of gastrointestinal structures, demonstrating body position.

31. A. Which radiographic position does Fig. 12-8 represent? _____

B. How could you determine this? _____

32. Which radiographic position does Fig. 12-9 represent?

_____

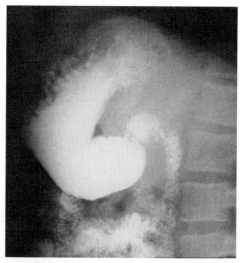

Fig. 12-9. Gastrointestinal radiograph demonstrating body position.

33. A. Which radiographic position does Fig. 12-10 represent? _____

   B. How could you determine this? _____

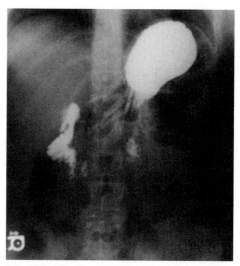

Fig. 12-10. Gastrointestinal radiograph demonstrating body position.

34. A. Fig. 12-11 represents a(n) _____ (anterior or posterior) oblique position.

   B. How could you determine this? _____

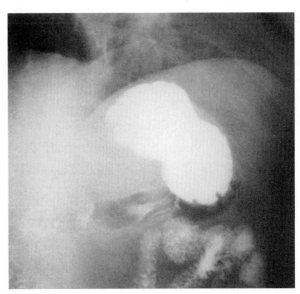

Fig. 12-11. Oblique radiograph of gastrointestinal structures.

   C. Which specific radiographic position does Fig. 12-12 represent? _____

   D. How could you determine this? _____

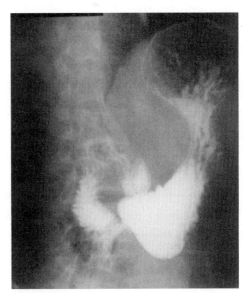

Fig. 12-12. Oblique radiograph of gastrointestinal structures.

35. The act of chewing is termed:

    A. Mastication   C. Aspiration

    B. Deglutition   D. Peristalsis

36. Which term describes food once it enters the stomach and is mixed with gastric fluids?

    _____

37. The churning or mixing activity of chyme in the small intestine is called:

    A. Peristalsis   C. Rhythmic segmentation

    B. Deglutition   D. Digestion

38. Which one of the following nutrients is not digested?

    A. Vitamins   C. Carbohydrates

    B. Lipids   D. Proteins

39. A high and transverse stomach indicates a _____ body type with the pyloric

    portion at the vertebral level of _____.

40. A _____ or _____ type of body habitus usually has
    a low and vertical stomach with the pyloric portion of the stomach at the vertebral level of

    _____.

41. What is the most common radiopaque contrast media used in the gastrointestinal system?

    _____

42. What type of radiolucent contrast medium is most commonly used for double-contrast gastrointestinal studies?

    _____

43. A. What is the ratio of barium to water for a thick mixture of barium sulfate? _____

    B. What is the ratio for a thin barium mixture? _____

44. When should a water-soluble contrast medium be used during an upper GI rather than barium sulfate?

    _____

45. Which one of the following conditions may prevent the use of water-soluble contrast agents for a geriatric patient?

    A. Bowel obstruction   C. Dehydration

    B. Chronic aspiration   D. Perforated ulcer

46. True/False: Water-soluble contrast agents pass through the gastrointestinal tract faster than barium sulfate.

47. True/False: Digital fluoroscopy does not require the use of image receptor cassettes.

48. Which of the cardinal principles of radiation protection is most effective in reducing exposure to the technologist

    during fluoroscopy? _____

49. Protective aprons of lead equivalency must be worn during fluoroscopy?

    A. 1.0 mm Pb/Eq
    C. 0.25 mm Pb/Eq
    B. 0.50 mm Pb/Eq
    D. 0.15 mm Pb/Eq

50. Which one of the following is the older term for GERD?

    A. Esophageal reflux
    C. Esophageal varices
    B. Barrett's esophagus
    D. Zenker's diverticulum

51. A large outpouching of the upper esophagus is termed:

    A. Zenker's diverticulum
    C. Barrett's esophagus
    B. Achalasia
    D. Esophageal varices

52. A phytobezoar is:

    A. An outpouching of the mucosal wall
    C. A rare tumor
    B. Trapped mass of hair in the stomach
    D. Trapped vegetable fiber in the stomach

53. What can be added to barium sulfate and swallowed to detect a radiolucent foreign body lodged in the esophagus?

    _____

54. What is the reason that the patient may be asked to swallow a mouthful of water drawn through a straw during an esophagogram?

    _____

55. How much rotation of the body should be used for an RAO esophagogram projection?

    _____

56. Why is an RAO position preferred rather than an LAO during an esophagogram?

    _____

57. Why is the AP projection of the esophagus not a preferred projection for the esophagogram series?

    _____

58. What criterion is used with ultrasound in determining whether a patient has HPS?

    A. Abnormally long pylorus
    C. Presence of air-fluid level in the duodenum
    B. Absence of rugae
    D. Antral muscle thickness exceeding 4 mm

59. Other than the esophagogram, what other imaging modality is performed to diagnose Barrett's esophagus?

    A. Computed tomography
    C. Magnetic resonance
    B. Nuclear medicine
    D. Sonography

60. Which upper GI position best demonstrates a possible gastric diverticulum in the posterior wall of the fundus of the stomach?

    _____

61. **Situation:** An upper GI series is performed on an asthenic patient. A radiograph of the RAO position reveals that the duodenal bulb and C loop are not in profile. The technologist rotated the patient 70 degrees. What modification of the position is required during the repeat exposure?

62. **Situation:** A radiograph taken during a double-contrast upper GI demonstrates that the fundus is barium filled and that the body is air filled. This was either an AP or a PA radiograph, which needs to be repeated. Which specific position does this radiograph represent?

63. **Situation:** A patient with a clinical history of cirrhosis of the liver with acute GI bleeding comes to the radiology department. What may be the most likely reason that an esophagram was ordered for this patient?

64. **Situation:** During an esophagram, the radiologist asks the patient to try to bear down as if having a bowel movement. What is this maneuver called, and why did the radiologist make such a request?

65. **Situation:** During an upper GI, the radiologist reports that she sees a "lucent-halo" sign in the duodenum. What form of pathology did the radiologist observe?

66. Which one of the following technical/positioning factors does not apply to a MD-Gastroview upper GI study?

    A. 125 kV

    B. Exposure made on expiration

    C. 40-inch (102-cm) SID

    D. Erect and recumbent positions performed

67. **Situation:** A radiograph of an upper GI is not labeled correctly, and the technologist is unsure which position was performed. A double-contrast GI study was completed with all positions performed recumbent. The radiograph demonstrates barium in the fundus and air in the body and pylorus and duodenal bulb in profile. Which position was performed?

68. Which one of the following shielding devices best reduces exposure to the lower torso of the fluoroscopist?

    A. Lead drape

    B. Bucky shield

    C. Lead gloves

    D. Grid

69. **Situation:** During an esophagogram, the radiologist remarks that Schatzki's ring is present. Which condition or disease process is indicated by the presence of this radiographic sign?

70. **Situation:** A patient comes to radiology with a clinical history of a possible trichobezoar. What is a trichobezoar and which radiographic procedure is best to diagnose it?

13 Lower Gastrointestinal System

CHAPTER OBJECTIVES

After you have successfully completed the activities in this chapter, you will be able to:

_____ 1. List three divisions of the small intestine and the major parts of the large intestine.

_____ 2. Identify the function, location, and pertinent anatomy of the small and large intestine.

_____ 3. Differentiate between the terms colon and large intestine.

_____ 4. On drawings and radiographs, identify specific anatomy of the lower gastrointestinal canal from the duodenum through the anus.

_____ 5. Identify the sectional differences that differentiate the large intestine from the small intestine.

_____ 6. List specific clinical indications and contraindications for a small bowel series and a barium enema examination.

_____ 7. Match specific types of pathology to the correct radiographic appearances and signs.

_____ 8. Identify patient preparation for a small bowel series and barium enema.

_____ 9. List five safety concerns that must be followed during a barium enema procedure.

_____ 10. Identify the radiographic procedure and sequence for a small bowel series.

_____ 11. Identify the purpose, clinical indications, and methodology for the enteroclysis, CT enteroclysis, computed tomography colonography, and the intubation small bowel method procedures.

_____ 12. Identify the patient preparation, room preparation, and fluoroscopic procedure for a barium enema.

_____ 13. Identify the purpose, clinical indications, and methodology for an evacuative proctogram.

_____ 14. Identify the correct procedure for inserting a rectal enema tube.

_____ 15. List specific information related to the routine positions or projections of a small bowel series and barium enema examination to include size and type of image receptor, central ray location, direction and angulation of the central ray, and the anatomy best demonstrated.

_____ 16. Identify the advantages, procedure, and positioning for an air-contrast barium enema.

_____ 17. Given various hypothetic situations, identify the correct modification of a position and/or exposure considerations to improve the radiographic image.

POSITIONING AND RADIOGRAPHIC TECHNIQUE

——— 1. Using a peer, position for routine and special projections for the small bowel and barium enema series.

——— 2. Critique and evaluate small bowel and barium enema series radiographs based on the five divisions of radiographic criteria: (1) anatomy demonstrated, (2) position, (3) collimation and CR, (4) exposure, and (5) anatomic side markers.

——— 3. Distinguish between acceptable and unacceptable small bowel and barium enema series radiographs resulting from exposure factors, motion, collimation, positioning, or other errors.

LEARNING EXERCISES

Complete the following review exercises after reading the associated pages in the textbook as indicated by each exercise. Answers to each review exercise are given at the end of the review exercises.

PART I: RADIOGRAPHIC ANATOMY
REVIEW EXERCISE A: Radiographic Anatomy of the Lower Gastrointestinal System (see textbook pp. 488-492)

1. A. How long is the average small bowel if removed and stretched out during autopsy?

_____

B. In a person with good muscle tone, the length of the entire small intestine is _____.

C. The average length of the large intestine is _____.

2. List the three divisions of the small intestine in descending order, starting with the widest division:

A. _____   B. _____   C. _____

3. Which division of the small intestine is the shortest? _____

4. In which two abdominal quadrants would the majority of the jejunum be found?

_____

5. Which division of the small intestine has a feathery or coiled-spring appearance during a small bowel series?

_____

6. Which division of the small intestine is the longest? _____

7. Which two aspects of the large intestine are not considered part of the colon?

_____

8. The colon is divided into _____ sections and has _____ flexures.

9. List the two functions of the ileocecal valve:

A. _____

B. _____

10. What is another term for the appendix? _____

11. Match the following aspects of the small and large intestine to their characteristics:

_____ 1. Jejunum

_____ 2. Duodenum

_____ 3. Ileum

_____ 4. Cecum

_____ 5. Appendix

_____ 6. Ascending colon

_____ 7. Descending colon

_____ 8. Transverse colon

_____ 9. Sigmoid colon

A. Longest aspect of the large intestine

B. Widest portion of the large intestine

C. A blind pouch inferior to the ileocecal valve

D. Aspect of small intestine that is the smallest in diameter but longest in length

E. Distal part; also called the iliac colon

F. Shortest aspect of small intestine

G. Lies in pelvis but possesses a wide freedom of motion

H. Makes up 40% of the small intestine

I. Found between the cecum and transverse colon

12. A. What is the term for the three bands of muscle that pull the large intestine into pouches?

_____

B. These pouches, or sacculations, seen along the large intestine wall are called

_____.

13. What is an older term for the mucosal folds found within the jejunum? _____

14. Identify the structures labeled on Figs. 13-1 and 13-2. Include secondary names in parentheses where indicated.

Fig. 13-1

A. _____ (___)

B. _____

C. _____

D. _____

E. ___ (_____) ___

F. _____

G. ___ (_____) ___

H. _____

I. _____

J. _____

K. _____

L. _____

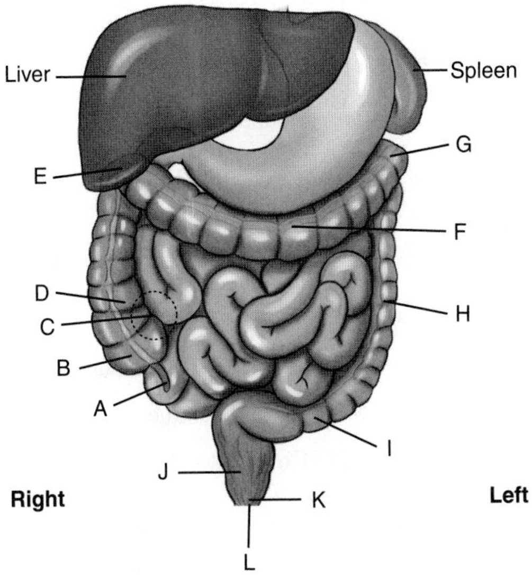

Fig. 13-1. Structures of the lower gastrointestinal tract, anterior view.

Fig. 13-2

M. _____

N. _____

O. _____

P. _____

Q. _____

R. _____

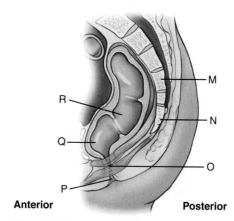

Fig. 13-2. Structures of the lower gastrointestinal tract, lateral view.

15. Which portion of the small intestine is located primarily to the left of the midline?

_____

16. Which portion of the small intestine is located primarily in the RLQ? _____

17. Which portion of the small intestine has the smoothest internal lining and does not present a feathery appearance when barium-filled? _____

18. Which aspect of the small intestine is most fixed in position? _____

19. In which quadrant does the terminal ileum connect with the large intestine? _____

20. Which muscular band marks the junction between the duodenum and jejunum?

_____

21. The widest portion of the large intestine is the _____.

22. Which flexure of the large intestine usually extends more superiorly? _____

23. Inflammation of the vermiform appendix is called _____.

24. Which of the following structures will fill with air during a double-contrast barium enema with the patient supine? (More than one answer may be correct.)

   A. Ascending colon   C. Rectum   E. Descending colon

   B. Transverse colon   D. Sigmoid colon

25. Which aspect of the GI tract is primarily responsible for digestion, absorption, and reabsorption?

   A. Small intestine   C. Large intestine

   B. Stomach   D. Colon

26. Which aspect of the GI tract is responsible for the synthesis and absorption of vitamins B and K and amino acids?

   A. Duodenum   C. Large intestine

   B. Jejunum   D. Stomach

27. Four types of digestive movements occurring in the large intestine are listed below. Which one of these movement types also occurs in the small intestine?

    A. Peristalsis   C. Mass peristalsis

    B. Haustral churning   D. Defecation

28. Identify the gastrointestinal structures labeled on Fig. 13-3.

    A. _____

    B. _____ (region)

    C. _____

    D. _____

    E. _____ (region)

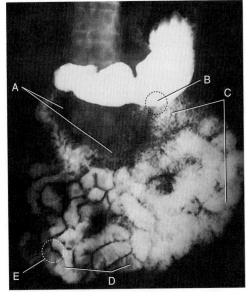

Fig. 13-3. Structure identification on a PA 30-minute small bowel radiograph.

29. Identify the gastrointestinal structures labeled on Fig. 13-4.

    A. _____

    B. _____

    C. _____

    D. _____

    E. _____

    F. _____

    G. _____

    H. _____

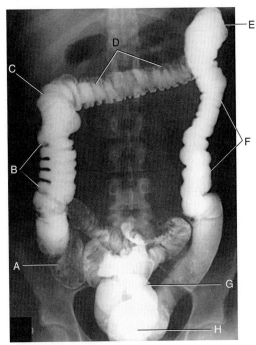

Fig. 13-4. Structure identification on an AP barium enema radiograph.

30. Classify the following structures as being **intraperitoneal, retroperitoneal**, or **infraperitoneal.**

———— 1. Cecum

———— 2. Ascending colon

———— 3. Transverse colon

———— 4. Descending colon

———— 5. Sigmoid colon

———— 6. Upper rectum

———— 7. Lower rectum

———— 8. C loop of duodenum

———— 9. Jejunum

———— 10. Ileum

A. Intraperitoneal

B. Retroperitoneal

C. Infraperitoneal

REVIEW EXERCISE B: Clinical Indications and Radiographic Procedures for the Small Bowel Series and Barium Enema (see textbook pp. 493-512)

1. Which of the following conditions pertains to a radiographic study of the small intestine?

A. May perform as a double-contrast media study

B. An enteroclysis procedure

C. Timing of the procedure is necessary

D. All of the above

2. List the two conditions that may prevent the use of barium sulfate during a small bowel series:

A. _____   B. _____

3. What type of patients should be given extra care when using a water-soluble contrast medium?

_____ and _____.

4. Match the following definitions or statements to the correct clinical indications for the small bowel series:

———— A. Common birth defect found in the ileum

———— B. Common parasitic infection of the small intestine

———— C. Obstruction of the small intestine

———— D. Patient with lactose or sucrose sensitivities

———— E. New growth

———— F. A form of sprue

———— G. Inflammation of the intestine

———— H. Form of inflammatory disease of the GI tract

1. Ileus

2. Neoplasm

3. Meckel's diverticulum

4. Malabsorption syndrome

5. Enteritis

6. Celiac disease

7. Regional enteritis

8. Giardiasis

5. Match the following pathologic conditions or diseases to the correct radiographic appearance:

_____ A. Circular staircase or herringbone sign

_____ B. Cobblestone appearance

_____ C. Apple core sign

_____ D. Dilation of the intestine with thickening of circular folds

_____ E. Large diverticulum of the ileum

_____ F. "Beak sign"

1. Adenocarcinoma

2. Meckel's diverticulum

3. Ileus

4. Giardiasis

5. Regional enteritis

6. Volvulus

6. Giardiasis is a condition acquired through:

A. Contaminated food

B. Contaminated water

C. Person-to-person contact

D. All of the above

7. Meckel's diverticulum is best diagnosed with which imaging modality?

A. Small bowel series

B. Enteroclysis

C. Magnetic resonance imaging

D. Nuclear medicine

8. Whipple's disease is a rare disorder of the:

A. Distal small intestine

B. Proximal small intestine

C. Proximal large intestine

D. Distal large intestine

9. How much barium sulfate is generally given to an adult patient for a small-bowel-only series?

_____

10. When is a small bowel series deemed completed? _____

11. How long does it usually take to complete an adult small bowel series? _____

12. When is the first radiograph generally taken during a small bowel series? _____

13. True/False: Fluoroscopy is sometimes used during a small bowel series to visualize the ileocecal valve.

14. The term enteroclysis describes what type of a small bowel study? _____

15. What two types of contrast media are used for an enteroclysis? _____

16. Which two pathologic conditions are best evaluated through an enteroclysis procedure?

_____

17. True/False: It takes approximately 12 hours for barium sulfate in a healthy adult, given orally, to reach the rectum.

18. The tip of the catheter is advanced to the _____ during an enteroclysis.

A. Duodenojejunal flexure (suspensory ligament)

B. C loop of duodenum

C. Pyloric sphincter

D. Ileocecal sphincter

19. What is the purpose of introducing methylcellulose during an enteroclysis? _____

20. A procedure to alleviate postoperative distention of a small intestine obstruction is called:

   A. Diagnostic intubation   C. Therapeutic intubation

   B. Enteroclysis   D. Small bowel series

21. What is the recommended patient preparation before a small bowel series? _____

22. Which position is recommended for small bowel radiographs? Why? _____

23. Match the following definitions or statements to the correct clinical indication for the barium enema procedure:

   _____ A. A twisting of a portion of the intestine on its own mesentery   1. Polyp

   _____ B. Outpouching of the mucosal wall   2. Diverticulum

   _____ C. Inflammatory condition of the large intestine   3. Intussusception

   _____ D. Severe form of colitis   4. Volvulus

   _____ E. Telescoping of one part of the intestine into another   5. Ulcerative colitis

   _____ F. Inward growth extending from the lumen of the intestinal wall   6. Colitis

24. Which type of patient usually experiences intussusception? _____

25. A condition of numerous herniations of the mucosal wall of the large intestine is called

   _____

26. Which one of the following pathologic conditions may produce a "tapered or corkscrew" radiographic sign during a barium enema?

   A. Diverticulosis   C. Volvulus

   B. Ulcerative colitis   D. Diverticulitis

27. Which one of the following conditions may produce the "cobblestone" radiographic sign during a barium enema?

   A. Ulcerative colitis   C. Diverticulosis

   B. Appendicitis   D. Adenocarcinoma

28. What is the most common form of carcinoma found in the large intestine?

   A. Simple-cell carcinoma   C. Annular carcinoma

   B. Basal cell carcinoma   D. Complex-cell carcinoma

29. True/False: Intestinal polyps and diverticula are very similar in structure.

30. True/False: Volvulus occurs more frequently in males than females.

31. True/False: The barium enema is a commonly recommended procedure for diagnosing possible acute appendicitis.

32. True/False: Any stool retained in the large intestine may require postponement of a barium enema study.

33. Which four conditions would prevent the use of a laxative cathartic before a barium enema procedure?

    A. _____   C. _____

    B. _____   D. _____

34. True/False: An example of an irritant cathartic is magnesium citrate.

35. List the three types of enema tips commonly used (all are considered single-use and disposable):

    A. _____   B. _____   C. _____

36. True/False: Synthetic latex enema tips or gloves do not cause problems for latex-sensitive patients.

37. What water temperature is recommended for barium enema mixtures? _____

38. To minimize spasm during a barium enema, _____ can be added to the contrast media mixture.

    A. Glucagon   C. Saline

    B. Lidocaine   D. Valium

39. What is the name of the patient position recommended for insertion of the rectal enema tip?

    _____

40. The initial insertion of the rectal enema tip should be pointed toward the:

    A. Symphysis pubis   C. Umbilicus

    B. Bladder   D. Tip of coccyx

41. Which one of the following procedures is most effective to demonstrate small polyps in the colon?

    A. Single-contrast barium enema   C. Enteroclysis

    B. Double-contrast barium enema   D. Evacuative proctogram

42. Which aspect of the large intestine must be demonstrated during evacuative proctography?

    A. Sigmoid colon   C. Anorectal angle

    B. Haustra   D. Rectal ligament

43. Which one of the following clinical conditions is best demonstrated with evacuative proctography?

    A. Intussusception   C. Rectal prolapse

    B. Volvulus   D. Diverticulosis

44. Which one of the following procedures uses the thickest mixture of barium sulfate?

    A. Single-contrast barium enema   C. Evacuative proctogram

    B. Double-contrast barium enema   D. Enteroclysis

45. Into which position is the patient placed for imaging during the evacuative proctogram?

    A. AP spine   C. Ventral decubitus

    B. Left or right lateral decubitus   D. Lateral

46. True/False: A special tapered enema tip is inserted into the stoma before a colostomy barium enema.

47. True/False: The enema bag should not be more than 36 inches (92 cm) above the table top before the beginning of the procedure.

48. True/False: The technologist should review the patient's chart before a barium enema to determine whether a sigmoidoscopy or colonoscopy was performed recently.

49. True/False: Both computed tomography and sonography may be performed to aid in diagnosing appendicitis.

50. True/False: Because of the density and the amount of barium within the large intestine, computed radiography should not be used during a barium enema.

51. Which one of the following statements is true in regard to CT enteroclysis?

    A. A duodenojejunal tube does not have to be inserted for the procedure

    B. 0.1% barium sulfate suspension is often instilled before the procedure

    C. Does not detect obstructions of the small intestine

    D. Is rarely performed today

52. Another term for CT colonography (CTC) is _____.

53. True/False: A cleansing bowel prep is not required before a CTC.

54. Why is oral contrast media sometimes given during a CTC?

    A. To detect small polyps

    B. To detect bleeding outside of the intestinal wall

    C. To mark or "tag" fecal matter

    D. Oral contrast never should be given before a CTC.

55. What is the chief disadvantage of a CT colonography (CTC)?

    A. Cannot remove polyps discovered during CTC

    B. Radiation dose to patient

    C. Inflating the large intestine with air may rupture the intestinal wall

    D. Procedure is painful for the patient

REVIEW EXERCISE C: Positioning of the Lower Gastrointestinal System (see textbook pp. 513-524)

1. True/False: Single-contrast barium enemas are performed commonly on patients with a clinical history of diverticulosis.

2. Which of the following projections is recommended to be taken during a small bowel series?

    A. Supine AP   C. Erect AP

    B. Left lateral decubitus   D. Prone PA

3. True/False: Shielding is not recommended during studies of the lower GI tract. _____

4. Due to faster transit time of barium from the stomach to the ileocecal valve in pediatric patients, how frequently should images be taken during a small bowel series to avoid missing critical anatomy and possible pathology?

5. True/False: If a retention-type enema tip is used, it should be removed after fluoroscopy is completed and before overhead projections are taken to better visualize the rectal region.

6. The _____ position is a recommended alternative for the lateral rectum projection during a double-contrast BE procedure.

7. What kV is recommended for a small bowel series (single contrast study)? _____

8. Where is the CR centered for the 15-minute radiograph during a small bowel series?

   A. Iliac crest   C. 2 inches (5 cm) above iliac crest

   B. Xiphoid process   D. ASIS

9. What are the breathing instructions for a projection taken during a small bowel series?

   _____

10. Generally, a small bowel series is complete once the contrast media reaches the _____.

11. Which type of patient habitus may require two 35- × 43-cm (14- × 17-inch) cross-wise cassettes for an AP barium enema projection?

    A. Hypersthenic   C. Hyposthenic

    B. Sthenic   D. Asthenic

12. Which projection(s) taken during a barium enema best demonstrate(s) the right colic flexure?

    _____

13. How much body rotation is required for oblique barium enema projections?

    _____

14. Which position should be performed if the patient cannot lie prone on the table to visualize the left colic flexure?

    _____

15. Which projection, taken during a double-contrast barium enema, produces an air-filled image of the right colic

    flexure, ascending colon, and cecum? _____

16. Where is the CR centered for a lateral projection of the rectum? _____

17. Which projection during a double-contrast barium enema series best demonstrates the descending colon for possible

    polyps? _____

18. Which aspect of the large intestine is best demonstrated with an AP axial projection?

    _____

19. What is the advantage of performing an AP axial oblique projection rather than an AP axial?

    _____

20. A. What is another term describing the AP and PA axial projections? _____

    B. What CR angle is required for the AP axial? _____

    C. What CR angle is required for the PA axial? _____

21. Which position is recommended for the postevacuation projection taken following a barium enema?

A. PA prone   C. AP erect

B. AP supine   D. Left lateral decubitus

22. What kV range is recommended for a postevacuation projection following a barium enema?

_____

23. A. What is the recommended kV range for oblique projections taken during a single-contrast barium enema study?

_____

    B. What is the recommended kV range for oblique projections taken during a double-contrast study?

_____

24. What medication can be given during a barium enema to minimize colonic spasm during a barium enema?

_____

REVIEW EXERCISE D: Problem Solving for Technical and Positioning Errors

1. **Situation:** A radiograph of a double-contrast barium enema projection reveals an obscured anatomic side marker. The technologist is unsure whether it is an AP or PA recumbent projection. The transverse colon is primarily filled with barium, with the ascending and descending colon containing a lesser amount. Which position does this radiograph represent?

_____

_____

2. **Situation:** A radiograph of a lateral decubitus projection taken during an air-contrast barium enema reveals that the upside aspect of the colon is overpenetrated. The following factors were used during this analog exposure: 120 kV, 30 mAs, 40-inch (102-cm) SID, and compensating filter for the air-filled aspect of the large intestine. Which one of these factors must be modified during the repeat exposure?

_____

_____

3. **Situation:** A radiograph of an AP axial barium enema projection of the rectosigmoid region reveals that there is considerable superimposition of the sigmoid colon and rectum. The following factors were used during this analog exposure: 120 kV, 20 mAs, 40-inch (102-cm) SID, 35° caudad CR angle, and collimation. Which one of these factors must be modified or corrected for the repeat exposure?

_____

_____

4. **Situation:** A barium enema study performed on a hypersthenic patient reveals that the majority of the radiographs demonstrate that the left colic flexure was cut off. What can be done during the repeat exposures to avoid this problem?

_____

_____

5. **Situation:** A technologist has inserted an air-contrast retention tip for a double-contrast BE study. He is not sure how much to inflate the retention balloon. Should he inflate it as much as the patient can tolerate, or is there a better alternative?

_____

_____

6. **Situation:** A student technologist is told to place the patient on the x-ray table in a Sims' position in preparation for the tip insertion for a barium enema. Describe how the patient should be positioned.

_____

_____

7. **Situation:** A patient with a clinical history of regional enteritis comes to the radiology department. What type of procedure would be most diagnostic for this condition?

_____

_____

8. **Situation:** A patient is referred to the radiology department for a presurgical small bowel series. What modification to the standard study needs to be made for this particular patient?

_____

_____

9. **Situation:** A patient comes to the radiology department for a small bowel series. However, because of a stroke, the patient is unable to swallow the contrast medium. What type of study should be performed for this patient?

_____

_____

10. **Situation:** An infant with a possible intussusception is brought to the emergency room. Which radiographic procedure may serve a therapeutic role in correcting this condition?

_____

_____

11. **Situation:** Before a barium enema, the technologist experienced difficulty in inserting the enema rectal tip (without causing significant pain for the patient). What should the technologist do to complete this task?

_____

_____

12. **Situation:** During the fluoroscopy aspect of a barium enema, the radiologist detects an unusual defect within the right colic flexure. She asks that the technologist provide the best images possible of this region. Which two projections will best demonstrate the right colic flexure?

_____

_____

13. **Situation:** A patient with a clinical history of possible enteritis comes to the radiology department. Which type of radiographic GI study would most likely be indicated for this condition? (Of course, this would have to be requested by the referring physician.)

_____

_____

14. **Situation:** A patient's clinical history includes possible giardiasis. What radiographic procedures would likely be indicated for this condition?

_____

_____

15. **Situation:** A patient is scheduled for a computed tomography colonography (CTC). What is the recommended patient preparation for this procedure?

_____

_____

PART II: LABORATORY EXERCISES

You must gain experience in positioning each part of the lower GI before performing the following exams on actual patients. You can get experience in positioning and radiographic evaluation of these projections by performing exercises using radiographic phantoms and practicing on other students (although you will not be taking actual exposures).

Laboratory Exercise A: Radiographic Evaluation

1. Evaluate and critique the radiographs produced during the previous experiments, additional radiographs of esophagrams and lower GI procedures provided by your instructor, or both. Evaluate each projection for the following points (check off when completed):

_____ Evaluate the completeness of the study. (Are all of the pertinent anatomic structures included on the radiograph?)

_____ Evaluate for positioning or centering errors (e.g., rotation, off centering).

_____ Evaluate for correct exposure considerations and possible motion. (Are the density and contrast of the images acceptable?)

_____ Determine whether markers and an acceptable degree of collimation and/or area shielding are visible on the images.

Laboratory Exercise B: Physical Positioning

On another person, simulate performing all routine and special projections of the lower GI as follows. Include the six steps listed in the following and described in the textbook. (Check off each when completed satisfactorily.)

Step 1. Appropriate size and type of image receptor (IR) with correct side markers

Step 2. Correct CR placement and centering of part to CR and/or IR

Step 3. Accurate collimation

Step 4. Area shielding of patient where advisable

Step 5. Use of proper immobilizing devices when needed

Step 6. Approximate correct exposure factors, breathing instructions where applicable, and initiating exposure

Projections	*Step 1*	*Step 2*	*Step 3*	*Step 4*	*Step 5*	*Step 6*
● PA 15- or 30-minute small bowel	___	___	___	___	___	___
● PA 1- or 2-hour small bowel	___	___	___	___	___	___
● PA or AP barium enema	___	___	___	___	___	___
● RAO and LAO barium enema	___	___	___	___	___	___
● LPO and RPO barium enema	___	___	___	___	___	___
● Right and left lateral decubitus	___	___	___	___	___	___
● AP and LPO axial	___	___	___	___	___	___
● PA and RAO axial	___	___	___	___	___	___
● Lateral rectum	___	___	___	___	___	___
● Ventral decubitus lateral rectum	___	___	___	___	___	___

SELF-TEST

MY SCORE = _____%

This self-test should be taken only after completing all of the readings, review exercises, and laboratory activities for a particular section. The purpose of this test is not only to provide a good learning exercise but also to serve as a strong indicator of what your final evaluation exam for this chapter will cover. It is strongly suggested that if you do not get at least a 90% to 95% grade on each self-test, you should review those areas in which you missed questions before going to your instructor for the final evaluation exam.

1. During life, how long is the entire small intestine?

   A. 15 to 18 feet (4.5 to 5.5 m)   C. 5 to 10 feet (1.5 to 3 m)

   B. 20 to 25 feet (6 to 7.5 m)   D. 30 to 40 feet (9 to 12 m)

2. Which aspect of the small intestine is considered the longest?

   A. Duodenum   C. Ileum

   B. Jejunum   D. Cecum

3. Which aspect of the small intestine possesses the smallest diameter?

   A. Ileum   C. Cecum

   B. Duodenum   D. Jejunum

4. The part of the intestine with a "feathery" and "coiled spring" appearance when filled with barium is the:

   A. Ileum   C. Jejunum

   B. Duodenum   D. Cecum

5. List the two aspects of the large intestine not considered part of the colon.

   A. _____   B. _____

6. What is the correct term for the appendix? _____

7. True/False: The rectum possesses two anteroposterior curves that have a direct impact on rectal enema tip insertions.

8. True/False: The small sacculations found within the jejunum are called haustra.

9. Which colic flexure (right or left) is located 1 to 2 inches (2.5 to 5 cm) higher or more superior in the abdomen?

   _____

10. What is the name for the band of muscular tissue found at the junction of the duodenum and jejunum?

    A. Valvulae conniventes   C. Duodenal flexure

    B. Haustra   D. Suspensory ligament of the duodenum

334

Chapter **13 Lower Gastrointestinal System: Self-Test**

11. Identify the labeled structures on the following radiographs (Figs. 13-5 and 13-6). Include secondary names where indicated by parentheses.

Fig. 13-5:

A. _____

B. _____

C. _____

D. _____

E. _____

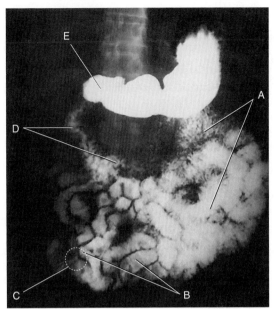

Fig. 13-5. Structure identification on a gastrointestinal radiograph.

Fig. 13-6

F. ____ (_____) ____

G. _____

H. _____

I. _____

J. _____

K. _____

L. ____ (_____) ____

M. _____

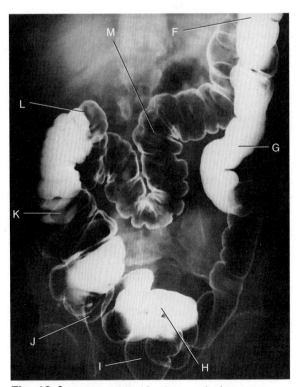

Fig. 13-6. Structure identification on a barium enema radiograph.

12. Which one of the following structures is intraperitoneal?

    A. Descending colon   C. Transverse colon

    B. Rectum   D. Ascending colon

13. Where does the reabsorption of inorganic salts occur in the gastrointestinal tract?

    A. Duodenum   C. Stomach

    B. Large intestine   D. Jejunum

14. Which one of the following digestive movements occurs in the small intestine?

    A. Haustral churning   C. Mass peristalsis

    B. Rhythmic segmentation   D. Mastication

15. Match each of the following pathologic conditions to its correct definition:

    _____ 1. Meckel's diverticulum

    _____ 2. Diverticulosis

    _____ 3. Enteritis

    _____ 4. Whipple's disease

    _____ 5. Polyp

    _____ 6. Malabsorption syndrome

    _____ 7. Diverticulitis

    _____ 8. Volvulus

    _____ 9. Intussusception

    _____ 10. Crohn's disease

    _____ 11. Ulcerative colitis

    _____ 12. Giardiasis

    _____ 13. Appendicitis

A. Telescoping of the bowel into another aspect of it

B. A new growth extending from mucosal wall

C. A twisting of the intestine on its own mesentery

D. Condition of small herniations present along the intestinal wall

E. Chronic inflammatory condition of small intestine

F. Outpouchings located in distal ileum

G. Unable to process certain nutrients

H. May be caused by cutting off blood supply to it or infection

I. Inflammation of the small intestine

J. Inflammation of small herniations in the intestinal wall

K. Caused by a flagellate protozoan

L. Disorder of proximal small intestine

M. Chronic inflammatory condition of the large intestine

16. Match the following radiographic appearances to the correct pathologic conditions:

_____ 1. A tapered or corkscrew appearance seen during a barium enema

_____ 2. Apple-core lesion

_____ 3. String sign

_____ 4. Dilation of the intestine with thickening of the circular folds

_____ 5. Stove-pipe appearance of colon

_____ 6. Mushroom-shaped dilation with a small amount of barium extending beyond it

_____ 7. Jagged or sawtooth appearance of the intestinal wall

_____ 8. Inward growth from intestinal wall

A. Ulcerative colitis

B. Diverticulosis

C. Intussusception

D. Volvulus

E. Regional enteritis

F. Polyp

G. Neoplasm

H. Giardiasis

17. _____ is a group of intestinal malabsorption diseases involving the inability to absorb certain proteins and dietary fat.

18. Which of the following imaging modalities/procedures is often performed to diagnose and may treat an intussusception?

A. Barium enema   C. Nuclear medicine scan

B. Enteroclysis   D. CT

19. True/False: The barium enema is recommended to diagnose acute appendicitis.

20. Why is the PA rather than AP recumbent position recommended for a small bowel series?

_____

21. What is the minimum amount of time a patient needs to remain NPO before a small bowel series?

_____

22. What is another term for a laxative? _____

23. Which type of rectal enema tip is ideal for the patient with a relaxed anal sphincter?

_____

24. True/False: Natural latex-based gloves are safe to be worn by all technologists.

25. What drug can be added to the barium sulfate mixture to minimize intestinal spasm during a barium enema?

_____

26. What breathing instructions should be given to the patient during insertion of the enema tip?

_____

27. Which one of the following disorders is best diagnosed during an evacuative proctogram?

   A. Regional enteritis   C. Volvulus

   B. Diverticulosis   D. Prolapse of rectum

28. Which type of health condition may restrict the use of glucagon during a barium enema?

   _____

29. Which region of the large intestine must be visualized during an evacuative proctogram study?

   A. Cecum   C. Ileocecal valve

   B. Anorectal angle   D. Left colic flexure

30. True/False: A small balloon retention catheter may be placed within the stoma of the colostomy to deliver contrast media during a barium enema.

31. Which oblique position, the LAO or RAO, best demonstrates the ascending colon and right colic flexure?

   _____

32. What is the average length of time in a routine small bowel series for the barium to pass through the ileocecal

   sphincter (healthy adult)? _____

33. Which one of the following commercial contrast media would be used during an evaluative proctogram?

   A. Hypaque   C. Gastroview

   B. Gastrografin   D. Anatrast

34. How much rotation of the body is required for the LAO position during a barium enema?

   _____

35. The CR and image receptor should be centered approximately _____ higher for the 15- or 30-minute small bowel image than for the later images.

36. The term *evacuative proctography* is sometimes used for a lower GI tract procedure. This procedure is also commonly

   called _____.

37. **Situation:** A patient is unable to lie prone on the radiographic table during a barium enema. Which specific projection

   best demonstrates the right colic flexure? _____

38. **Situation:** A patient is scheduled for a double-contrast barium enema. During the fluoroscopy phase of the study, the radiologist detects a possible polyp in the lower descending colon. Which specific projection best demonstrates this region of the colon?

   _____

   _____

39. **Situation:** A patient with a clinical history of a rectocele comes to the radiology department. Which radiographic procedure will best diagnose this condition?

   _____

40. True/False: A PA axial oblique (RAO) barium enema projection is an optional projection to demonstrate the right colic flexure.

41. True/False: For a hypersthenic type of patient, a 35- × 43-cm (14- × 17-inch) IR placed lengthwise and centered correctly generally includes the entire barium-filled large intestine on one IR.

42. What are the patient shielding recommendations during a barium enema?

_____

43. A. The RAO projection best demonstrates the _____ (right or left) colic flexure

with the CR and image receptor centered to the level of _____.

B. The LAO projection best demonstrates the (right or left) colic flexure with the CR and image receptor centered

to the level of _____.

44. **Situation:** During a barium enema, a possible polyp is seen in the left colic flexure. Which of the following projections will best demonstrate it?

A. RPO   C. RAO

B. AP axial   D. PA

45. **Situation:** A patient has a clinical history of regional enteritis. Which of the following procedures is most often performed for this condition?

A. Intubation small bowel series   C. Enteroclysis

B. Single-contrast barium enema   D. Double-contrast barium enema

46. **Situation:** A patient comes to the radiology department with a clinical history of Meckel's diverticulum. Which imaging modality is most often performed for this condition?

_____

47. **Situation:** A patient comes to the radiology department with a clinical history of giardiasis. She is scheduled for a barium enema procedure. Which of the following precautions must be followed during the procedure?

A. Wear gloves   C. Wear eye protection

B. Wear surgical mask   D. All of the above

48. True/False: The transit time of barium through the small intestine of the pediatric patient is usually less than that required for an adult.

14 Urinary System and Venipuncture

CHAPTER OBJECTIVES

After you have successfully completed the activities in this chapter, you will be able to:

_____ 1. Identify the location and pertinent anatomy of the urinary system to include the adrenal glands.

_____ 2. Identify specific structures of the macroscopic and microscopic anatomy and physiology of the kidney.

_____ 3. Identify the orientation of the kidneys, ureters, and urinary bladder with respect to the peritoneum and other structures of the abdomen.

_____ 4. List the primary functions of the urinary system.

_____ 5. Describe the spatial relationship between the male and female reproductive system and the urinary system.

_____ 6. On drawings and radiographs, identify specific anatomy of the urinary system.

_____ 7. Identify key lab values and drug concerns that must be verified before intravenous injections of contrast media.

_____ 8. Identify characteristics specific to either ionic or nonionic contrast media.

_____ 9. Describe the two categories of contrast media reactions and the symptoms specific to each type of reaction.

_____ 10. Differentiate among mild, moderate, and severe levels of systemic contrast media reactions.

_____ 11. Identify the steps and safety measures to be followed during a venipuncture procedure.

_____ 12. List safety measures to be followed before and during the injection of an iodinated contrast media.

_____ 13. Define specific urinary pathologic terminology and indicators.

_____ 14. Match specific types of urinary pathology to the correct radiographic appearances and signs.

_____ 15. List the purpose, contraindications, and high-risk patient conditions for intravenous urography.

_____ 16. Identify two methods used to enhance pelvicaliceal filling during intravenous urography and contraindications for their use.

_____ 17. Explain the difference between a nephrogram and a nephrotomogram.

_____ 18. Identify specific aspects related to the retrograde urogram and how this procedure differs from an intravenous urogram (IVU).

_____ 19. Identify specific aspects related to the retrograde cystogram.

_____ 20. Identify specific aspects related to the retrograde urethrogram.

_____ 21. List specific information related to the routine and special projections for excretory urography, retrograde urography, cystography, urethrography, and voiding cystourethrography to include size and type of image receptor (IR), central ray location, direction and angulation of central ray, and anatomy best visualized.

_____ 22. Given various hypothetic situations, identify the correct modification of a position and/or exposure factors to improve the radiographic image.

POSITIONING AND RADIOGRAPHIC TECHNIQUE

_____ 1. Using a peer, position for routine and special projections for an intravenous urogram procedure.

_____ 2. Critique and evaluate urinary study radiographs based on the five divisions of radiographic criteria: (1) anatomy demonstrated, (2) position, (3) collimation and CR, (4) exposure, and (5) anatomic side markers.

_____ 3. Distinguish between acceptable and unacceptable urinary study radiographs based on exposure considerations, motion, collimation, positioning, or other errors.

LEARNING EXERCISES

Complete the following review exercises after reading the associated pages in the textbook as indicated by each exercise. Answers to each review exercise are given at the end of the review exercises.

PART I: RADIOGRAPHIC ANATOMY
REVIEW EXERCISE A: Radiographic Anatomy of the Urinary System (see textbook pp. 526-532)

1. The kidneys and ureters are located in the _____ space.

   A. Intraperitoneal   C. Extraperitoneal

   B. Infraperitoneal   D. Retroperitoneal

2. The _____ glands are located directly superior to the kidneys.

3. Which structures create a 20° angle between the upper pole and lower pole of the kidney?

   _____

4. What is the specific name for the mass of fat that surrounds each kidney? _____

5. What degree of rotation from supine is required to place the kidneys parallel to the IR?

   _____

6. Which two landmarks can be palpated to locate the kidneys? _____

7. Which term describes an abnormal drop of the kidneys when the patient is placed erect?

   _____

8. List the three functions of the urinary system:

   A. _____

   B. _____

   C. _____

9. A buildup of nitrogenous waste in the blood is called:

   A. Hemotoxicity   C. Sepsis

   B. Uremia   D. Renotoxicity

10. The longitudinal fissure found along the central medial border of the kidney is called the

    _____.

11. The peripheral or outer portion of the kidney is called the _____.

12. The term that describes the total functioning portion of the kidney is _____.

13. The microscopic functional and structural unit of the kidney is the _____.

14. True/False: The efferent arterioles carry blood to the glomeruli.

15. What is another (older) name for the glomerular capsule? _____

16. True/False: The glomerular capsule and proximal and distal convoluted tubules are located in the medulla of the kidney.

17. Which structure of the medulla is made up of a collection of tubules that drain into the minor calyx?

    _____

18. Identify the renal structures labeled on Fig. 14-1:

    A. _____

    B. _____

    C. _____

    D. _____

    E. _____ (region)

    F. _____ (region)

    G. _____

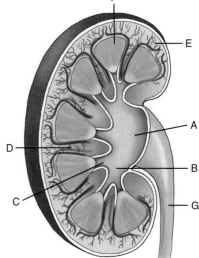

Fig. 14-1. Cross-section of a kidney.

19. Identify the structures making up a nephron and collecting duct (Fig. 14-2). For each structure, indicate with a check mark whether it is located in the cortex or medulla portion of the kidney.

Structure	Cortex	Medulla
A. _____	_____	_____
B. _____	_____	_____
C. _____	_____	_____
D. _____	_____	_____
E. _____	_____	_____
F. _____	_____	_____
G. _____	_____	_____
H. _____	_____	_____
I. _____	_____	_____

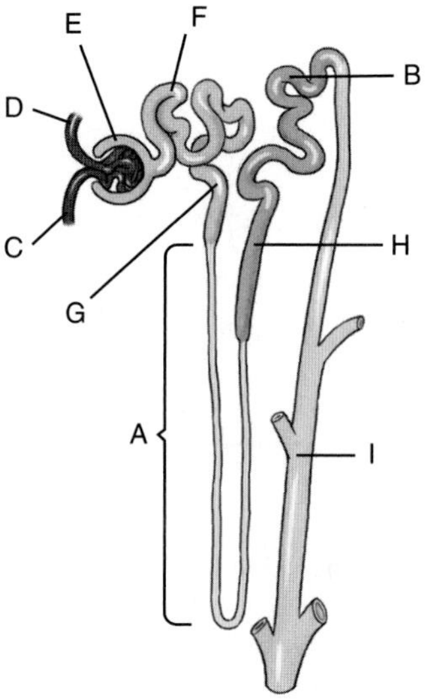

Fig. 14-2. Structures of a nephron and collecting duct.

20. Which two processes move urine through the ureters to the bladder?

    A. _____   B. _____

21. Which one of the following structures is located most anterior as compared with the others?

    A. Proximal ureters   C. Urinary bladder

    B. Kidneys   D. Suprarenal glands

22. What is the name of the junction found between the distal ureters and urinary bladder?

    _____

23. What is the name of the inner, posterior region of the bladder formed by the two ureters entering and the urethra exiting?

    _____

24. What is the name of the small gland found just inferior to the male bladder?

    _____

25. The total capacity for the average adult bladder is:

    A. 100 to 200 mL   C. 350 to 500 mL

    B. 200 to 300 mL   D. 500 to 700 mL

26. Which one of the following structures is considered to be most posterior?

    A. Ovaries   C. Vagina

    B. Urethra   D. Kidneys

27. Identify the urinary structures labeled on Fig. 14-3:

A. _____

B. _____

C. _____

D. _____

E. _____

F. _____

G. _____

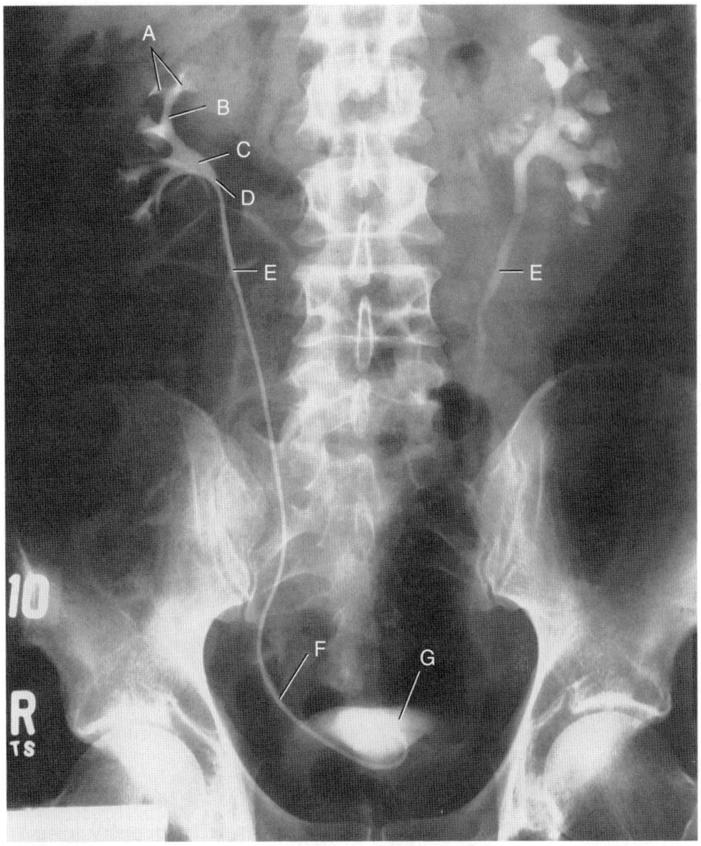

Fig. 14-3. AP retrograde urogram radiograph.

PART II: RADIOGRAPHIC POSITIONING, CONTRAST MEDIA, AND PATHOLOGY
REVIEW EXERCISE B: Venipuncture (see textbook pp. 533-537)

1. Intravenous contrast media may be administered by either:

A. _____

B. _____

2. True/False: The patient (or legal guardian) must sign an informed consent form before a venipuncture procedure is performed on a pediatric patient.

3. For most IVUs, veins in the _____ are recommended for venipuncture.

A. Iliac fossa   C. Axillary fossa

B. Anterior, carpal region   D. Antecubital fossa

4. The most common size of needle used for bolus injections on adults is:

A. 23 to 25 gauge   C. 18 to 22 gauge

B. 14 to 16 gauge   D. 28 gauge

5. The two most common types of needles used for bolus injection of contrast media are

   _____ and _____

6. In the correct order, list the six steps followed during a venipuncture procedure as listed and described in the textbook (pp. 535-537):

   1. _____

   2. _____

   3. _____

   4. _____

   5. _____

   6. _____

7. True/False: The bevel of the needle needs to be facing downward during the actual puncture into a vein.

8. True/False: If extravasation occurs during the puncture, the technologist should slightly retract the needle and then push it forward again.

9. True/False: If unsuccessful during the initial puncture, a new needle should be used during the second attempt.

10. True/False: The radiologist is responsible for documenting all aspects of the venipuncture procedure in the patient's chart.

REVIEW EXERCISE C: Contrast Media and Urography (see textbook pp. 538-542)

1. The two major types of iodinated contrast media used for urography are ionic and nonionic. Indicate whether each of the following characteristics applies to ionic (I) or nonionic (N) contrast media:

   _____ A. Uses a parent compound of a benzoic acid

   _____ B. Will not significantly increase the osmolality of the blood plasma

   _____ C. Incorporates sodium or meglumine to increase solubility of the contrast media

   _____ D. Creates a hypertonic condition in the blood plasma

   _____ E. Is more expensive

   _____ F. Produces less severe reactions

   _____ G. Is a near-isotonic solution

   _____ H. Poses a greater risk for disrupting homeostasis

   _____ I. Uses a parent compound of an amide or glucose group

   _____ J. May increase the severity of side effects

2. Which one of the following compounds is a common anion found in ionic contrast media?

   A. Diatrizoate or iothalamate   C. Benzoic acid

   B. Sodium or meglumine   D. None of the above

3. Any disruption in the physiologic functions of the body that may lead to a contrast media reaction is the basis for the:

   A. Homeostasis theory   C. Vasovagal theory

   B. Anaphylactoid theory   D. Chemotoxic theory

4. An expected outcome to the introduction of contrast media is described as a _____.

5. The normal creatinine level for an adult should range between _____.

6. Normal BUN levels for an adult should range between _____.

7. A. Metformin hydrochloride is a drug that is taken for the management of _____.

   B. The American College of Radiology recommends that metformin be withheld for

      _____ hours after a contrast medium procedure and resumed only if kidney function is again determined to be within normal limits.

8. The leakage of contrast media from a vessel into the surrounding soft tissues is called

   _____.

9. List the two general categories of contrast media reactions:

   A. _____

   B. _____

10. Which type of reaction is a true allergic response to iodinated contrast media?

    _____

11. Which type of reaction is caused by the stimulation of the vagus nerve by introduction of a contrast medium,

    which causes heart rate and blood pressure to fall? _____

12. True/False: Vasovagal reactions are not considered to be life threatening.

13. Matching: Match the following symptoms to the correct category of systemic contrast media reaction. (More than one symptom may apply to a type of reaction.)

_____ A. Brachycardia (<50 beats/minute)   1. Mild

_____ B. Tachycardia (>100 beats/minute)   2. Moderate

_____ C. Angioedema   3. Severe

_____ D. Lightheadedness

_____ E. Hypotension (systolic blood pressure <80 mm Hg)

_____ F. Temporary renal failure

_____ G. Laryngeal swelling

_____ H. Cardiac arrest

_____ I. Mild hives

14. True/False: Mild-level contrast media reactions do not usually require medication or medical assistance.

15. True/False: Urticaria is the formal term for excessive vomiting.

16. A temporary failure of the renal system is an example of a(n) _____ reaction.

A. Mild   C. Severe

B. Moderate   D. Local

17. Matching: For each of the following symptoms, identify the type (1-5) of contrast media reactions (may be used more than once):

_____ A. Convulsions   1. Side effect

_____ B. Metallic taste   2. Mild systemic

_____ C. Angioedema   3. Moderate systemic

_____ D. Bradycardia   4. Severe systemic

_____ E. Itching   5. Local

_____ F. Vomiting

_____ G. Temporary hot flash

_____ H. Respiratory arrest

_____ I. Pulmonary edema

_____ J. Extravasation

_____ K. Severe urticaria

18. What should the technologist do first when a patient is experiencing either a moderate or a severe level contrast media reaction? _____

19. What is the primary purpose of the premedication procedure before an iodinated contrast media procedure?

_____

20. Which of the following drugs is often given to the patient as part of the premedication procedure?

    A. Epinephrine   C. Combination of Benadryl and prednisone
    B. Valium   D. Lasix

21. Which type of patient is a likely candidate for the premedication procedure before a contrast media study?

    A. Elderly patient   C. Pediatric patient
    B. Asthmatic patient   D. Patient with hypertension

22. In addition to notifying a nurse or physician when contrast media has extravasated into the soft tissues, what should the technologist first do to increase reabsorption?

_____

23. True/False: Tissue inflammation from extravasated contrast media peaks 1 to 2 hours after the incident.

24. True/False: Acute renal failure may occur 48 hours after an iodinated contrast media procedure.

25. List 10 contraindications that may prevent a patient from having a contrast media procedure performed.

    A. _____   F. _____

    B. _____   G. _____

    C. _____   H. _____

    D. _____   I. _____

    E. _____   J. _____

REVIEW EXERCISE D: Radiographic Procedures, Pathologic Terms, and Clinical Indications (see textbook pp. 542-553)

1. A trademark name for a diuretic drug is _____.

2. A. Why is the term IVP incorrect in describing a radiographic examination of the kidneys, ureters, and bladder after intravenous injection of contrast media?

   _____

   B. What is the correct term and correct abbreviation for the exam described in question A?

   _____

3. Which specific aspect of the kidney is visualized during an IVU? _____

4. Which one of the following conditions is a common pathologic indication for an IVU?

    A. Sickle cell anemia   C. Hematuria

    B. Multiple myeloma   D. Anuria

5. Which one of the following conditions is described as a rare tumor of the kidney?

    A. Pheochromocytoma   C. Melanoma

    B. Multiple myeloma   D. Renal cell carcinoma

6. Matching: Match each of the following urinary pathologic terms to its correct definition:

_____ A. Pneumouria	1. Passage of large volume of urine
_____ B. Urinary reflux	2. Presence of glucose in urine
_____ C. Uremia	3. Excess urea and creatinine in the blood
_____ D. Anuria	4. Diminished amount of urine being excreted
_____ E. Polyuria	5. Presence of gas in urine
_____ F. Micturition	6. Indicated by presence of uremia, oliguria, or anuria
_____ G. Retention	7. Constant or frequent involuntary passage of urine
_____ H. Oliguria	8. Backward return flow of urine
_____ I. Glucosuria	9. Absence of a functioning kidney
_____ J. Urinary incontinence	10. Complete cessation of urinary secretion
_____ K. Renal agenesis	11. Act of voiding
_____ L. Acute renal failure	12. Inability to void

7. Match each of the following descriptions to the correct disorder:

_____ A. Enlargement of the prostate gland

_____ B. Fusion of the lower poles of kidneys during the development of the fetus

_____ C. Inflammation of the capillary loops of the glomeruli of the kidneys

_____ D. Artificial opening between the urinary bladder and aspects of the large intestine

_____ E. A large stone that grows and completely fills the renal pelvis

_____ F. Increased blood pressure to the kidneys due to atherosclerosis

_____ G. Normal kidney that fails to ascend into the abdomen but remains in the pelvis

_____ H. Multiple cysts in one or both kidneys

1. Vesicorectal fistula
2. Renal hypertension
3. Ectopic kidney
4. Horseshoe kidney
5. Staghorn calculus
6. Polycystic kidney disease
7. Benign prostatic hyperplasia
8. Glomerulonephritis

8. Match each of the following radiographic appearances to the correct disorder:

_____ A. Rapid excretion of contrast media

_____ B. Mucosal changes within bladder

_____ C. Bilateral, small kidneys with blunted calyces

_____ D. Irregular appearance of renal parenchyma or collecting system

_____ E. Signs of abnormal fluid collections

_____ F. Abnormal rotation of the kidney

_____ G. Elevated or indented floor of bladder

_____ H. Signs of obstruction of urinary system

1. Malrotation
2. Vesicorectal fistula
3. Renal cell carcinoma
4. BPH
5. Renal hypertension
6. Renal calculi
7. Cystitis
8. Chronic Bright disease

9. A condition characterized by regions or areas of subcutaneous swelling caused by allergic reaction to food or drugs is termed _____.

10. Contraction of the muscles within the walls of the bronchi and bronchioles, producing a restriction of air passing through them, is a condition called _____.

11. Loss of consciousness resulting from reduced cerebral blood flow is termed _____.

12. An eruption of wheals (hives) often caused by a hypersensitivity to food or drugs is a condition termed

_____.

13. What type of renal calculi is often associated with chronic urinary tract infections?

   _____

14. True/False: The patient should void before an IVU to prevent possible rupture of the bladder if compression is applied.

15. What is the primary purpose of ureteric compression? _____

16. List the six conditions that could contraindicate the use of ureteric compression:

   A. _____   D. _____

   B. _____   E. _____

   C. _____   F. _____

17. When does the timing for an IVU exam start? _____

18. List the routine five-step imaging sequence for a routine IVU:

   A. _____   D. _____

   B. _____   E. _____

   C. _____

19. What is the primary difference between a standard and a hypertensive IVU? _____

20. In which department are most retrograde urograms performed? _____

21. True/False: A retrograde urogram examines the anatomy and function of the pelvicaliceal system.

22. True/False: The Brodney clamp is used for male and female retrograde cystourethrograms.

23. Which of the following involves a direct introduction of the contrast media into the structure being studied?

   A. Retrograde urogram   C. Retrograde urethrogram
   B. Retrograde cystogram   D. All of the above

24. Which of the following alternative imaging modalities is *not* routinely being used to diagnose renal calculi?

   A. Nuclear medicine   C. Magnetic resonance imaging
   B. Sonography   D. Computed tomography

25. True/False: Urinary studies on pediatric patients should be scheduled early in the morning to minimize the risk for dehydration.

26. True/False: The number of retrograde urography procedures for urethral calculi has been reduced as a result of the increased use of CT.

27. Exposure factors used during a CT procedure can be adjusted to compensate for a decrease or increase in body

   size according to _____ and _____.

28. True/False: The patient does not require extensive bowel preparation before a CT scan for renal calculi.

29. Which imaging modality is used to detect subtle tissue changes following a renal transplant?

   A. MRI

   C. Radiography-IVU

   B. CT

   D. Nuclear medicine

30. True/False: Nuclear medicine is highly effective in demonstrating signs of vesicoureteral reflux.

REVIEW EXERCISE E: Radiographic Positioning of the Urinary System (see textbook pp. 553-560)

1. How will an enlarged prostate gland appear on a postvoid radiograph taken during an IVU?

   _____

2. Where should the pneumatic paddle be placed for the ureteric compression phase of an IVU?

   _____

3. What can be done to enhance filling of the calyces of the kidney if ureteric compression is contraindicated?

   _____

4. A retrograde pyelogram is primarily a nonfunctional study of the _____.

5. What are the four reasons a scout projection is taken before the injection of contrast media for an IVU?

   A. _____   C. _____

   B. _____   D. _____

6. What specific anatomy is examined during a retrograde ureterogram?

   A. Primarily the ureters

   C. Entire urinary system

   B. Primarily the renal pelvis and calyces

   D. Urinary bladder

7. Which specific position is recommended for a male patient during a voiding cystourethrogram?

   _____

8. What kV range (analog and digital) is recommended for an IVU? _____

9. True/False: There is a change in SID recommendations when placing a patient erect versus supine for an IVU AP projection.

10. True/False: Male and female patients should have the gonads shielded for an AP scout projection.

11. True/False: Tomograms taken during an IVU with an exposure angle of 10° or less are called zonography.

12. How many tomograms (zonograms) are usually produced during a routine IVU?

   _____

13. At what stage of an IVU is the renal parenchyma best seen?

   A. 5 minutes after injection

   C. After the postvoid projection

   B. 10 minutes after injection

   D. Within 1 minute after injection

14. Where is the CR centered for a nephrotomogram?

   A. At xiphoid process

   C. At iliac crest

   B. Midway between xiphoid process and iliac crest

   D. At axillary costal margin

15. Which specific position, taken during an IVU, places the left kidney parallel to the IR?

   _____

16. How much obliquity is required for the LPO/RPO projections taken during an IVU?

   _____

17. Which position best demonstrates possible nephroptosis? _____

18. What CR angle is used for the AP projection taken during a cystogram?

   A. 20° to 25° caudad

   C. 10° to 15° caudad

   B. 5° to 10° cephalad

   D. 30° to 40° caudad

19. True/False: Contrast media should never be injected into the bladder under pressure but should be allowed to fill slowly by gravity in the presence of an attendant.

REVIEW EXERCISE F: Problem Solving for Technical and Positioning Errors

1. **Situation:** A radiograph of an AP scout projection of the abdomen, taken during an IVU, reveals that the symphysis pubis is cut off slightly. The patient is too large to include the entire abdomen on a 35- × 43-cm (14- × 17-inch) IR. What should the technologist do in this situation?

   _____

   _____

2. **Situation:** A nephrogram is ordered as part of an IVU study. When the nephrogram image is processed, there is a minimal amount of contrast media within the renal parenchyma and the calyces are beginning to fill with contrast media. What specific problem led to this radiographic outcome?

   _____

   _____

3. **Situation:** A 45° RPO radiograph taken during an IVU reveals that the left kidney is foreshortened. What modification is needed to improve this image during the repeat exposure?

   _____

   _____

4. **Situation:** An AP projection taken during the compression phase of an IVU reveals that the majority of the contrast media has left the collecting system of the kidneys. The technologist placed the pneumatic paddles near the umbilicus and ensured that they were inflated. What can the technologist do to ensure better retention of contrast media in the collecting system during the compression phase of future IVUs?

   _____

   _____

5. **Situation:** An AP axial projection radiograph taken during a cystogram reveals that the floor of the bladder is superimposed over the symphysis pubis. What can the technologist do to correct this problem during the repeat exposure?

_____

_____

6. **Situation:** A patient comes to the radiology department for an IVU. While taking the clinical history, the technologist learns the patient has renal hypertension. How must the technologist modify the IVU imaging sequence to accommodate this patient's condition?

_____

_____

7. **Situation:** A patient comes to the radiology department for an IVU. The AP scout reveals an abnormal density near the lumbar spine that the radiologist suspects is an abdominal aortic aneurysm. What should the technologist do about the ureteric compression phase of the study that is part of the procedure protocol?

_____

_____

8. **Situation:** A patient comes to the radiology department for an IVU. The patient history indicates that he may have an enlarged prostate gland. Which projection will best demonstrate this condition?

_____

_____

9. **Situation:** A patient with a history of bladder calculi comes to the radiology department. A retrograde cystogram has been ordered. During the interview, the patient reports that he had a severe reaction to contrast media in the past. What other imaging modality(-ies) can be performed to best diagnose this condition?

_____

_____

10. **Situation:** The same patient described in question 9 may also have calculi in the kidney. What is the preferred imaging modality for this situation when iodinated contrast media cannot be used?

_____

_____

11. **Situation:** A patient comes to the radiology department for an IVU. As the patient's clinical history is being reviewed, it is discovered that he is diabetic. What additional question(s) should the patient be asked during the interview before the procedure?

_____

_____

12. **Situation:** During an IVU, the patient complains of a metallic taste and has a sudden urge to urinate. What action should the technologist take?

_____

_____

13. **Situation:** While reviewing the chart of a patient scheduled for an IVU, the technologist discovers that the BUN of the patient is 15 mg/100 mL with a creatinine level of 1.3 mg/dL. Can this patient safely undergo an IVU?

_____

_____

PART III: LABORATORY EXERCISES

Although it is impossible to duplicate many aspects of urinary studies on a phantom in the lab, evaluation of actual radiographs and physical positioning is possible. You can get experience in positioning and radiographic evaluation of these projections by performing exercises using radiographic phantoms and practicing on other students (although you will not be taking actual exposures). Technologists must learn the positioning routine, room setup, and fluoroscopy procedure for their particular facility.

Laboratory Exercise A: Radiographic Evaluation

1. Using actual radiographs of IVU, cystogram, and retrograde urogram procedures provided by your instructor, evaluate each position for the following points (check off when completed):

_____ Evaluate the completeness of the study. (Are all pertinent anatomic structures included on the radiograph?)

_____ Evaluate for positioning or centering errors (e.g., rotation, off centering).

_____ Evaluate for correct exposure factors and possible motion. (Is the contrast medium properly penetrated?)

_____ Determine whether patient rotation is correct for specific positions.

_____ Determine whether anatomic side markers and an acceptable degree of collimation and/or area shielding are visible on the images.

Laboratory Exercise B: Physical Positioning

On another person, simulate performing all routine and special projections of the IVU as follows. Include the six steps listed below and described in the textbook. (Check off each when completed satisfactorily.)

Step 1. Appropriate size and type of image receptor with correct side markers

Step 2. Correct CR placement and centering of part to CR and/or image receptor

Step 3. Accurate collimation

Step 4. Area shielding of patient where advisable

Step 5. Use of proper immobilizing devices when needed

Step 6. Approximate correct exposure factors, breathing instructions where applicable, and initiating exposure

Projections	Step 1	Step 2	Step 3	Step 4	Step 5	Step 6
● AP scout	_____	_____	_____	_____	_____	_____
● LPO and RPO	_____	_____	_____	_____	_____	_____
● AP cystogram	_____	_____	_____	_____	_____	_____
● Lateral cystogram	_____	_____	_____	_____	_____	_____

SELF-TEST

This self-test should be taken only after completing all of the readings, review exercises, and laboratory activities for a particular section. The purpose of this test is not only to provide a good learning exercise but also to serve as a strong indicator of what your final evaluation exam for this chapter will cover. It is strongly suggested that if you do not get at least a 90% to 95% grade on each self-test, you should review those areas in which you missed questions before going to your instructor for the final evaluation exam.

1. The kidneys are _____ structures.

   A. Retroperitoneal   B. Intraperitoneal   C. Infraperitoneal   D. Extraperitoneal

2. The ureters enter the _____ aspect of the bladder.

   A. Lateral   B. Anterolateral   C. Posterolateral   D. Superolateral

3. The ureters lie on the _____ (anterior or posterior) surface of each psoas major muscle.

4. The kidneys lie at a _____ angle in relation to the coronal plane.

5. An abnormal drop of more than _____ inches, or

   _____ cm, in the position of the kidneys when the patient is erect indicates a condition termed *nephroptosis*.

6. The buildup of nitrogenous waste in the blood creates a condition called _____.

7. How much urine is normally produced by the kidneys in 24 hours?

   A. 2.5 L   B. 180 L   C. 0.5 L   D. 1.5 L

8. The renal veins connect directly to the:

   A. Abdominal aorta   C. Azygos vein

   B. Superior mesenteric vein   D. Inferior vena cava

9. The 8 to 18 conical masses found within the renal medulla are called the _____.

10. The major calyces of the kidney unite to form the _____.

11. The microscopic unit of the kidney (of which there are more than 1 million in each kidney) is called the

   _____.

12. True/False: About 50% of the glomerular filtrate processed by the nephron is reabsorbed into the kidney's venous system.

13. True/False: The loop of Henle and collecting tubules are located primarily in the medulla of the kidney.

14. The three constricted points along the length of the ureters where a kidney stone is most likely to lodge are:

    A. _____   B. _____   C. _____

15. The inner, posterior triangular aspect of the bladder that is attached to the floor of the pelvis is called the

    _____.

16. True/False: The retrograde ureterogram demonstrates the ureters, renal pelvis, and major and minor calyces.

17. Identify the structures labeled on this radiograph (Fig. 14-4):

    A. _____

    B. _____

    C. _____

    D. _____

    E. _____

    F. _____

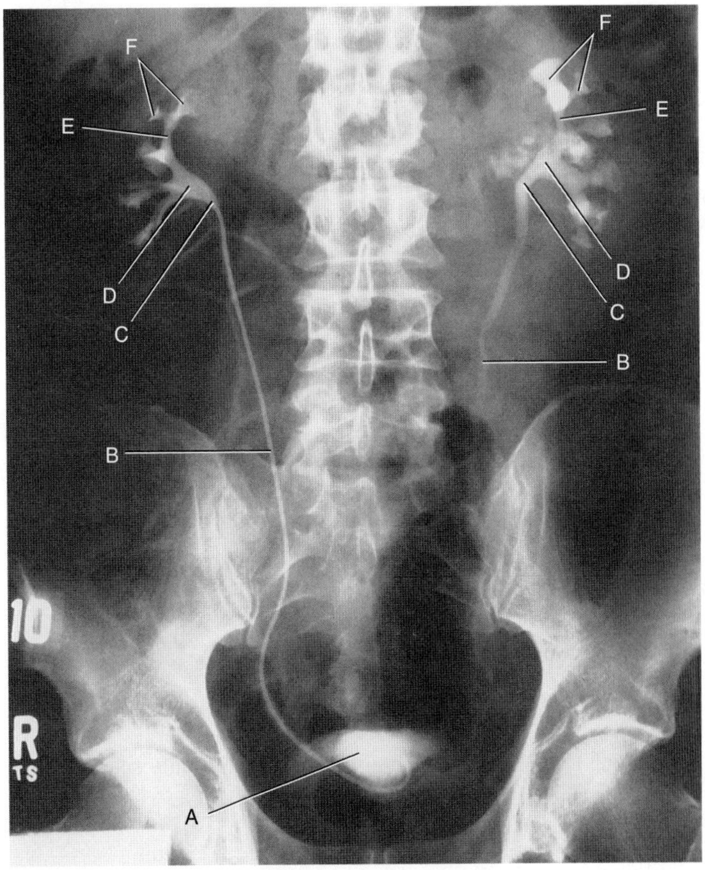

Fig. 14-4. Radiograph of the urinary system.

18. The term describing the radiographic procedure demonstrated on the radiograph in Fig. 14-4

    is _____.

19. Under what circumstances should a pregnant patient have an IVU performed? _____

20. List the two classes of iodinated contrast media used for urinary studies: _____ and

    _____.

21. Match the following characteristics to the correct type of iodinated contrast media:

_____ A. Dissociates into two separate ions once injected   I. Ionic

_____ B. Possesses low osmolality   N. Nonionic

_____ C. Uses a salt as its cation

_____ D. Parent compound is a carboxyl group

_____ E. Less expensive of the two types

_____ F. Produces a less severe contrast media reaction

_____ G. Diatrizoate is a common anion

_____ H. Does not contain a cation

_____ I. Creates a hypertonic condition in blood plasma

_____ J. Creates a near isotonic solution

22. The normal range of creatinine in an adult is:
    A. 2.0 to 3.4 mg/dL
    B. 0.6 to 1.5 mg/dL
    C. 8 to 25 mg/100 mL
    D. 0.1 to 1.25 mg/dL

23. How long must a patient be withheld from taking metformin after an iodinated contrast media procedure?
    A. 48 hours
    B. 2 hours
    C. 24 hours
    D. 72 hours

24. Hot flashes are classified as a(n):
    A. Side effect
    B. Local reaction
    C. Moderate systemic reaction
    D. Severe systemic reaction

25. Which one of the following veins is not normally selected for venipuncture during an IVU?
    A. Basilic
    B. Cephalic
    C. Axillary
    D. Median cubital

26. At what angle is the needle advanced into the vein during venipuncture? _____

27. How long should the venipuncture site be cleaned with an alcohol wipe before needle insertion?
    A. 10 seconds
    B. 15 seconds
    C. 20 seconds
    D. 30 seconds

28. How high should the tourniquet be placed above the puncture site?
    A. 1 to 2 inches (2.5 to 5 cm)
    B. 3 to 4 inches (8 to 10 cm)
    C. 4 to 6 inches (10 to 15 cm)
    D. ½ inch (1.25 cm)

29. Which one of the following conditions is considered high risk for an iodinated contrast media procedure?

   A. Hematuria

   B. Pheochromocytoma

   C. Diabetes mellitus

   D. Hypertension

30. What is the normal range for a patient's BUN?

   A. 0.1 to 3.0 mg/100 mL

   B. 3.5 to 5.0 mg/100 mL

   C. 5.0 to 7.5 mg/100 mL

   D. 8 to 25 mg/100 mL

31. What is the best course of action for a patient experiencing a mild systemic contrast media reaction?

   A. Observe and reassure patient

   B. Call for immediate medical attention

   C. Inform your supervisor

   D. Inform the referring physician

32. Which of the following is a symptom of a vasovagal reaction?

   A. Itching

   B. Angioedema

   C. Cardiac arrhythmias

   D. Urticaria

33. A true allergic reaction to iodinated contrast agents is classified as a(n):

   A. Mild

   B. Vasovagal reaction

   C. Anaphylactic reaction

   D. Local reaction

34. Tachycardia (>100 beats/minute) is a symptom of a(n) _____ type of reaction.

   A. Side effect

   B. Severe systemic

   C. Moderate systemic

   D. Local

35. Brachycardia (<50 beats/minute) is a symptom of a(n) _____ type of syste mic reaction.

   A. Mild

   B. Moderate

   C. Severe

   D. Organ-specific

36. Which of the following drugs may be given to minimize the risk for acute renal failure following a contrast media procedure?

   A. Prednisone

   B. Corticosteroid

   C. Benadryl

   D. Lasix

37. Metformin is a drug given to patients with:

   A. Sensitivity to iodine

   B. Diabetes

   C. Acute renal failure

   D. Chronic renal failure

38. Which one of the following drugs can be given as part of the premedication protocol before an iodinated contrast media procedure?

   A. Prednisone

   B. Zantac

   C. Cipro

   D. Pentobarbital

39. Excretion of a diminished amount of urine in relation to the fluid intake is the general definition for:

   A. Polyuria

   B. Proteinuria

   C. Oliguria

   D. Nephroptosis

40. Constant or frequent involuntary passage of urine is termed:

    A. Micturition
    B. Urinary reflux
    C. Retention
    D. Urinary incontinence

41. The absence of a functioning kidney is called:

    A. Renal agenesis
    B. Renal failure
    C. Nephroptosis
    D. Oliguria

42. Complete cessation of urinary secretion by the kidneys is termed:

    A. Micturition
    B. Anuria
    C. Urinary incontinence
    D. Chronic renal failure

43. True/False: Adult forms of polycystic disease are inherent.

44. Hypernephroma is another term for:

    A. Renal cell carcinoma
    B. Wilms' tumor
    C. Hydronephrosis
    D. Renal hypertension

45. Extravasation is classified as a(n) _____ reaction.

    A. Local
    B. Mild
    C. Moderate
    D. Severe

46. Laryngeal swelling is classified as a:

    A. Side effect
    B. Mild level reaction
    C. Moderate level reaction
    D. Severe level reaction

47. True/False: Bladder carcinoma is three times more common in males than females.

48. Which one of the following conditions may produce hydronephrosis?

    A. Renal obstruction
    B. Glomerulonephritis
    C. Renal hypertension
    D. BPH

49. Which one of the following disorders is an example of a congenital anomaly of the urinary system?

    A. Ectopic kidney
    B. Pyelonephritis
    C. Urinary tract infection
    D. BPH

50. True/False: The patient should void before the IVU to prevent dilution of the contrast media in the bladder.

51. Which one of the following conditions would contraindicate the use of ureteric compression?

    A. Hematuria
    B. Ureteric calculi
    C. Urinary tract infection
    D. Multiple myeloma

52. Typically, at what timing sequence during an IVU are the oblique projections taken?

    _____

53. Which projection(s) best demonstrate(s) the renal parenchyma? When should it (they) be taken?

    _____

54. Which procedure may require a Brodney clamp? _____

55. Which specific body position places the right kidney parallel to the IR? _____.

56. **Situation:** An AP projection taken during a retrograde cystogram reveals that the symphysis pubis is superimposed over the floor of the bladder. What can be done during the repeat exposure to correct this problem?

_____

_____

57. **Situation:** Before the beginning of an IVU, the radiologist requests a nephrogram be taken as part of the study. At what point of the study should this projection be taken?

_____

_____

58. **Situation:** A patient comes to the radiology department for an IVU after abdominal surgery the day before. The IVU protocol requires that ureteric compression be used. What else can be done to achieve the same goal without using compression?

_____

_____

59. **Situation:** A radiograph of a RPO position taken during an IVU reveals that the left kidney is foreshortened and superimposed over the spine. What is the positioning error that led to this radiographic outcome?

_____

_____

15 Trauma, Mobile, and Surgical Radiography

This chapter has been divided into the following four sections:

1. **Mobile X-Ray Equipment and Radiation Protection.** Understanding the various types of mobile x-ray and fluoroscopy equipment used in trauma radiography (including use in surgery) is essential for technologists. Knowing and following safe radiation protection practices for workers around mobile equipment is especially important because of the unshielded environments where mobile equipment is generally used (such as in the emergency room, in surgery, or in patients' rooms).

2. **Trauma Positioning Principles and Fracture Terminology.** Technologists should know the more common fracture terms included in this chapter to better understand patient histories and to ensure that the most appropriate projections are taken to demonstrate these fracture sites.

3. **Trauma and Mobile Positioning and Procedures.** This section describes specific positioning for each body part in which the patient cannot be moved from the supine position. Adaptation of CR angles and IR placement as required is demonstrated and described for each body part.

4. **Surgical Radiography.** This section describes the role and responsibilities of the radiologic technologist in performing imaging in the surgical suite. Included are the following: essential surgical terminology, surgical radiographic equipment, various orthopedic fixation devices, and common surgical procedures that require radiographic support.

CHAPTER OBJECTIVES

After you have successfully completed the activities of this chapter, you will be able to:

_____ 1. Describe the two primary types of mobile radiographic units and their operating principles.

_____ 2. Explain the features, operating principles, and uses of mobile fluoroscopy units.

_____ 3. Describe the difference in exposure field levels with different orientations of the x-ray tube and intensifiers with the C-arm.

_____ 4. Explain why the AP projection orientation of the C-arm is not recommended.

_____ 5. Explain the three positioning principles that must be observed during trauma radiography.

_____ 6. Define and apply terms for specific types of fractures and soft tissue injuries.

_____ 7. List the projections taken for a postreduction study of the limbs, including open and closed reductions.

_____ 8. List projections for trauma and mobile procedures of the chest, bony thorax, and abdomen.

_____ 9. List projections for trauma and mobile procedures for various parts of the upper and lower limbs.

_____ 10. List projections for trauma and mobile procedures of the cervical, thoracic, and lumbar spine.

_____ 11. List trauma and mobile procedures for the skull and facial bones.

_____ 12. List the essential attributes of an effective surgical technologist.

_____ 13. Describe the role of the various members of the surgical team.

_____ 14. Differentiate between sterile and nonsterile environments in the surgical suite.

_____ 15. Define asepsis and describe methods and procedures to protect the integrity of the sterile environment.

_____ 16. Describe surgical attire that must be worn by the technologist before entering the operating suite, presurgical area, and recovery.

_____ 17. Explain the preparation, cleaning, and safe use of radiographic equipment in surgery.

_____ 18. Describe common radiographic procedures performed in surgery, including required equipment, the role of the technologist, and surgical equipment and devices used during the procedure.

_____ 19. Match common surgical terms, orthopedic devices, and procedures to their correct definitions.

LEARNING EXERCISES

The following review exercises should be completed only after careful study of the associated pages in the textbook as indicated by each exercise. Answers to each review exercise are given at the end of this workbook.

REVIEW EXERCISE A: Mobile X-Ray Equipment and Radiation Protection (see textbook pp. 564-569)

1. List the two primary types of mobile x-ray units:

   A. _____   B. _____

2. True/False: A fully charged battery-powered mobile unit has a driving range of up to 10 miles on level ground.

3. With battery-powered types, how long does recharging take if the batteries are fully discharged?

   _____

4. Which type of mobile unit is lighter in weight? _____

5. What is the common term for a mobile fluoroscopy unit? _____

6. What are the two primary components of a mobile fluoroscopy unit (located on each end of the structure from which it gets its name)?

   A. _____   B. _____

7. Why shouldn't the mobile fluoroscopy unit be placed in the AP projection ("tube on top" position)?

   _____

8. A. With the tube and intensifier in a horizontal position, at which side of the patient should the surgeon stand if he or she must remain near the patient—the x-ray tube side or the intensifier side?

   _____

   B. Why? _____

9. Of the two monitors found on most mobile fluoroscopy units, which one is generally considered the "active"

monitor—the right or the left? _____

10. True/False: Image orientation on the mobile fluoroscopy monitors must be determined by the operator before the patient is brought into the room.

11. True/False: All mobile digital fluoroscopy units have the ability to magnify the image on the monitor during fluoroscopy.

12. A 30° C-arm tilt from the vertical perspective will increase exposure to the head and neck regions of the operator

by a factor of _____

13. True/False: AEC exposure systems are not feasible with mobile fluoroscopy.

14. Name the feature that allows an image to be held on the monitor while also providing continuous fluoroscopy

imaging. _____

For questions 15 to 19, review exposure field information on Figs. 15-1 and 15-2. (Also see the same exposure field drawings and charts in Chapter 15 of the textbook.)

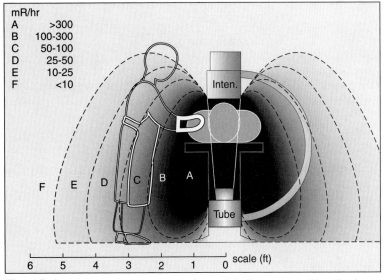

Fig. 15-1. Occupational exposure during mobile fluoroscopy, PA projection.

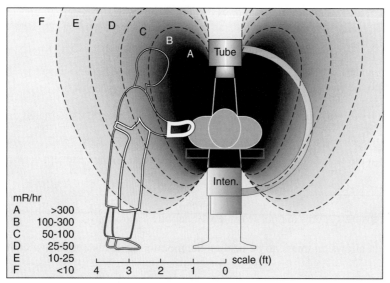

Fig. 15-2. Occupational exposure during mobile fluoroscopy, AP projection.

15. **Situation:** The C-arm is in position for a PA projection. What exposure field range would the operator receive at waist level standing 3 feet from the patient?

   A. 20 to 25 mR/hour

   B. 25 to 50 mR/hour

   C. 50 to 100 mR/hour

   D. 100 to 300 mR/hour

16. Approximately how much exposure at waist level would the operator receive with 5 minutes of fluoroscopy exposure standing 3 feet from the patient? (Hint: First convert mR/hour to mR/minute by dividing by 60; then multiply by minutes of fluoroscopy time.)

   A. 5 mR

   B. 60 mR

   C. 25 mR

   D. 2 mR

17. If a technologist receives 50 mR/hour standing 3 feet from the mobile fluoroscopy unit, what would be the exposure rate if he or she moved back to a distance of 4 feet?

   A. 10 mR/hour

   B. 25 mR/hour

   C. 100 mR/hour

   D. No significant difference

18. A technologist standing 1 foot from a mobile fluoroscopy unit is receiving approximately 400 mR/hour. What is the *total* exposure to the technologist if the procedure takes 10 minutes of fluoroscopy time to complete?

_____

19. **Situation:** An operator receives 25 mR/hour to the facial and neck region with the C-arm in position for a PA projection (intensifier on top). Approximately how much would the operator receive at the same distance if the C-arm were reversed to an AP projection position (tube on top)?

    A. 25 to 50 mR/hour

    B. 50 to 100 mR/hour

    C. 100 to 300 mR/hour

    D. 300 to 500 mR/hour

20. True/False: The intermittent mode used during mobile fluoroscopy procedures is helpful during procedures to produce brighter images, but it results in significantly increased patient exposure.

REVIEW EXERCISE B: Trauma Positioning Principles and Fracture Terminology (see textbook pp. 570-576)

1. Which single term best describes the primary difference between trauma positions and standard positioning?

    _____

2. What should be done to achieve specific projections if the patient cannot move because of trauma?

    _____

3. What is the minimum number of projections generally required for any trauma study?

    _____

4. How many joints must be included for an initial study of a long bone? _____

5. True/False: A follow-up postreduction radiograph of the middle portion of long bones should be collimated closely to the fracture region.

6. True/False: Mobile CT units are available for use in emergency and surgical situations.

7. True/False: Nuclear medicine is effective in diagnosing certain emergency conditions such as pulmonary emboli.

8. True/False: For trauma patients who cannot be moved for conventional diagnostic imaging, other modalities, such as ultrasound or nuclear medicine, may be used rather than trying to move the patient into specific positions.

9. List the two terms for describing displacement of a bone from a joint:

    A. _____   B. _____

10. List the four regions of the body most commonly dislocated during trauma:

    A. _____   C. _____

    B. _____   D. _____

11. What is the correct term for a partial dislocation? _____

12. A forced wrenching or twisting of a joint that results in a tearing of supporting ligaments is a

_____.

13. An injury in which there is no fracture or breaking of the skin is called a _____.

14. What is the correct term that describes the relationship of the long axes of fracture fragments?

_____

15. Which term describes a type of fracture in which the fracture fragment ends are overlapped and not in contact?

_____

16. A. Which term describes the angulation of a distal fracture fragment toward the midline?

_____

B. Would this fracture angulation be described as a medial or lateral apex? _____

17. What is the primary difference between a simple and compound fracture?

_____

18. List two types of incomplete fractures:

A. _____   B. _____

19. Which type of comminuted fracture produces several wedge-shaped separate fragments?

_____

20. What is the name of the fracture in which one fragment is driven into the other?

_____

21. List the secondary name for the following fractures:

A. Hutchinson's fracture: _____

B. Baseball fracture: _____

C. Compound fracture: _____

D. Depressed fracture: _____

E. Simple fracture: _____

22. True/False: An avulsion fracture is the same as a chip fracture.

23. What type of reduction fracture does not require surgery? _____

24. Match each of the following types of fractures to its correct definition. (Use each choice only once.)

_____ 1. Greenstick   A. Fracture of proximal half of ulna with dislocation of radial head

_____ 2. Comminuted   B. Fracture of the base of the first metacarpal

_____ 3. Monteggia   C. Fracture of the pedicles of C2

_____ 4. Boxer's   D. Fracture of distal radius with anterior displacement

_____ 5. Smith's   E. Complete fracture of distal fibula, frequently with fracture of medial malleolus

_____ 6. Hutchinson's F. Fracture of lateral malleolus, medial malleolus, and distal posterior tip of tibia

_____ 7. Bennett's   G. Incomplete fracture with broken cortex on one side of bone only

_____ 8. Avulsion   H. Fracture resulting in multiple (two or more) fragments

_____ 9. Depressed   I. Fracture of distal fifth metacarpal

_____ 10. Stellate   J. Intraarticular fracture of radial styloid process

_____ 11. Trimalleolar K. Fracture of distal radius with posterior displacement

_____ 12. Compression L. Indented fracture of the skull

_____ 13. Pott's   M. Fracture due to a severe stress to a tendon

_____ 14. Colles'   N. Fracture with fracture lines radiating from center point

_____ 15. Hangman's   O. Fracture producing a reduced height of the anterior vertebral body

25. A. Fig. 15-3 illustrates which specific "named fracture"? _____

   B. Which bone is most commonly fractured, and which displacement commonly

   occurs with this fracture? _____

   C. Describe the type of injury or fall that commonly results in this type of fracture.

   _____

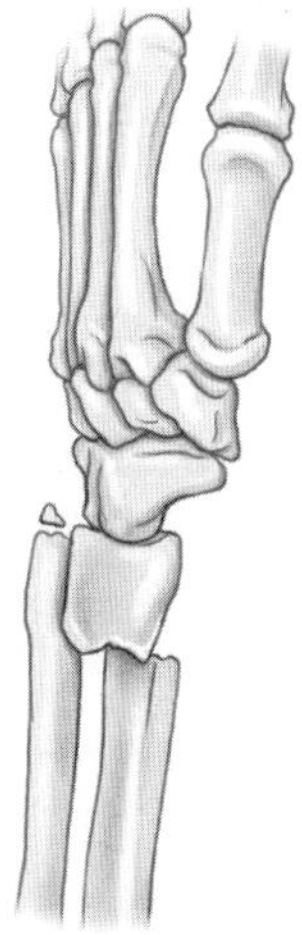

Fig. 15-3.

26. A. Fig. 15-4 illustrates which specific "named" fracture? _____

B. Which bone(s) is (are) commonly fractured with this type of fracture?

_____

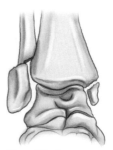

Fig. 15-4.

REVIEW EXERCISE C: Trauma and Mobile Positioning and Procedures (see textbook pp. 577-598)

1. How is the CR centered and aligned in relationship to the sternum for an AP portable projection of the chest?

_____

2. A. 35- × 43-cm (14- × 17-inch) IR should be placed _____ (crosswise or lengthwise) for an AP portable chest on an average or large patient.

B. Why? _____

3. True/False: Focused grids are recommended for mobile chest projections.

4. Which position can be used to replace the RAO of the sternum for the patient who cannot lie prone on the table

but can be rotated into a semisupine position? _____

5. How must the grid be aligned to prevent grid cutoff when angling the CR mediolaterally for an oblique projection of the sternum when the patient cannot be rotated or moved at all from the supine position?

_____

6. Other than the straight AP, what other projection of the ribs can be taken for the supine immobile patient who

cannot be rotated into an oblique position? _____

7. Which one of the following positions or projections will best demonstrate free intraabdominal air on the patient who cannot stand or sit erect?

A. Left lateral decubitus   C. Right lateral decubitus

B. AP KUB   D. Dorsal decubitus

8. Which one of the following projections of the abdomen will most effectively demonstrate a possible abdominal aortic aneurysm?

A. Left lateral decubitus   C. Right lateral decubitus

B. AP KUB   D. Dorsal decubitus

9. What is the disadvantage of performing a PA rather than an AP projection of the thumb?

_____

10. Which projections are taken for a postreduction study (casted) of the wrist? _____

11. **Situation:** A study of a fractured wrist was taken with the following analog exposure factors: 60 kV, 10 mAs, detail screens. A fiberglass cast is placed on the wrist, and a postreduction study is ordered. Which one of the following techniques would be ideal for the postreduction study?

   A. 70 kV and 10 mAs   C. 65 kV and 10 mAs

   B. 80 kV and 10 mAs   D. 55 kV and 15 mAs

12. True/False: A PA horizontal beam projection of the elbow can be taken for a patient with multiple injuries.

13. True/False: For a trauma lateral projection of the elbow, the CR must be kept parallel to the interepicondylar plane.

14. **Situation:** A patient with a possible fracture of the proximal humerus enters the emergency room. Because of multiple injuries, the patient is unable to stand or sit erect. What positioning routine should be performed to diagnose the extent of the injury?

_____

15. **Situation:** A patient with a possible dislocation of the proximal humerus enters the emergency room. Because of multiple injuries, the patient is unable to stand or sit erect. In addition to a routine AP projection, what second projection demonstrates whether it is an anterior or posterior dislocation?

_____

16. A scapular Y projection taken AP supine for a trauma patient usually requires a _____ degree rotation of the body away from the image receptor.

   A. 25 to 30   B. 45   C. 50 to 60   D. 70

17. How much CR angulation should be used for an AP axial projection of the clavicle on a hypersthenic patient?

   A. 10°   B. 15°   C. 20°   D. 25°

18. To ensure that the joints are opened up for an AP projection of the foot, how is the CR aligned?

   A. Perpendicular to the long axis of the tibia

   B. Perpendicular to the plantar surface

   C. 10° posteriorly from perpendicular to plantar surface

   D. 10° posteriorly from perpendicular to dorsal surface

19. **Situation:** An orthopedic surgeon orders a mortise projection of the ankle, but the patient has a severely fractured ankle and cannot rotate the ankle medially for the mortise projection. What can the technologist do to provide this projection without rotating the ankle?

_____

20. **Situation:** A patient with a possible dislocation of the patella enters the emergency room. What type of positioning routine should be performed on this patient that would safely demonstrate the patella?

_____

21. **Situation:** A patient with a possible fracture of the proximal tibia and fibula enters the emergency room. The routine AP and lateral projections are inconclusive. Because of severe pain, the patient is unable to rotate the leg from the AP position. What position or projection could be performed that would provide an unobstructed view of the fibular head and neck?

_____

22. Which one of the following projections would be performed on a trauma patient to provide a lateral view of the proximal femur?

A. Danelius-Miller method   C. Waters method

B. Fuchs method   D. Ottonello method

23. How must the IR and grid be positioned for the inferosuperior (axiolateral) projection for the hip?

_____

24. Which of the following projections demonstrates the odontoid process for the trauma patient who is unable to open the mouth yet can extend the skull and neck? (Subluxation and fracture have been ruled out.)

A. Vertebral arch projection   C. Judd method

B. AP axial   D. Fuchs method

25. **Situation:** A patient with injuries suffered in a motor vehicle accident enters the emergency room. The ER physician orders a lateral C-spine projection to rule out a fracture or dislocation. Because of the thickness of the shoulders, C6-C7 is not visualized. What additional projection can be taken safely to demonstrate this region of the spine?

_____

26. **Situation:** A patient with a possible C2 fracture enters the emergency room on a backboard. The AP projection does not demonstrate C2. In addition, the patient cannot open his mouth because of a mandible fracture. Which projection can be performed safely to demonstrate this region of the spine?

A. Swimmer's method   C. Vertebral arch projection

B. Judd method   D. 35° to 40° cephalad axial projection

27. Which projection will best demonstrate (with only minimal distortion) the pedicles of the cervical spine on a

severely injured patient? _____

28. Identify the two CR angles for the AP axial trauma oblique projections of the cervical spine:

A. _____ lateromedial   B. _____ cephalad

29. True/False: A grid must be used with the AP axial trauma oblique projection for the cervical spine to reduce scatter radiation reaching the IR.

30. **Situation:** A patient with a possible basilar skull fracture enters the emergency room. The ER physician wants a projection that best demonstrates a sphenoid effusion. The patient cannot stand or sit erect. Which one of the following projections would achieve this goal?

A. AP skull   C. Horizontal beam lateral skull

B. Lateral recumbent skull   D. Modified Waters projection

31. Which one of the following projections of the skull would project the petrous ridges in the lower one-third of the orbits on a supine trauma patient?

    A. AP skull, CR 0° to OML
             C. AP skull, CR 15° cephalad to OML

    B. AP skull, CR 15° caudad to OML
          D. AP skull, CR 30° caudad to OML

32. True/False: The CR should not exceed a 30° caudad angle for the AP axial projection of the cranium to avoid excessive distortion of the cranial bones.

33. True/False: AP projections of the skull and facial bones will increase exposure to the thyroid gland as compared with PA projections.

34. How is the CR angled and where is it centered for the AP acanthioparietal (reverse Waters) projection of the facial bones?

_____

35. What type of CR angulation is required for the trauma version of an axiolateral projection of the mandible?

_____

36. **Situation:** A patient with a Monteggia fracture enters the emergency room. Which one of the following positioning routines should be performed on this patient?

    A. AP and lateral thumb
             C. AP and horizontal beam lateral lower leg

    B. PA and horizontal beam lateral wrist
       D. PA or AP and horizontal beam lateral forearm

37. **Situation:** A patient with a possible greenstick fracture enters the emergency room. What age group does this type of fracture usually affect?

    A. Pediatric
             C. Middle age

    B. Young adult
           D. Elderly

38. **Situation:** A patient with a possible Pott's fracture enters the emergency room. Which one of the following positioning routines should be performed on this patient?

    A. AP and horizontal beam lateral lower leg
     C. AP and lateral thumb

    B. PA and horizontal beam lateral wrist
      D. Three projections of the hand

39. **Situation:** A patient is struck directly on the patella with a heavy object, shattering it. The resultant fracture most likely would be described as a:

    A. Burst fracture
             C. Stellate fracture

    B. Compression fracture
        D. Smith's fracture

REVIEW EXERCISE D: Surgical Radiography (pp. 599-618)

1. List the four essential attributes of the successful surgical technologist:

    A. _____
        C. _____

    B. _____
        D. _____

2. Match the following roles to the correct member of the surgical team:

_____ 1. Scrub

_____ 2. Surgical assistant

_____ 3. Certified surgical

_____ 4. Surgeon

_____ 5. Circulator

_____ 6. Anesthesiologist

A. Individual who assists the surgeon

B. Health professional who prepares the OR by supplying it with the appropriate supplies and instruments

C. Individual who has the responsibility of technologist ensuring the safety of the patient and monitoring physiologic functions and fluid levels of the patient during surgery

D. Individual who has primary responsibility for the surgical procedure and the well-being of the patient before, during, and immediately after surgery

E. Individual who prepares the sterile field, scrubs, and gowns the members of the surgical team, and prepares and sterilizes the instruments before the surgical procedure

F. Individual who assists in the OR by to the needs of the scrubbed members within the sterile field before, during, and after the surgical procedure

3. True/False: The technologist may violate the sterile environment in surgery if wearing sterile gloves, mask, and surgical scrubs.

4. True/False: The surgeon is responsible to maintain a safe radiation environment for all personnel in the OR.

5. True/False: The technologist has a moral and ethical responsibility to report any violations of the sterile field during surgery even if it was not noticed by another member of the surgical team.

6. Surgical _____ is the absence of infectious organisms.

7. _____ consists of the practice and procedures to minimize the level of infectious agents present in the surgical environment.

   A. Asepsis   C. Sterile practice

   B. OSHA standards   D. Surgical asepsis

8. Which parts of a sterile gown are considered sterile?

   A. From the top of the shoulders to the knee

   B. The sleeves and waist region

   C. The shoulders to the level of the sterile field, as well as the sleeve from the cuff to just above the elbow

   D. The entire surgical gown

9. True/False: The entire OR table is considered to be sterile.

10. List the three measures that can be taken to maintain the sterile field when operating a mobile fluoroscopy unit in a surgical suite:

   A. _____

   B. _____

   C. _____

11. True/False: Soft (canvas) shoes should be worn in surgery.

12. True/False: The pliable nose stripe on the surgical mask helps prevent fogging of eye glasses.

13. True/False: Protective eyewear is not required to be worn by the technologist during most surgical procedures.

14. True/False: Sterile gloves must be worn when handling a contaminated IR in surgery.

15. What type of equipment cleaner should not be used in surgery? _____

16. What is the primary disadvantage of using the "boost" feature during a mobile fluoroscopic procedure?

_____

17. What is the primary advantage of using the "boost" feature during a mobile fluoroscopic procedure?

_____

18. Which cardinal rule is most effective in reducing occupational exposure? _____

19. List the three terms describing the cardinal rules of radiation protection:

   A. _____   B. _____   C. _____

20. Which one of the following measures is most effective (and practical) in limiting exposure with mobile fluoroscopy?

   A. Limit C-arm procedures to surgery cases only.

   B. Prevent nonradiologists from using the C-arm.

   C. Use intermittent or "foot-tapping" fluoroscopy.

   D. Limit all fluoroscopy procedures to no more than 10 minutes.

21. What anatomy is examined during an operative (immediate) cholangiogram? _____

22. What is the common name for the special tray device that holds the IR and grid during an operative cholangiogram?

_____

23. How must the IR and grid be aligned if the OR table is tilted during an operative cholangiogram?

_____

24. On the average, how much contrast media is injected during an operative cholangiogram?

_____

25. List the three advantages to laparoscopic cholecystectomy over traditional cholecystectomy:

   A. _____

   B. _____

   C. _____

26. Identify the anatomy of the biliary system labeled on this operative cholangiogram (Fig. 15-5).

A. _____

B. _____

C. _____

D. _____

E. _____

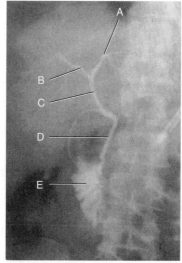

Fig. 15-5. Radiograph of an operative cholangiogram procedure.

27. A radiographic examination of the pelvicaliceal system only during surgery is termed:

    A. Retrograde ureterogram

    B. Antegrade pyelogram

    C. Nephrostomy

    D. Retrograde pyelogram

28. In what position is the patient placed during retrograde urography?

    A. Sims' position

    B. Modified lithotomy position

    C. Trendelenburg position

    D. Fowler's position

29. Which of the following orthopedic procedures is considered nonsurgical?

    A. Open reduction

    B. External fixation

    C. Closed reduction

    D. Internal fixation

30. Which of the following orthopedic devices is classified as an external fixator?

    A. Intramedullary nail

    B. Cerclage wire

    C. Semitubular plate

    D. Ilizarov device

31. Which of the following orthopedic devices is often used during a hip pinning?

    A. Cannulated screw assembly

    B. Ilizarov device

    C. Kirschner wire

    D. Semitubular plate

32. Which of the following devices is often used to reduce femoral, tibial, and humeral shaft fractures?

    A. Intramedullary nail

    B. Cerclage wire

    C. Ilizarov device

    D. Compression screw

33. What is the name of the newer type of prosthetic device to replace a defective hip joint?

    _____

34. A surgical procedure performed to alleviate pain caused by bony neural impingement involving the spine is

    termed _____.

35. What is the name of the device used to stabilize the vertebral body in lieu of traditional spinal fusion?

    _____

36. In what position is the patient placed during most cervical laminectomies? _____

37. List the two internal fixators commonly used during scoliosis surgery:

    A. _____   B. _____

38. Match each of the following surgical terms and devices to its correct definition:

_____ A. Orthopedic wire that tightens around fracture site to reduce shortening of limb

_____ B. Narrow, orthopedic screw designed to enter and fix cortical bone

_____ C. Large screw used in internal fixation of nondisplaced fractures of proximal femur

_____ D. Fabricated (artificial) substitute for a diseased or missing anatomic part

_____ E. Isolation drape that separates the sterile field from the nonsterile environment

_____ F. Soaking of moisture through a sterile or nonsterile drape, cover, or protective barrier

_____ G. Unthreaded (smooth) or threaded metallic wire used to reduce fractures of wrist (carpals) and individual bones of the hands and feet

_____ H. Orthopedic screw designed to enter and fix porous and spongy bone

_____ I. Creation of an artificial joint to correct ankylosis

_____ J. Electrohydraulic shock waves used to break apart calcifications in the urinary system

1. Arthroplasty

2. Cancellous screw

3. Cannulated screw

4. Cerclage wire

5. Cortical screw

6. ESWL

7. Kirschner wire

8. Prosthesis

9. Shower curtain

10. Strike through

39. Which type of pathology is addressed through a vertebroplasty?

A. Compression fracture of the vertebral body

B. Herniated intervertebral disk

C. Scoliosis

D. Spondylolysis

Directions: This self-test should be taken only after completing all of the readings, review exercises, and laboratory activities for a particular section. The purpose of this test is not only to provide a good learning exercise but also to serve as a strong indicator of what your final evaluation exam will be. It is strongly suggested that if you do not receive at least a 90% to 95% grade on this self-test, you should review those areas in which you missed questions before going to your instructor for the final evaluation exam for this chapter.

1. From the list of possible fracture types below, indicate which fracture is represented on each drawing or radiograph by writing in the correct term where indicated (A through I):

- Single (closed) fracture
- Compound (open) fracture
- Torus fracture
- Greenstick fracture
- Plastic fracture
- Transverse fracture
- Oblique fracture
- Spiral fracture
- Comminuted fracture
- Impacted fracture
- Baseball (mallet) fracture
- Barton fracture
- Bennett's fracture
- Colles' fracture
- Monteggia fracture
- Nursemaids' elbow fracture
- Pott's fracture
- Avulsion fracture
- Chip fracture
- Compression fracture
- Stellate fracture
- Tuft fracture

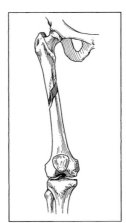 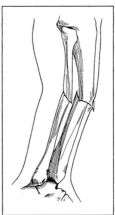 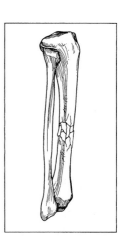

A. _____ B. _____ C. _____

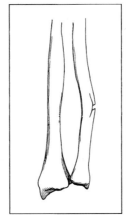 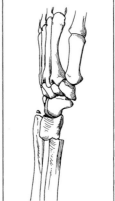 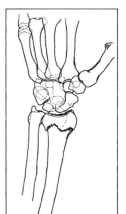

D. _____ E. _____ F. _____

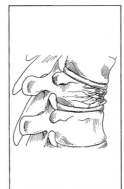 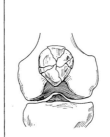 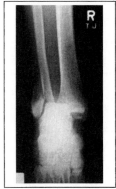

G. _____ H. _____ I. _____

2. A battery-powered, battery-operated mobile x-ray unit can climb a maximum incline of:

A. 7°   C. 12°

B. 10°   D. 15°

3. Which type of mobile radiography x-ray unit is self-propelled? _____

4. Which type of mobile x-ray unit is lighter weight? _____

5. True/False: C-arms are most generally stationary fluoroscopy units used in surgery.

6. True/False: The C-arm fluoroscopy unit can be rotated a minimum of 180°.

7. True/False: The AP projection with the x-ray tube placed directly above the anatomy during a C-arm procedure is recommended to minimize OID.

8. True/False: Digital C-arm units can store images on videotape or computer hard disk memory.

9. What is the term for the process of holding one image on the C-arm monitor while also providing continuous

fluoroscopy? _____

10. Match each of the following types of fracture to its correct definition (using each answer only once):

_____ A. Fracture through the pedicles of C2   1. Nursemaids' elbow

_____ B. Fracture of proximal half of ulna with dislocation of radial head   2. Bennett's

_____ C. Fracture due to a disease process   3. Baseball

_____ D. Fracture resulting in an isolated bone fragment   4. Pathologic

_____ E. Subluxation of the radial head on a child   5. Hangman's

_____ F. Fracture along base of first metacarpal   6. Hutchinson's

_____ G. Fracture of distal phalanx with finger extended   7. Stress or fatigue

_____ H. Also called a March fracture   8. Chip

_____ I. Also called a chauffeur's fracture   9. Monteggia

11. True/False: Any trauma study requires at least two projections as close to 90° opposite from each other as possible.

12. True/False: On an initial study of a long bone, both joints should be included for each projection.

13. True/False: Collimation on trauma cases can lead to cutoff of key anatomy and pathology, therefore it should be limited to the size of the IR.

14. The technologist must be at least _____ from the x-ray tube during a mobile radiographic procedure.

A. 2 feet/0.6 m   C. 6 feet/1.8 m

B. 4 feet/1.3 m   D. 8 feet/2.4 m

15. True/False: Wearing a protective lead apron is optional if the technologist is at least 8 feet/2.4 m from both the x-ray tube and patient during a mobile radiographic procedure.

16. True/False: The exposure dose is greater on the image intensifier side than on the x-ray tube side with the C-arm in the horizontal configuration.

17. True/False: A 30° tilt of C-arm from the vertical perspective will increase the dose by a factor of three to the head and neck region.

18. What should be the final step that the technologist takes before returning a trauma patient to the ER following a radiographic procedure?

    A. Review patient history
           C. Check patient armband/identification

    B. Review examination requisition
          D. Ensure side rails are up on the patient cart

19. True/False: Angiography of the aortic arch for the trauma patient has declined due to the increased use of CT angiography.

20. A. What is the correct term for the displacement of a bone from a joint? _____

    B. What is the correct term for a partial displacement? _____

21. Which one of the following terms describes a poor alignment between the ends of a fractured bone?

    A. Dislocation
           C. Apex angulation

    B. Lack of apposition
          D. Anatomic apposition

22. Which one of the following terms describes a bending of a distal fracture away from the midline?

    A. Valgus angulation
          C. Apex angulation

    B. Varus angulation
          D. Bayonet apposition

23. **Situation:** A technologist using a C-arm fluoroscope receives 125 mR/hour standing 2 feet (0.6 meters) from the patient. What is the exposure rate if the technologist moves to a distance of 6 feet (1.8 meters)?

    A. Less than 10 mR/hour
         C. 30 to 50 mR/hour

    B. 15 to 30 mR/hour
          D. 50 to 75 mR/hour

24. **Situation:** A technologist receives 30 mR/hour during a C-arm fluoroscopic procedure. What is the total exposure dose if the procedure takes 8 minutes of fluoroscopy time? _____

25. Radiologists often use the Salter-Harris system to classify _____ fractures.

    A. Pathologic
         C. Stellate

    B. Trimalleolar
         D. Epiphyseal

26. **Situation:** A patient with a possible pleural effusion in the right lung enters the emergency room. The patient is unable to stand or sit erect. What position would best demonstrate this condition?

    A. Right lateral decubitus
         C. Dorsal decubitus

    B. AP supine
          D. Semierect AP

27. Where is the CR centered for an AP semierect projection of the chest? _____

28. **Situation:** A patient with a crushing injury to the thorax enters the emergency room. The patient is on a backboard and cannot be moved. Which projections can be performed to determine whether the sternum is fractured?

29. **Situation:** A patient with possible ascites enters the emergency room. The patient is unable to stand or sit erect. Which one of the following positions would best demonstrate this condition?

A. AP supine KUB

B. Dorsal decubitus

C. Left lateral decubitus

D. Prone KUB

30. What is the minimum number of projections required for a postreduction study of the wrist?

_____

31. How is the CR aligned for a trauma lateral projection of the elbow? _____

32. Which lateral projection would best demonstrate the mid-to-distal humerus without rotating the limb?

_____

33. How much rotation of the body, from a supine position, is generally required for a lateromedial scapula projection

with a trauma patient who can be turned up partially on her side? _____

34. To ensure that the CR is aligned properly for an AP trauma projection of the foot, the CR is angled:

_____

35. **Situation:** A patient with a possible fracture of the ankle enters the emergency room. The patient cannot rotate the lower limb. What can be done to provide the orthopedic surgeon with a mortise projection of the ankle?

_____

36. **Situation:** Following a postreduction of a fractured tibia/fibula, a postreduction study is ordered. A fiberglass cast was placed on the fractured leg. The original technique was 70 kV at 4 mAs (film/screen system). How much should the technologist increase their factors from the original technique?

_____

37. Which one of the following projections demonstrates the C1-C2 vertebra if the patient cannot open his mouth?

A. 35° to 40° cephalad, AP axial projection

B. Swimmer's lateral

C. 15° to 20° cephalad, AP axial projection

D. Articular pillar projection

38. **Situation:** A patient with a possible fracture of the cervical spine pedicles enters the emergency room. Which one of the following projections will best demonstrate this region of the spine without moving the patient?

A. Perform a swimmer's lateral

B. Perform an articular pillar projection

C. Perform a Fuchs method

D. Perform AP axial trauma oblique projections

39. What is the name of the device on the x-ray tube mount that permits compound angles of the x-ray tube?

A. C-arm

B. Trunnion

C. Angle brace

D. Tube angle stop

40. Which one of the following facial bone projections will best demonstrate air-fluid levels in the maxillary sinuses for a patient unable to stand or sit erect?

    A. AP acanthioparietal   C. AP modified acanthioparietal

    B. Trauma, horizontal beam lateral   D. AP axial

41. A. On a horizontal beam lateral trauma skull projection, should the IR be placed lengthwise or crosswise to the

    patient? _____

    B. Where should the CR be centered for this lateral skull projection? _____

42. **Situation:** A patient with a possible compression fracture of the lumbar spine enters the emergency room. Which specific projection of the lumbar spine series would best demonstrate this fracture?

    A. AP   C. Lateral

    B. LPO and RPO   D. AP L5-S1 projection

43. **Situation:** A patient with a possible Barton fracture comes to the radiology department. Which one of the following positioning routines would best demonstrate this?

    A. AP or PA and lateral wrist   C. AP and lateral foot

    B. AP, mortise, and lateral ankle   D. AP and lateral lower leg

44. **Situation:** A patient enters the ER with a possible radial head dislocation. The arm is immobilized with the elbow flexed 90°. Which one of the following projections will best demonstrate the radial head free of superimposition of the ulna without having to extend the elbow?

    A. AP partial flexion   C. Jones method

    B. Trauma axiolateral projection   D. Lateromedial projection

45. For successful surgical radiographic exposures, clear communication must be established between the surgeon, technologist, and:

    A. Scrub   C. Circulator

    B. CST   D. Anesthesiologist

46. CST is the acronym for _____.

47. Suctioning, tying, and clamping blood vessels, as well as assisting in cutting and suturing tissues, are the general duties of the:

    A. CST   C. Surgical assistant

    B. Circulator   D. Scrub

48. The absence of infectious organisms is the definition for:

    A. Surgical cleanliness   C. Asepsis

    B. Sepsis   D. Surgical sterility

49. What portion(s) of the OR table is (are) considered sterile:

    A. Only the level of the tabletop

    B. Entire table

    C. Tabletop and half of the base

    D. None of the table

50. True/False: Scrubs worn in radiology may be also worn in surgery.

51. True/False: Scrub covers must be removed before entering the surgical suite.

52. True/False: The technologist can wear nonsterile gloves when handling the IR and surgical cover following a procedure.

53. Imaging equipment permanently stored in surgery must be cleaned at least:
    A. Daily   C. Monthly
    B. Bimonthly   D. Weekly

54. Which one of the following techniques will best reduce dose to the surgical team during a C-arm procedure?
    A. Use boost function whenever possible.
    B. Place tube in vertical position above patient.
    C. Use intermittent fluoroscopy.
    D. Lower kV as low as possible.

55. What is the primary benefit of the "pulse mode" on a digital C-arm unit?

    _____

56. **Situation:** An image taken during an operative cholangiogram reveals that the biliary ducts are superimposed over the spine. The surgeon wants the ducts projected away from the spine. Which one of the following positions may eliminate this problem during the repeat exposure?
    A. Shallow RPO   C. AP
    B. Shallow LPO   D. Horizontal beam lateral

57. True/False: Laparoscopic cholecystectomy is not suited for every patient and condition.

58. Retrograde urography is a _____ (nonfunctional or functional) examination of the urinary system.

59. A retrograde pyelogram is a specific radiographic examination of the _____ system.

60. ORIF is the abbreviation for _____.

61. Which one of the following devices helps maintain the sterile environment in surgery during a C-arm guided hip pinning?

    A. Shower curtain   C. Cassette cover

    B. Mylar shield   D. Good cleaning of equipment before procedure

62. Which one of the following orthopedic devices is used to stabilize a midfemoral shaft fracture?

    A. Austin-Moore prosthesis   C. Interbody fusion cages

    B. Intramedullary rod   D. Cannulated screw

63. Which one of the following devices is an example of an external fixator?

    A. Interbody fusion cage   C. Modular bipolar prosthesis

    B. Thompson prosthesis   D. Ilizarov device

64. Which one of the following procedures does *not* require the use of mobile fluoroscopy?

   A. Hip pinning

   B. Intramedullary rod insertion

   C. Open reduction of tibia

   D. All of the above require fluoroscopic guidance

65. Which of the following devices can be used for spinal fusion surgery rather than the use of a pedicle screw?

   A. Austin-Moore prosthesis

   B. Cannulated screw

   C. Dynamic compression plate

   D. Interbody fusion cage

66. Which spinal procedure may require the use of Harrington or Luque rods?

   A. Scoliosis corrective surgery

   B. Microdiscectomy

   C. Spinal fusion

   D. All of the above

67. An unthreaded (smooth) or threaded metallic wire used to reduce fractures of the wrist (carpals) is called

   _____

68. A special OR table used for hip pinnings and other orthopedic procedures to provide traction to the involved limb

   is termed _____.

69. DHS is an abbreviation for _____.

16 | Pediatric Radiography

Positioning considerations are unique to pediatric radiography and present a definite challenge for all technologists. Children cannot be handled and positioned like miniature adults. They have special needs and require patience and understanding. Their anatomic makeup is vastly different from that of adults, especially the skeletal system. The bony development (ossification) of children goes through specific growth stages from infancy to adolescence. These need to be understood by technologists so that the appearance of the normal growth stages can be recognized. Examples of normal bone development patterns at various ages are included in this chapter and the textbook.

The routine and optional projections and positions are much different for children than adults. You need to know and understand these differences to be able to visualize the essential anatomy of children of various ages.

The most obvious differences for children when compared with adults are the methods of positioning and immobility. Small children cannot simply be instructed to hold still in certain positions or hold their breath during the exposure. You will need to learn how to relate to children and communicate with them to gain their cooperation without forceful immobilization.

Special immobilization techniques need to be learned along with the use of various types of commonly available immobilization equipment. Specialized restraining devices available in many departments will be explained and demonstrated in this chapter.

Radiation protection for these small patients must also be a major concern because the younger the child, the more sensitive the tissues are to radiation. Thus accurate collimation and gonadal shielding are absolutely essential. High-speed IR should also be used, and repeats must be minimized. Keeping all child doses as low as possible is even more important than in adult radiography. Therefore careful study of this chapter and related clinical experience are essential before you attempt a radiographic examination on a small child or infant. As a student, you may have limited opportunity to observe and assist with pediatric patients during your training. This makes learning and mastering the information provided in this chapter of the textbook and this workbook-laboratory manual even more important.

CHAPTER OBJECTIVES

After you have successfully completed the activities of this chapter, you will be able to:

_____ 1. List the steps and process of the technologist's introduction to the child and parent and the potential role of the parent during the child's examination.

_____ 2. Define the term *nonaccidental trauma (NAT)* and describe the role of technologists if they suspect child abuse based on individual state guidelines.

_____ 3. Identify the more common commercial immobilization devices and explain their function.

_____ 4. List the most common types of ancillary devices used for immobilization.

_____ 5. List the four steps of "mummifying" an infant. Perform this procedure on a simulated patient.

_____ 6. Define terms relating to bone development or ossification and identify the radiographic appearance and the normal stages of development of secondary growth centers.

_____ 7. Identify methods of reducing patient and guardian doses and repeat exposures during pediatric procedures.

_____ 8. Identify alternative imaging modalities and procedures performed on pediatric patients.

_____ 9. List the common clinical indications for radiographic examinations of the pediatric chest, upper and lower limbs, pelvis and hips, skull, and abdomen.

_____ 10. For select forms of pathology of the pediatric skeletal system, determine whether manual exposure factors would increase, decrease, or remain the same.

_____ 11. Describe positioning, technical factors, shielding requirements, and immobilization techniques for procedures of the chest, skeletal system, and abdomen.

_____ 12. List general patient preparation requirements for procedures of the pediatric abdomen, including specific minimum patient preparation requirements for the upper GI, lower GI, and genitourinary procedures.

_____ 13. List the types and quantities of contrast media based on age as recommended for upper GI, lower GI, and genitourinary procedures.

_____ 14. Using an articulated pediatric mannequin, correctly immobilize and position a patient.

_____ 15. Using gonadal shielding, perform examinations of the chest, abdomen, upper limb, lower limb, pelvis and hips, and skull.

_____ 16. According to established evaluation criteria, critique and evaluate radiographs provided by your instructor for each of the previously mentioned examinations.

_____ 17. Discriminate between acceptable and unacceptable radiographs and describe how positioning or technical errors can be corrected.

LEARNING EXERCISES

The following review exercises should be completed only after careful study of the associated pages in the textbook as indicated by each exercise. Answers to each review exercise are given at the end of this workbook.

PART I: INTRODUCTION TO PEDIATRIC RADIOGRAPHY
REVIEW EXERCISE A: Immobilization, Ossification, Radiation Protection, Pre-exam Preparation, and Clinical Indications (see textbook pp. 620-630)

1. List the two important general factors that produce a successful pediatric radiographic procedure:

   A. _____

   B. _____

2. List the three possible roles for the parent during a pediatric procedure:

   A. _____

   B. _____

   C. _____

3. True/False: Parents should never be in the radiographic room with their child.

4. True/False: The technologist should always use as short an exposure time as possible during pediatric procedures.

5. True/False: The parent has the right to refuse the use of immobilization devices.

6. A device with an adjustable type of bicycle seat and two clear plastic body clamps is called

   _____.

7. For what is the immobilization device described in question 6 most commonly used?

   _____

8. Why is tape is not recommended for immobilization purposes on children?

   _____

9. When adhesive tape is used to immobilize a child (if not placed directly over the parts to be radiographed), what two methods are used to prevent the adhesive tape from injuring the skin?

   A. _____

   B. _____

10. Briefly describe the four steps for "mummifying" a child:

    1. _____

    2. _____

    3. _____

    4. _____

11. Primary centers of bone formation (ossification) involving the midshafts of long bones are called

    _____.

12. Secondary centers of ossification of the long bones are called _____.

13. The area in which bone growth in length occurs is termed the _____.

14. At approximately what age does the skeleton reach full ossification?
    A. 12 years old   C. 25 years old
    B. 18 years old   D. 40 years old

15. At approximately what age does the epiphysis of the fibular apex first become clearly visible?
    A. 1 or 2 years old   C. 5 or 6 years old
    B. 3 or 4 years old   D. 12 years old

16. True/False: Battered child syndrome (BCS) is the current term for child abuse.

17. True/False: The technologist is responsible for reporting potential signs of child abuse to the police.

18. What are five of the six specific classifications of child abuse?

   1. _____

   2. _____

   3. _____

   4. _____

   5. _____

19. How can rib fractures be a radiographic indication of child abuse?

   _____

20. List three safeguards to help reduce repeat exposures during pediatric procedures:

   A. _____   B. _____   C. _____

21. Other than gonadal shielding, what three safeguards can be used to reduce the patient dose during pediatric procedures?

   A. _____   B. _____   C. _____

22. Sometimes a primary technologist and assisting technologist work together. Match each of the following duties with the correct technologist.

   _____ 1. Initiates exposures   A. Primary technologist

   _____ 2. Positions the patient   B. Assisting technologist

   _____ 3. Processes the images

   _____ 4. Positions the tube and collimates

   _____ 5. Sets exposure factors

   _____ 6. Instructs the parents

23. True/False: Clothing, bandages, and diapers generally do not need to be removed from the regions being radiographed on pediatric patients because they do not cause artifacts on the radiographs (as long as metallic fasteners are not present).

24. True/False: Renal CT scans have largely replaced intravenous urography studies for children.

25. Increasing kV and _____, dose *can* be reduced to the pediatric patient during a CT scan.

   A. mA   C. Scan resolution

   B. Region of body scanned D. Pitch ratio

26. True/False: Multiphase CT examinations are necessary for most pediatric studies.

27. Beyond radiography, what other imaging modality is used to diagnose congenital hip dislocations in the newborn?

  A. Sonography C. Nuclear medicine

  B. CT D. MRI

28. Which one of the following imaging modalities is most effective in diagnosing pyloric stenosis in children?

  A. Sonography C. Functional MRI

  B. Spiral/helical CT D. Nuclear medicine

29. Functional MRI has been used to detect disorders in all the following conditions except:

  A. Autism C. Hydrocephalus

  B. Tourette's syndrome D. Attention deficient hyperactivity disorder

30. Match each of the following pathologic disorders of the pediatric chest with the best definition or description. (Use each choice only once.)

  _____ A. Meconium aspiration

  _____ B. Hyaline membrane disease

  _____ C. Neonate Graves' disease

  _____ D. Epiglottitis

  _____ E. Cystic fibrosis

  _____ F. Croup

  _____ G. Hemoptysis

  1. Bacterial infection can lead to closure of the upper airway

  2. Also known as respiratory distress syndrome

  3. Inherited disease leading to clogging of bronchi

  4. May develop during stressful births

  5. Viral infection leading to labored breathing and dry cough

  6. Coughing up blood

  7. A form of hyperthyroidism

31. Match each of the following pathologic disorders of the pediatric skeletal system to the best definition or description:

  _____ A. Meningocele

  _____ B. Köhler's bone disease

  _____ C. Craniostenosis

  _____ D. Talipes equinus

  _____ E. Osteogenesis imperfecta

  _____ F. Achondroplasia

  _____ G. Myelocele

  _____ H. Osteochondrosis

  1. Decreased bone formation at growth plates

  2. Abnormally soft bones

  3. Spinal cord protrudes through an opening

  4. Prematurely closed cranial sutures

  5. Disease of epiphyseal and growth plate

  6. Protrusion of meninges through opening

  7. Inflammation of navicular in the foot

  8. Congenital deformity of the foot

32. Match each of the following clinical indications of the pediatric abdomen to the best definition or description:

_____ A. Ileus   1. May result in repeated, forceful vomiting

_____ B. Pyloric stenosis   2. Characterized by absence of rhythmic contractions of large intestine

_____ C. NEC   3. Condition characterized by absence of an opening in an organ

_____ D. Atresias   4. Cancer of the kidney of embryonal origin

_____ E. Hypospadias   5. Obstruction caused by lack of contractile movement of the intestinal wall

_____ F. Hirschsprung disease   6. Inflammation of the inner lining of the intestine

_____ G. Wilms' tumor   7. Congenital defect in male urethra

33. Indicate whether the following pathologic conditions require that manual exposure factors be increased (+), decreased (−), or remain the same (0):

_____ A. Idiopathic juvenile osteoporosis

_____ B. Osteogenesis imperfecta

_____ C. Osteomalacia

34. What is meconium?

A. Pancreatic enzymes   C. Dark green secretion of the liver and intestinal glands mixed with amniotic fluid

B. Blood and lymph   D. Pus and dead blood cells

35. True/False: Malignant bone tumors are rare in young children.

PART II: RADIOGRAPHIC POSITIONING
REVIEW EXERCISE B: Pediatric Positioning of the Chest, Skeletal System, and Skull (see textbook pp. 631-642)

1. True/False: If available, the Pigg-O-Stat should be used rather than relying on parental assistance during a pediatric chest examination.

2. Complete the following technical factors for an AP or PA pediatric chest:

A. Grid or nongrid? _____   D. SID, AP supine chest: _____

B. kV range (analog and digital): _____   E. SID, PA erect chest: _____

C. Image receptor—lengthwise or crosswise? _____

3. What kV range (analog and digital) is generally used for a lateral chest? _____

4. Should a grid be used for a 2-year-old lateral chest? _____

5. The Pigg-O-Stat can be used effectively for an erect PA and lateral chest from infancy to approximately

_____ years of age.

6. When should a chest exposure be initiated for a crying child? _____

7. Which radiographic structures are evaluated to determine rotation on a PA projection of the chest?

_____

8. How is the x-ray tube aligned for a lateral projection of the chest if the patient is on a Tam-em board?

_____

9. True/False: A well-inspired, erect chest radiograph taken on a young pediatric patient will visualize only six to seven ribs above the diaphragm.

10. True/False: The entire upper limb is commonly included on an infant rather than individual exposures of specific parts of the upper limb.

11. True/False: Except for survey exams, individual projections of the elbow, wrist, and shoulder should generally be taken on older children rather than including these regions on a single projection.

12. Match the following pathologic indicators with the correct radiographic procedure:

_____ A. Atelectasis   1. Chest

_____ B. Köhler's disease   2. Upper or lower limb

_____ C. Cystic fibrosis

_____ D. Talipes

_____ E. RDS

13. Which single radiographic position provides a lateral projection of bilateral lower limbs for the nontraumatic

pediatric patient? _____

14. Which radiographic projections (and method) are performed for the infant with congenital club feet?

_____

15. True/False: It is important to place the foot into true AP and lateral positions when performing a clubfoot study.

16. True/False: It is possible to provide gonadal shielding for both male and female pediatric patients for AP and lateral projections of the hips.

17. What size image receptor should be used for a skull routine on a 6-year-old patient?

_____

18. Which one of the following CR angulations places the petrous ridges in the lower one-third of the orbits with an AP reverse Caldwell projection of the skull?
    A. 15° cephalad to OML   C. CR perpendicular to OML
    B. 15° caudad to OML   D. 30° cephalad to OML

19. Which one of the following clinical indicators would apply to a pediatric skull series?
    A. Osteomyelitis   C. Craniostenosis
    B. CHD   D. Hyaline membrane disease

20. Which skull positioning line is placed perpendicular to the film for an AP Towne 30° caudal projection of the skull?

    A. IOML   C. MML

    B. OML   D. AML

21. True/False: Parental assistance for skull radiography is preferred rather than using head clamps and a mummy wrap on a pediatric patient.

22. True/False: Children more than 5 years of age can usually hold their breath after a practice session.

23. Correct centering for the following can be achieved by placing the central ray at the level of which structure or landmark?

    A. AP, PA, or lateral chest: _____

    B. AP abdomen (infants and small children): _____

    C. AP supine abdomen (older children): _____

    D. AP skull: _____

REVIEW EXERCISE C: Positioning of the Pediatric Abdomen and Contrast Media Procedures (see textbook pp. 643-661)

1. A backward flow of urine from the bladder into the ureters and kidneys is called

   _____.

2. True/False: Small retention enema tips can be used on infants during a barium enema to help barium retention.

3. What type of contrast media is recommended for reducing an intussusception?

   _____

4. What is the maximum height of the barium enema bag above the tabletop before the beginning of the procedure?

   _____

5. True/False: The chest and abdomen are generally almost equal in circumference in the newborn.

6. True/False: Bony landmarks in infants are easy to palpate and locate.

7. True/False: It is difficult to distinguish the small bowel from the large bowel on a plain abdomen on an infant.

8. True/False: The radiographic contrast on a pediatric abdominal radiograph is high compared with that of an adult abdominal radiograph.

9. Complete the recommended NPO fasting before the following pediatric contrast media procedures:

    A. 1-year-old upper GI: _____   C. Infant lower GI: _____

    B. 2-month-old upper GI: _____   D. Pediatric IVU: _____

10. List five conditions that contraindicate the use of laxatives or enemas in preparation for a lower GI study:

A. _____

B. _____

C. _____

D. _____

E. _____

11. Place an X next to the clinical indicators that apply for an AP abdomen (KUB).

_____ A. Croup   _____ E. Mastoiditis

_____ B. NEC   _____ F. Hepatomegaly

_____ C. Intussusception   _____ G. Appendicitis

_____ D. Foreign body localization   _____ H. Hydrocephalus

12. Where is the CR centered for an erect abdomen on a small child? _____

13. A. What is the minimum kV (analog and digital) for an AP abdomen projection of a newborn without a grid?

_____

B. A grid is required for a pediatric AP abdomen if the abdomen measures more than _____ cm.

14. Which one of the following projections of the abdomen best demonstrates the prevertebral region?

A. AP supine KUB   C. Dorsal decubitus abdomen

B. PA prone KUB   D. AP erect abdomen

15. A malignant tumor of the kidney common in children under the age of 5 years is:

A. Wilms' tumor   B. Adenocarcinoma   C. Ewing's sarcoma   D. Teratoma

16. What is the most common clinical indication for a voiding cystourethrogram?

_____

17. Which one of the following conditions is caused by inflammation of the inner lining of the large or small bowel, resulting in tissue death?

A. NEC   B. CHD

C. Intussusception   D. Meconium ileus

18. Which of the following procedures or projections should be performed for a possible meconium ileus?

A. IVU procedure   B. Barium enema

C. AP supine abdomen   D. AP erect abdomen

19. True/False: A piece of lead vinyl can be placed beneath the child's lower pelvis during conventional fluoroscopy to reduce the gonadal/mean bone marrow dose.

20. How much barium should be given to each of the following patients for an upper GI series?

A. Newborn to 1 year old: _____

C. 3 to 10 years old: _____

B. 1 to 3 years old: _____

D. Over 10 years old: _____

21. What may be the only recourse if a pediatric patient refuses to drink barium for an upper GI series?

_____

22. True/False: The transit time of the contrast media for reaching the cecum during a small bowel series on a 3-year-old child is approximately 2 hours.

23. True/False: Latex enema tips should be used for barium enemas for children under the age of 1 year.

24. Which projections are frequently performed during a VCUG on a pediatric patient?

_____

25. True/False: A radionuclide study for vesicourethral reflux provides a smaller patient dose compared with a fluoroscopic voiding cystourethrogram.

REVIEW EXERCISE D: Problem Solving and Analysis

1. **Situation:** A young child is sent to the radiology department for a skull series. The guardian states that she is willing to hold her child during the exposures; however, the guardian is 8 months pregnant. What should the technologist do next?

A. Place a 0.5-mm lead apron on the guardian and allow her to hold her child.

B. The technologist should hold the child during each exposure and have the guardian wait outside.

C. Have another (nonradiology) health professional hold the child and have the guardian wait outside the room.

D. Have a radiography student hold the child and have the guardian wait outside the room.

2. **Situation:** A 3-year-old child comes to the radiology department for an erect abdomen examination. He is unable to hold still for the exposures. Which immobilization device should be used for this patient?

A. Tam-em board

C. Plexiglas hold-down paddle

B. Pigg-O-Stat

D. Have another technologist hold child

3. **Situation:** A child comes to the radiology department with possible croup. Which one of the following procedures best demonstrates this condition?

A. AP and lateral upper airway

C. PA and lateral chest

B. Erect abdomen

D. Sinus series

4. **Situation:** A newborn is diagnosed with RDS. Which one of the following procedures is commonly performed for this condition?

A. Abdomen

C. CT of head

B. Functional MRI

D. Chest

5. **Situation:** A child comes to the radiology department with a clinical history of Legg-Calvé-Perthes disease. Which one of the following projections best demonstrates this condition?

A. PA and lateral chest

C. AP and lateral hip

B. Supine and erect abdomen

D. AP and lateral bilateral lower limbs

6. **Situation:** A child comes to the radiology department with a clinical history of Köhler bone disease. Which one of the following radiographic routines demonstrates this condition?

   A. Foot

   B. Shoulder

   C. Lumbar spine

   D. Cervical spine

7. **Situation:** A child comes to radiology with a clinical history of talipes equinovarus. Which of the following positioning routines and/or methods is often performed for this condition?

   A. Coyle method

   B. Erect AP knee projections

   C. AP and lateral foot—Kite method

   D. AP and lateral hip

8. **Situation:** Which radiographic procedure is often performed for Hirschsprung disease?

   A. Upper GI

   B. MRI

   C. Cystourethrography

   D. Barium enema

9. **Situation:** Which radiographic procedure is often performed for pyloric stenosis?

   A. Barium enema

   B. Evacuative proctography

   C. Enteroclysis

   D. Upper GI

10. Which one of the following modalities is most effective in detecting signs of autism?

    A. fMRI

    B. Ultrasound

    C. Spiral CT

    D. Nuclear medicine

PART III: LABORATORY EXERCISES

Exercises A and B need to be carried out in a radiographic laboratory or a general diagnostic room in the radiology department. General immobilization paraphernalia must be available (i.e., tape, sheets or large towels, sandbags, various sizes and shapes of positioning sponge blocks, retention bands, head clamps, stockinettes, and Ace bandages). More common commercial immobilization devices, such as the Tam-em board or the Pigg-O-Stat (or similar devices), are optional if available. At least one of these devices should be made available for student use.

Exercise C can be carried out in a classroom or any room in which illuminators (view boxes) are available.

Laboratory Exercise A: Immobilization

For this section you will need some type of large articulated doll or mannequin to use as your patient. The doll should have arms and legs that are flexible (similar to those of a child). This does not need to be a phantom-like doll because radiographs will not be taken, but it will be used to simulate immobilization techniques and positioning for various body parts.

Check off each of the following activities as you complete them:

_____ 1. Complete the four steps of "mummifying."

_____ 2. Immobilize your patient correctly with the Velcro straps to restrain the upper and lower limbs and across the pelvic region.

Pigg-O-Stat (if available):

Laboratory Exercise B: Physical Positioning

This section again requires the use of a large articulated pediatric mannequin. Practice the following projections or positions until you can perform them accurately and without hesitation. Place a check mark by each activity when you have achieved it.

Include the details listed in the following as you simulate the routine projections for each exam that follows. Assume that the patient will not cooperate and forceful immobilization is required. Use suggested immobilization techniques.

_____ Correct size and type of image receptor (appropriate for size of "patient")

_____ Correct centering of part to image receptor

_____ Correct SID and location and angle of central ray

_____ Selection of appropriate restraining devices and application of the same

_____ Correct placement of markers

_____ Correct use of contact gonadal shield

_____ Accurate collimation to body part of interest

_____ Approximate correct exposure factors

	Examination	_Immobilization_
_____	1. AP chest, supine	Tam-em board or sandbags and/or stockinette and "Ace" bandages
_____	2. Lateral chest, patient	Sandbags and tape; or retention band recumbent in lateral position

If Tam-em board is available:

_____	3. Lateral chest, patient supine, horizontal beam CR	Tam-em board

If Pigg-O-Stat is available:

_____	4. PA chest erect, 72-inch (183-cm) SID	Pigg-O-Stat
_____	5. Lateral chest erect, 72-inch	Pigg-O-Stat (183-cm) SID
_____	6. AP abdomen, erect	Pigg-O-Stat
_____	7. AP abdomen, supine	Tam-em board; or tape, sandbags, and retention band
_____	8. AP and lateral upper limb	Tape, sandbags, and/or retention to band (from shoulder to hand)
_____	9. AP and lateral lower limb	Tape, sandbags, and/or retention band (from hips to feet)
_____	10. AP and lateral feet (such as follow-up exams for clubfeet)	Sitting on pad using tape
_____	11. AP pelvis and hips	Tape and sandbags and/or retention band
_____	12. Lateral hips	Tape and sandbags and/or retention band
_____	13. AP skull, 15° AP and 30° Towne	Head clamps or tape for head. Mummification and sandbags or retention band for limbs and body
_____	14. Lateral skull, turned into lateral position	Head clamps or tape for head. Mummification and sandbags or retention band for limbs and body
_____	15. Lateral skull, horizontal beam in supine	Tam-em board and tape for head position

Laboratory Exercise C: Anatomy Review and Critique Radiographs of the Abdomen

Use the radiographs provided by your instructor. These should include optimal-quality and less-than-optimal quality radiographs of each of the following: chest, supine and erect abdomen, AP and lateral upper limb, AP and lateral pelvis and hips, AP and lateral lower limb, and AP and lateral skull radiographs.

Radiographs of the pelvis and upper and lower limbs of patients of various ages should be included to demonstrate the normal ossification or growth stages from infancy to adolescence.

Place a check mark by each of the following steps when completed:

_____ 1. Examine normal stages of growth by the appearance of the epiphyses in the pelvis and the long bones of the upper and lower limbs. Estimate the approximate age of the patient by the appearance of such epiphyses.

_____ 2. Critique each radiograph based on evaluation criteria provided for each projection in the textbook. Pediatric radiographs require a wider range of acceptable positioning criteria than for adults. Part centering and specific central ray locations are not as critical for pediatric radiographs because multiple anatomic parts or bones are included on one IR. This is possible because detailed views of joint areas are not as important because these secondary growth areas are not yet fully developed. Thus complete limbs can be included on one film.

The following criteria guidelines can be used and checked as each radiograph is evaluated. Determine the corrections or adjustments in positioning or exposure factors necessary to bring those less-than-optimal radiographs up to a more desirable standard.

Radiographs

1	2	3	4	5	6

Criteria Guidelines

a. Correct image receptor size as appropriate for age and size of patient?

b. Correct orientation of part to image receptor?

c. Acceptable alignment and/or centering of part to image receptor?

d. Correct collimation and correct CR angle where appropriate (such as for an AP skull)?

e. Evidence of gonadal shield correctly placed (if this should be visible)?

f. Pertinent anatomy well visualized?

g. Evidence of motion?

h. Optimal exposure (density and/or contrast)?

i. Patient ID with date and side markers visible without superimposing essential anatomy?

Directions: This self-test should be taken only after completing all of the readings, review exercises, and laboratory activities for a particular section. The purpose of this test is not only to provide a good learning exercise but also to serve as a strong indicator of what your final evaluation exam will be. It is strongly suggested that if you do not receive at least a 90% to 95% grade on this self-test, you should review those areas in which you missed questions before going to your instructor for the final evaluation exam for this chapter.

1. At what age can most children be talked through a radiographic examination without purposeful immobilization?

   A. 1 year　　　　　　　　C. 3 years

   B. 18 months　　　　　　D. 5 years

2. At the first meeting between the technologist and the patient (accompanied by an adult), which of the following generally should *not* be discussed?

   A. Introduce yourself.

   B. Take the necessary time to explain what you will be doing.

   C. Discuss the possible forceful immobilization that will be needed if the child will not cooperate.

   D. Describe the total amount of radiation the patient will receive with that specific exam if it has to be repeated because of a lack of cooperation.

   E. All of these steps must be taken.

3. Which of the following is *not* the name of a known commercially available immobilization device?

   A. Posi-Tot　　　　　　　C. Pigg-O-Stat

   B. Tam-em board　　　　　D. Hold-em Tiger

4. The most suitable immobilization device for erect chests and/or the abdomen is the:

   A. Posi-Tot　　　　　　　C. Pigg-O-Stat

   B. Tam-em board　　　　　D. Hold-em Tiger

5. List the three factors that reduce the number of repeat exposures with pediatric patients:

   A. _____　　　B. _____　　　C. _____

6. Which immobilization device or method should be used for an erect 1-year-old chest procedure? Assume these devices are available.

   A. Tam-em board　　　　　C. Pigg-O-Stat

   B. Hold-down paddle　　　D. Parent holding child

7. Two common terms for the classic metaphyseal lesion (CML), which may indicate child abuse, are

   _____ and _____.

8. If child abuse is suspected by the technologist, he or she should:

   A. Ask the parent when the abuse occurred

   B. Report the abuse immediately to the necessary state officials as required by the state

   C. Refuse to do the examination or touch the child until a physician has examined the patient

   D. Do none of the above

9. Complete the following related to ossification by matching the correct term with the description. (More than one choice per blank may be used.)

   E = Epiphysis   D = Diaphysis   EP = Epiphyseal plate

   _____ 1. Primary centers

   _____ 2. Secondary centers

   _____ 3. Space between primary and secondary centers

   _____ 4. Occurs before birth

   _____ 5. Continues to change from birth to maturity

10. Which one of the following procedures can be performed to diagnose possible genetic fetal abnormalities?

    A. Nuclear medicine fetal scan   C. Functional MRI

    B. Spiral/helical CT   D. 3-D ultrasound

11. Which of the following procedures can be performed to evaluate children for attention deficient hyperactivity disorder?

    A. Spiral/helical CT   C. 3-D ultrasound

    B. Functional MRI   D. Nuclear medicine

12. Match each of the following conditions to its correct definition or statement. (Use each choice only once.)

    _____ A. Croup

    _____ B. Congenital goiter

    _____ C. Epiglottitis

    _____ D. Osteochondrosis

    _____ E. Osteogenesis imperfecta

    _____ F. Salter-Harris facture

    _____ G. Osteomalacia

    _____ H. Hirschsprung disease

    _____ I. Wilms' tumor

    _____ J. Neuroblastoma

    _____ K. Pyelonephritis

    _____ L. Atresia

    _____ M. Craniostenosis

    1. Tumor that usually occurs in children younger than 5

    2. Group of diseases affecting the epiphyseal growth plates

    3. Fracture involving the epiphyseal plate

    4. A common condition in children between the ages of 1 to 3, caused by a viral infection

    5. Premature closure of the skull sutures

    6. Second-most common form of cancer in children younger than 5 years of age

    7. Bacterial infection of the upper airway that may be fatal if untreated

    8. Congenital defect in which an opening into an organ is missing

    9. Enlarged thyroid at birth

    10. Bacterial infection of the kidney

    11. Also known as *congenital megacolon*

    12. Also known as *rickets*

    13. Inherited condition that produces very fragile bones

403

13. Indicate whether the following pathologic conditions require that manual exposure factors be increased (+), decreased (−), or remain the same (0):

_____ A. Idiopathic juvenile osteoporosis

_____ B. Osteomalacia

_____ C. Osteogenesis imperfecta

14. Which of the following imaging modalities is effective in detecting signs of attention deficit hyperactivity disorder (ADHD)?

A. CT 　　　　　　　　　　C. Nuclear medicine

B. Sonography 　　　　　　D. Functional MRI

15. Which one of the following techniques helps to remove the scapulae from the lung fields during chest radiography?

A. Make exposure on the second inspiration 　　　C. Extend arms upward

B. Extend the chin 　　　　　　　　　　　　　D. Place arms behind the patient's back

16. What is the kV range (analog and digital) for a pediatric study of the upper limb? _____

17. True/False: A hand routine for a 7-year-old would be the same as for an adult patient.

18. True/False: For a bone survey of a young child, both limbs are commonly radiographed for comparison.

19. Which radiographic technique or method is performed to radiographically study congenital clubfoot?

_____

20. Where is gonadal shielding placed for a bilateral hip study on a female pediatric patient?

_____

21. Match the following examinations with the clinical indicators with which they are most likely associated. (Answers may be used more than once.)

_____ A. Intussusception 　　　　　　　1. Chest

_____ B. NEC 　　　　　　　　　　　　2. Abdomen

_____ C. Atelectasis 　　　　　　　　　3. Upper and lower limbs

_____ D. Premature closure of fontanelles 　4. Pelvis and hips

_____ E. CHD 　　　　　　　　　　　　5. Skull

_____ F. Cystic fibrosis

_____ G. Meconium ileus

_____ H. Legg-Calvé-Perthes disease

_____ I. Hemoptysis

_____ J. Bronchiectasis

_____ K. Hyaline membrane disease

22. How much is the CR angled to the OML for an AP axial (Towne) projection of the skull?

    A. 15°   C. 25°

    B. None   D. 30°

23. Where is the CR centered for a lateral projection of the pediatric skull?

    A. At the EAM   C. 1 inch (2.5 cm) above the EAM

    B. Midway between the glabella and inion   D. ¾ inch (2 cm) anterior and superior to the EAM

24. The NPO fasting period for a 6-month-old infant before an upper GI is:

    A. 4 hours   C. 1 hour

    B. 3 hours   D. 6 hours

25. Other than preventing artifacts in the bowel, what is the other reason that solid food is withheld for 4 hours before a pediatric IVU?

    _____

26. Which one of the following conditions would contraindicate the use of laxatives before a contrast media procedure?

    A. Gastritis   C. Appendicitis

    B. Blood in stool   D. Diverticulosis

27. Where is the CR centered for a KUB on:

    A. An 8-year-old child? _____

    B. A 3-month-old infant? _____

28. Where is the CR centered for a PA and lateral pediatric chest projection? _____

29. What is the recommended amount of barium given to an 8-year-old child having an upper GI?

    _____

30. How is barium instilled into the large bowel for a barium enema study on an infant?

    _____

31. What is the bowel prep for a pediatric voiding cystourethrogram (VCUG)? _____

32. When is urinary reflux most likely to occur during a VCUG? _____

33. For a young pediatric small bowel study, the barium normally reaches the ileocecal region in _____ hour(s).

34. A VCUG on a child is most commonly performed to evaluate for (A) _____ and is

    generally scheduled to be completed (B) _____ (before or after) an IVU or ultrasound study of the kidneys.

35. True/False: Gonadal shielding should only be used in supine positions because of the difficulty in keeping the shield in place.

36. True/False: There should be no attempt to straighten out the abnormal alignment of the foot during a clubfoot study.

37. **Situation:** Which radiographic procedure is commonly performed for epiglottitis?

    A. Sinus series

    B. AP and lateral upper airway

    C. CT of the chest

    D. Functional MRI

38. **Situation:** Which of the following radiographic routines and/or procedures best demonstrates Osgood-Schlatter disease?

    A. Barium enema

    B. AP and lateral hip

    C. Upper GI

    D. AP and lateral knee

39. **Situation:** A 2-year-old child comes to the radiology department for a routine chest examination. While removing the child's shirt, you notice a human bite mark on the upper arm. What should you do next?

    A. Call hospital security.

    B. Inform the supervisor or physician.

    C. Interview the parents about the injury.

    D. Interview the child about the injury.

40. Which of the following conditions can be diagnosed prenatally with sonography?

    A. Tourette's syndrome

    B. Vesicoureteral reflux

    C. Spina bifida

    D. Autism

17 Angiography and Interventional Procedures

This chapter, which includes extensive detailed and somewhat complex anatomy and procedural information, is an excellent introduction to angiography and interventional procedures. It provides effective preparation and a good overview for the additional clinical training and experience that a cardiovascular technologist will need.

CHAPTER OBJECTIVES

After you have successfully completed the activities of this chapter, you will be able to:

_____ 1. List the divisions and components of the circulatory system.

_____ 2. List the three functions of the cardiovascular system.

_____ 3. On drawings, identify the components of the pulmonary and general systemic circulation.

_____ 4. Identify the four chambers of the heart, associated valves, and coronary circulation.

_____ 5. List and identify the four arteries supplying blood to the brain and the three branches arising from the aortic arch.

_____ 6. List the major branches of the external and internal carotid arteries and the primary divisions of the brain supplied by each.

_____ 7. On drawings, identify the major veins of the neck draining blood from the head and neck region.

_____ 8. List the major venous sinuses found in the cranium.

_____ 9. List the four segments of the thoracic aorta and describe the three common variations of the aortic arch.

_____ 10. List and identify the five major branches of the abdominal aorta.

_____ 11. List and identify the major abdominal veins.

_____ 12. List and identify the major arteries and veins of the upper and lower limbs.

_____ 13. List four functions of the lymphatic portion of the circulatory system.

_____ 14. Identify the six steps for the Seldinger technique.

_____ 15. Identify the equipment generally found in an angiographic room.

_____ 16. Identify the clinical indications, contraindications, and general procedure for cerebral angiography.

_____ 17. Identify the indications, catheterization technique, and general procedure for thoracic and abdominal angiography.

_____ 18. Identify the clinical indications, contraindications, and general procedure for peripheral angiography.

_____ 19. Identify specific examples of vascular and nonvascular interventional procedures.

Complete the following review exercises after reading the associated pages in the textbook as indicated by each exercise. Answers to each review exercise are given at the end of this workbook.

REVIEW EXERCISE A: Anatomy of Vascular System, Pulmonary and Systemic Circulation, and Cerebral Arteries and Veins (see textbook pp. 654-660)

1. List the two major divisions or components of the circulatory system:

   A. _____   B. _____

2. List the body system or part supplied by the following four divisions of the circulatory system:

   A. Cardio _____   C. Pulmonary _____

   B. Vascular _____   D. Systemic _____

3. List the three functions of the cardiovascular system:

   A. _____

   B. _____

   C. _____

4. Identify the major components of the general cardiovascular circulation as labeled on Fig. 17-1:

   A. _____

   B. _____

   C. _____

   D. _____

   E. _____

   F. _____

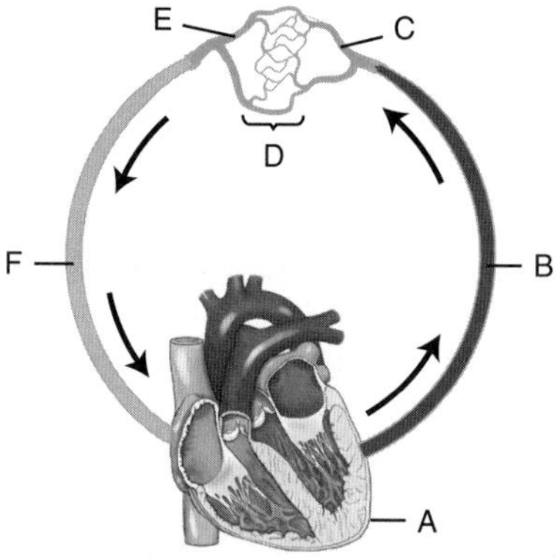

Fig. 17-1. Components of cardio-vascular circulation.

5. Which of the six general components of the circulatory system, identified in question 4, carry oxygenated blood to body tissue? _____

6. Which of the six general components of the circulatory system carry deoxygenated blood?

   _____

7. For each of the following three blood components, list the function and the common term (unless no other term exists):

	Common term	*Function*
1. Erythrocytes	A. _____	B. _____
2. Leukocytes	A. _____	B. _____
3. Platelets	A. (no other term given)	B. _____

8. Plasma, the liquid portion of blood, consists of (A) _____ % water and (B) _____ % plasma protein and salts, nutrients, and oxygen.

9. Identify the chambers of the heart and the associated blood vessels (arteries and veins) as labeled on Fig. 17-2:

   A. _____ (chamber)

   B. _____ (chamber)

   C. _____ (chamber)

   D. _____

   E. _____

   F. _____

   G. _____

   H. _____

   I. _____

   J. _____ (chamber)

   K. _____

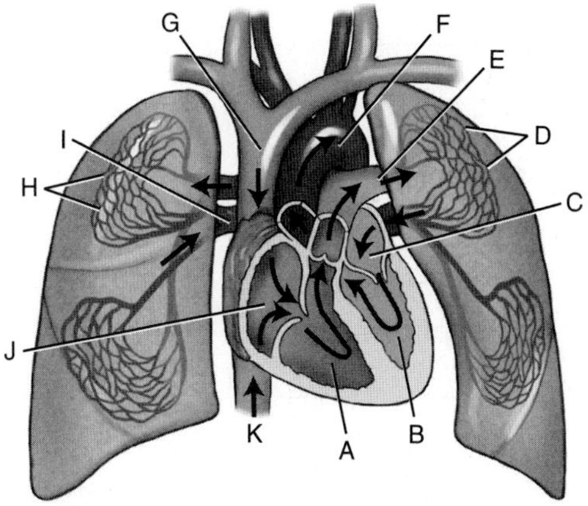

Fig. 17-2. Heart and pulmonary circulation (frontal view).

Questions 10 and 11 also relate to Fig. 17-2.

10. In general, arteries carry oxygenated blood, and veins carry deoxygenated blood. The exceptions to these rules are:

    A. The _____, which carry deoxygenated blood to the lungs

    B. The _____, which carry oxygenated blood back to the left atrium of the heart

11. A. Blood from the upper body returns to the heart through the _____.

    B. Blood from the abdomen and the lower limbs returns through the _____.

    C. Both of these major veins enter the _____ of the heart.

12. Identify the four major valves between the following heart chambers and associated vessels:

    A. Between right atrium and right ventricle: _____

    B. Between right ventricle and pulmonary arteries: _____

    C. Between left atrium and left ventricle: _____

    D. Between left ventricle and aorta: _____

13. A. The arteries that deliver blood to the heart muscle are the _____.

    B. These arteries originate at the _____.

14. List the three major branches of the coronary sinus:

    A. _____   B. _____   C. _____

15. Identify the labeled arteries on this drawing (Fig. 17-3):

    A. _____

    B. _____

    C. _____

    D. _____

    E. _____

    F. _____

    G. _____

    H. _____

    I. _____

    J. _____

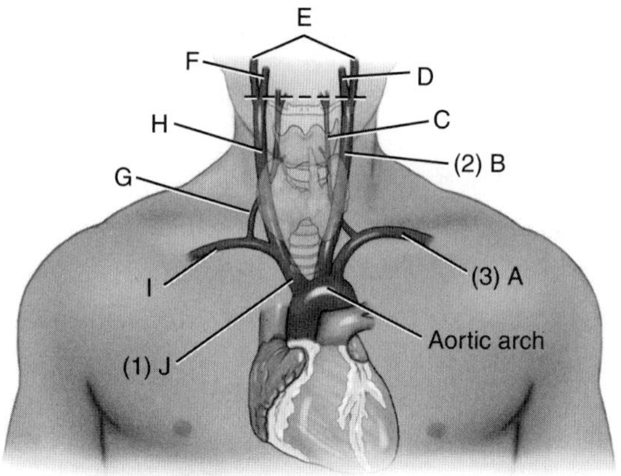

Fig. 17-3. Arterial branches of the aortic arch.

16. List the four major arteries supplying blood to the brain (important radiographically on a four-vessel angiogram):

    A. _____   C. _____

    B. _____   D. _____

17. List the three major branches of arteries arising from the arch of the aorta that supply the brain with blood:

    A. _____   B. _____   C. _____

18. True/False: The brachiocephalic artery bifurcates to form the right common and right vertebral arteries.

19. True/False: The level for bifurcation of the common carotid artery into the internal and external carotid arteries is at the level of C3-C4.

20. Any injection of the common carotid inferior to the bifurcation would result in filling both the

    _____ and _____ arteries.

21. What is the name of the S-shaped portion of the internal carotid artery near the petrous portion of the temporal bone?

    A. Carotid sinus   C. Carotid body

    B. Carotid canal   D. Carotid siphon

22. List the two end branches of the internal carotid artery:

    A. _____   B. _____

23. The _____ artery supplies much of the forebrain with blood.

24. The _____ supply the posterior circulation of the brain.

25. The two vertebral arteries unite to form the single _____ artery.

26. Which of the two major branches of each internal carotid artery (anterior cerebral or middle cerebral arteries) supply the lateral aspects of the cerebral hemispheres? _____

27. The anterior and middle cerebral arteries superimpose one another to a greater extent on the _____ (lateral or frontal) view.

28. Identify which one of the four drawings below (Fig. 17-4) demonstrates each of the following:

    1. Middle cerebral artery and branches of the internal carotid artery _____

    2. Anterior cerebral artery and branches of the internal carotid artery _____

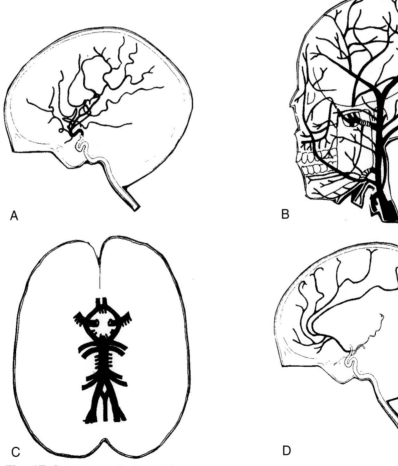

Fig. 17-4. Major cerebral arterial systems.

29. The posterior brain circulation communicates with the anterior circulation at the base of the brain in an arterial circle configuration called the arterial circle (Fig. 17-5). Identify the five arteries, or branches, that make up the **arterial circle** (circle of Willis) (labeled 1 through 5 on this drawing):

1. _____

2. _____

3. _____

4. _____

5. _____

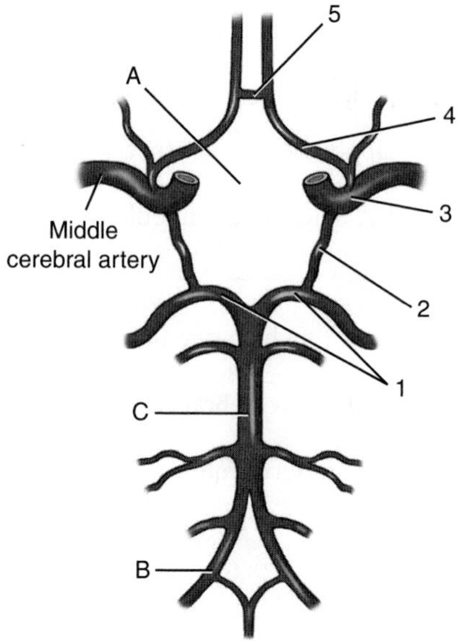

6. A. Name the gland (labeled A) located in the center of the arterial circle

   (circle of Willis): _____

   B. The right and left _____ enter the cranium through the foramen magnum.

   C. They then unite to form this single _____ artery.

Fig. 17-5. Structure identification of the arterial circle (circle of Willis).

30. List the three pairs of major veins draining the head, face, and neck region:

    A. _____

    B. _____

    C. _____

31. A. The three pairs of major veins, described in question 30, join the subclavian vein to form the

    _____ vein.

    B. This vein joins the equivalent vein on the other side to form the _____, which

    returns blood to the _____ of the heart.

32. True/False: The venous sinuses found in the brain are situated between layers of the dura mater.

33. True/False: All veins found in the brain possess no valves and are extremely thin.

34. Which of the following venous sinuses flow(s) posteriorly to drain into the straight sinus?
    A. Superior sagittal sinus   C. Straight sinus
    B. Inferior sagittal sinus   D. Sigmoid sinus

35. Which bony landmark signifies the location of the confluence of venous sinuses?

    A. Foramen magnum

    B. Petrous portion of temporal bone

    C. Internal occipital protuberance

    D. Sella turcica

REVIEW EXERCISE B: Anatomy of Thoracic and Abdominal Arteries and Veins, Portal System, Upper and Lower Limb Arteries and Veins, and Lymphatic System (see textbook pp. 661-665)

1. List the four segments of the thoracic section of the aorta as labeled on Fig. 17-6:

    A. _____

    B. _____

    C. _____

    D. _____

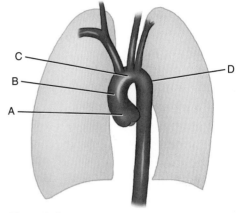

Fig. 17-6. Four segments of the aorta.

2. List the three common variations of the aortic arch that may be visualized during thoracic angiography and are demonstrated in Fig. 17-7:

    A. _____

    B. _____

    C. _____

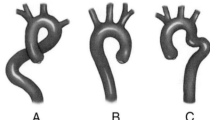

Fig. 17-7. Variations of the aortic arch.

3. Which one of the following veins receives blood from the intercostal, bronchial, esophageal, and phrenic veins?

    A. Pulmonary veins

    B. Azygos vein

    C. Inferior vena cava

    D. Superior vena cava

4. List the five major branches of the abdominal aorta, labeled 1 through 5 on Fig. 17-8 (listed in order from most superior to most inferior):

   1. _____

   2. _____

   3. _____

   4. _____

   5. _____

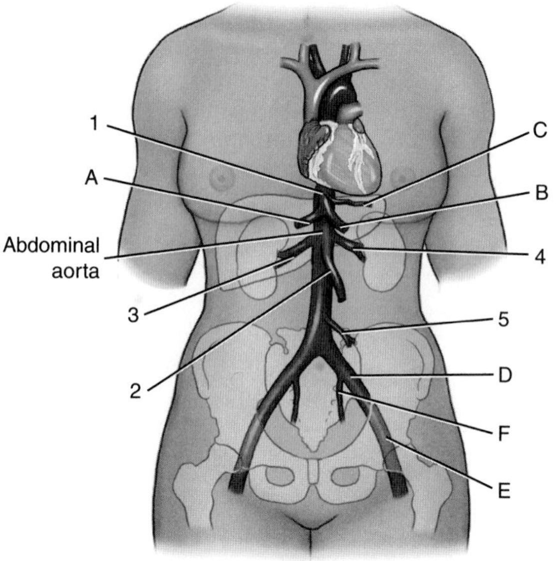

Fig. 17-8. Branches and divisions of the abdominal aorta.

5. At what approximate level does the descending aorta pass through the diaphragm to become the abdominal aorta?

   A. T9   C. L2

   B. T12   D. L3

6. List the three organs supplied with blood from the celiac artery, labeled A through C:

   A. _____

   B. _____

   C. _____

List the divisions of the abdominal aorta as it enters the pelvic region, labeled D through F (Fig. 17-8):

   D. _____

   E. _____

   F. _____

7. The distal abdominal aorta bifurcates at the approximate level of the _____ vertebra.

8. Venous blood is returned to the heart from structures below the diaphragm through the inferior vena cava. Identify the major venous tributaries to the inferior vena cava, as labeled on Fig. 17-9:

A. _____

B. _____

C. _____

D. _____

E. Inferior vena cava

F. _____

G. _____

H. _____

I. _____

J. _____

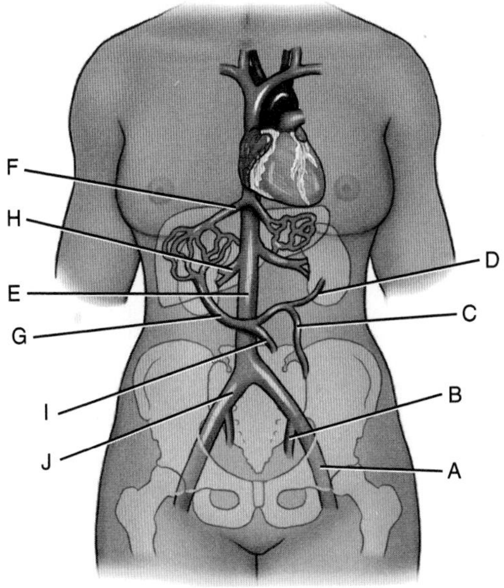

Fig. 17-9. Tributaries to the inferior vena cava.

9. Identify the following veins (A, B, D, and E) that make up the hepatic portal system, as labeled on Fig. 17-10. (Hint: A and B are the two major veins that unite to form the hepatic portal vein [C].)

A. _____

B. _____

C. _____

D. _____ drain "filtered" blood from the liver and return it to the:

E. _____

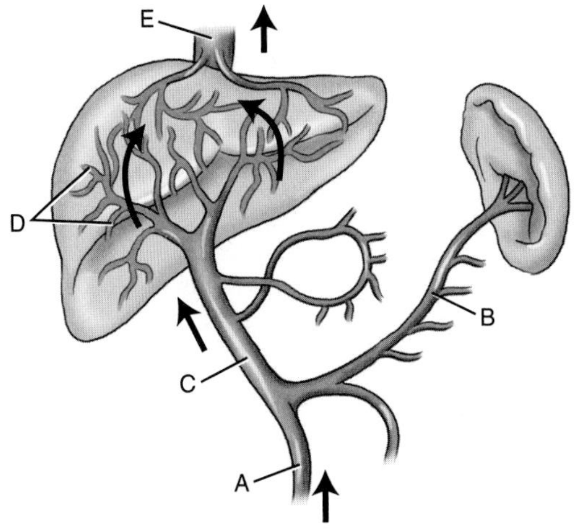

Fig. 17-10. Hepatic portal system.

10. Identify the following upper limb arteries (Fig. 17-11):

On the right side of the body, (A) the _____ artery gives rise to

(B) the _____ artery.

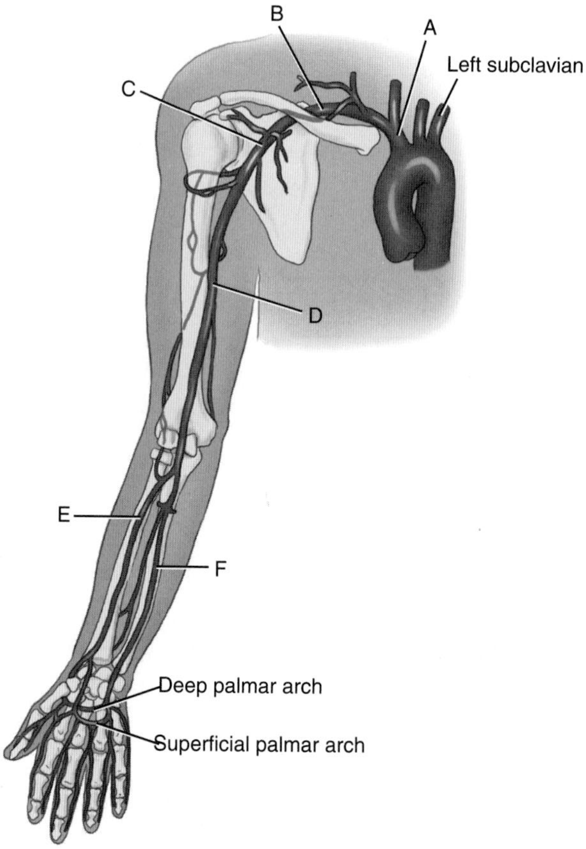

Identify the following primary arteries of the upper limb, labeled C through F.

C. _____

D. _____

E. _____

F. _____

Fig. 17-11. Upper limb arteries.

11. Identify the upper limb veins labeled on Fig. 17-12. The venous system of the upper and lower limbs may be divided into two sets. For the upper limb these begin with:

A. _____ and

B. _____, which form two parallel drainage channels.

Identify the veins returning blood to the heart, labeled C through G in Fig. 17-12:

C. _____

D. _____

E. _____

F. _____

G. _____

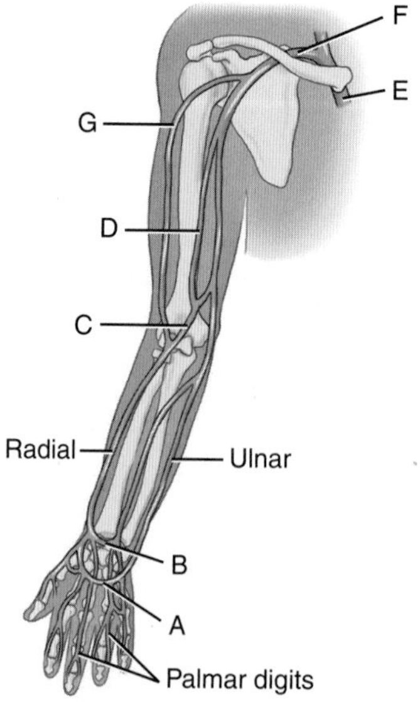

Fig. 17-12. Upper limb veins.

12. The vein most commonly used to draw blood at the elbow is the _____. (Hint: This is one of the veins [A-G] identified in Fig. 17-12 on p. 418.)

Lower Limb Arteries (Fig. 17-13)

13. Identify the following: The lower limb arterial system begins at the

   A. _____ artery and continues as the

   B. _____ artery and it divides into the

   C. _____ and

   D. _____ arteries in the area of the proximal and midfemur. At the knee, the femoral artery becomes the

   E. _____ artery, which continues into the foot as the

   F. _____ artery.

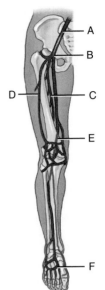

Fig. 17-13. Lower limb arteries.

Lower Limb Veins (Fig. 17-14)

14. Identify the following labeled veins of the lower limb:

   A. _____

   B. _____

   C. _____

   D. _____

   E. _____

   F. _____

   G. _____

   H. _____

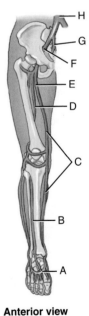

Anterior view
Fig. 17-14. Lower limb veins.

15. The longest vein in the body is the _____ of the lower limb. (Hint: This is one of the labeled veins in Fig. 17-14.)

16. Which duct in the lymphatic system receives interstitial fluid from the left side of the body, lower limbs, pelvis, and abdomen, and drains this fluid into the left subclavian vein? _____

17. List the four functions of the lymphatic system:

    A. _____

    B. _____

    C. _____

    D. _____

18. True/False: Lymphatic fluid moves in two directions—toward and away from tissues.

19. True/False: There are thousands of lymph nodes in the body.

20. The general term describing radiographic examination of the lymphatic vessels and nodes following injection of contrast media is _____.

21. Which imaging modality is replacing the procedure identified in question 20?

REVIEW EXERCISE C: Angiographic Procedures, Equipment, and Supplies (see textbook pp. 670-677)

1. Which of the following individuals is (are) not normally part of the angiographic team?

   A. Scrub nurse/technologist   C. Technologist

   B. Respiratory therapist   D. Radiologist

2. A common method or technique of introducing a needle and/or catheter into the blood vessel for angiographic procedures is called the _____.

3. In the correct order, list the six steps to the technique identified in question 2.

   A. _____   D. _____

   B. _____   E. _____

   C. _____   F. _____

4. In addition to the method listed above, what is another technique for accessing a vessel during angiography?

   _____

5. Which one of the following is not a common risk or complication of angiography?

   A. Embolus formation   C. Hypertension

   B. Dissection of a vessel   D. Contrast media reaction

6. Which one of the following vessels is preferred for arterial vessel access for the majority of angiographic procedures?

   A. Femoral artery   C. Axillary artery

   B. Brachial artery   D. Common carotid artery

7. What is the primary purpose of premedicating the patient before an angiographic procedure?

   A. Reduce the risk for bleeding   C. Help the patient relax

   B. Reduce the risk for infection   D. All of the above

8. What type of contrast media is used for most angiographic procedures? _____

9. List the six most common complications associated with angiography:

   1. _____

   2. _____

   3. _____

   4. _____

   5. _____

   6. _____

10. Generally, where is the femoral artery punctured during an arterial catheterization procedure?

   A. Just superior to the inguinal ligament   C. At the midpoint of the inguinal ligament

   B. Just inferior to the inguinal ligament   D. 2 inches superior to the popliteal artery

11. What is the minimum amount of time a patient should remain on bed rest following an invasive angiographic procedure?

   A. 1 hour   C. 4 hours

   B. 3 hours   D. 6 hours

12. At what degree angle should the head of the bed or stretcher be elevated following an invasive angiographic procedure?

   A. 10°   C. 20°

   B. 15°   D. 30°

13. True/False: Most pediatric angiographic procedures require heavy sedation.

14. True/False: Angiographic rooms need to be considerably larger than conventional radiographic rooms.

15. Outlets for _____ and _____ should be located on the room walls near the work area.

16. The two types of digital fluoroscopy and image acquisition systems include:

   A. _____

   B. _____

17. True/False: The analog-to-digital conversion type of angiographic system does not require an image intensifier tube.

18. True/False: The use of digital and/or digital subtraction angiography (DSA), as part of a PAC system, can eliminate the need for hard-copy images.

19. List three post-processing options with digital imaging to improve or modify the image:

    A. _____

    B. _____

    C. _____

20. Flow rate for an automatic electromechanical injector is affected by viscosity of contrast media, injector pressure,

    and _____ and _____ of the catheter.

21. The two purposes of the heating device on an electromechanical injector are:

    A. _____

    B. _____

22. True/False: Multislice CT can produce thinner slices and increase resolution of CTA images.

23. True/False: Computed tomography angiography (CTA) does not require the use of iodinated contrast media to demonstrate vascular structures.

24. True/False: Nuclear medicine complements other angiographic modalities even though it provides little anatomic detail.

25. True/False: Color duplex ultrasound is effective in demonstrating thrombus formation in the circle of Willis in the adult.

26. True/False: Magnetic resonance angiography (MRA) does not require the use of any type of contrast media or vessel puncture.

27. True/False: Magnetic resonance angiography requires the use of special contrast media to demonstrate vasculature.

28. True/False: Rotational angiography units move around the anatomy up to 360° during the procedure.

29. True/False: Carbon dioxide is recommended instead of iodinated contrast media for carotid angiography.

30. True/False: Gadolinium is recommended for renal angiography for patients with known renal disease.

REVIEW EXERCISE D: Angiography and Interventional Procedures (see textbook pp. 678-685)

1. List the five common clinical indicators for cerebral angiography:

   A. _____   D. _____

   B. _____   E. _____

   C. _____

2. The point of bifurcation is of special interest to the radiologist; at this point, the internal carotid artery is more

_____ (medial or lateral) when compared with the external carotid on an AP projection.

3. List four vessels commonly demonstrated during cerebral angiography:

A. _____

B. _____

C. _____

D. _____

4. List the three phases of cerebral circulation that can be visualized during cerebral angiography:

A. _____   B. _____   C. _____

5. List five specific pathologies that are common indications for thoracic and pulmonary angiography:

A. _____

B. _____

C. _____

D. _____

E. _____

6. True/False: Pulmonary arteriography for pulmonary emboli is the preferred imaging modality.

7. Which vessel is most often catheterized for a pulmonary angiogram?

A. Femoral vein   C. Subclavian vein

B. Femoral artery   D. Axillary artery

8. The preferred puncture site for a thoracic aortogram is the:

A. Femoral vein   C. Pulmonary artery

B. Pulmonary vein   D. Femoral artery

9. The preferred puncture site for a pulmonary arteriogram is:

A. Femoral vein   C. Pulmonary artery

B. Pulmonary vein   D. Femoral artery

10. What is the average amount of contrast media injected during a thoracic angiogram?

A. 5 to 8 mL   C. 20 to 25 mL

B. 10 to 15 mL   D. 30 to 50 mL

11. To prevent superimposition of the aortic arch with surrounding structures during a thoracic aortogram, a

_____ ° LAO is often performed.

A. 5 to 10   C. 45

B. 15 to 20   D. 60

12. Coronary angiography is typically a study of the:

A. Coronary arteries   C. Coronary veins

B. Aortic arch   D. Chambers of the heart

13. Which vessel is commonly catheterized for access to the right side of the heart? _____

14. The average imaging rate during angiocardiography is:

A. 2 to 3 frames per second   C. 15 to 30 frames per second

B. 8 to 10 frames per second   D. 45 to 60 frames per second

15. Which one of the following terms describes the pumping efficiency of the left ventricle?

A. Ejection fraction   C. Ejection coefficient

B. Systolic contraction ratio   D. Myocardial perfusion ratio

16. The term for an angiographic study of the superior and inferior vena cava is _____.

17. List five common clinical indicators for abdominal angiography:

A. _____

B. _____

C. _____

D. _____

E. _____

18. The common puncture site for selective abdominal angiography is the _____ using the Seldinger technique.

19. Superselective abdominal angiography can be performed to visualize specific branches (and associated organs) of the abdominal aorta. Which three branches are most commonly catheterized for this purpose?

A. _____

B. _____

C. _____

20. True/False: Venograms are rarely performed today because of increased use of color duplex ultrasound.

21. To study the left upper limb arteries, the catheter is passed from the aortic arch into the:

A. Left common carotid   C. Left vertebral artery

B. Left brachiocephalic vein   D. Left subclavian artery

22. True/False: Respiration is suspended for the angiographic imaging of the lower limb.

23. Define interventional imaging procedures:

_____

24. Interventional procedures are considered a benefit to patients because of:

    A. Increased cost of the procedures   C. Longer recovery times

    B. Shorter hospital stays   D. A poor second choice to surgery

25. True/False: Interventional angiographic procedures are used primarily for providing diagnostic information and secondarily for treatment of disease.

26. True/False: Interventional imaging procedures are most commonly performed in surgery.

27. How can uterine fibroid embolization help prevent the need for a patient to undergo a hysterectomy?

28. Which of the following procedures serves as a palliative measure for colonic strictures owing to inoperable neoplastic disease?

    A. Percutaneous biliary drainage (PBD)   C. Percutaneous abdominal drainage

    B. Enteric stenting   D. Nephrostomy

29. Indicate whether the following interventional procedures are vascular or nonvascular procedures:

    _____ 1. Percutaneous transluminal angioplasty (PTA)   A. Vascular procedure

    _____ 2. Infusion therapy   B. Nonvascular procedure

    _____ 3. Percutaneous biliary drainage (PBD)

    _____ 4. Percutaneous gastrostomy

    _____ 5. Stent placement

    _____ 6. Embolization

    _____ 7. Percutaneous abdominal drainage

    _____ 8. Nephrostomy

    _____ 9. Thrombolysis

    _____ 10. Percutaneous needle biopsy

    _____ 11. Kyphoplasty

    _____ 12. Transjugular intrahepatic portosystemic shunt (TIPS)

30. How is the hepatic portal system accessed during a TIPS procedure? _____

31. What type of medication can be used during infusion therapy to control bleeding?

    _____

32. What type of catheter is often used to retrieve urethral stones? _____

33. What is the name of the vertebroplasty procedure performed to restore the collapsed portion of a vertebral body?

_____

34. What specific device is placed within the collapsed vertebrae to restore their height and structure for the TIPS procedure identified in question 30? _____

35. What type of catheter is used for transluminal angioplasty? _____

36. What is the correct term describing the interventional procedure for dissolving a blood clot?

_____

37. Which one of the following pathologic indications is most common for performing a percutaneous biliary drainage (PBD)?

   A. Biliary obstruction   C. Posttraumatic biliary leakage
   B. Suppurative cholangitis   D. Unresectable malignant disease

38. True/False: Percutaneous abdominal drainage procedures have a success rate of only 50%.

39. True/False: Percutaneous gastrostomy is performed primarily for patients who are unable to eat orally.

40. Which of the following processes "ablate" tumor tissue during radiofrequency ablation (RFA)?

   A. Freezing   C. Low-intensity gamma radiation
   B. Chemical dissolving tissue D. Heating

SELF-TEST

MY SCORE = _____%

Directions: This self-test should be taken only after completing all of the readings, review exercises, and laboratory activities for a particular section. The purpose of this test is not only to provide a good learning exercise but also to serve as a strong indicator of what your final evaluation exam will be. It is strongly suggested that if you do not receive at least a 90% to 95% grade on this self-test, you should review those areas in which you missed questions before going to your instructor for the final evaluation exam for this chapter.

1. The two arteries that deliver blood to the heart muscle are:
   - A. Right and left pulmonary veins
   - B. Right and left brachiocephalic arteries
   - C. Right and left pulmonary arteries
   - D. Right and left coronary arteries

2. Which of the following arteries does not originate directly from the arch of the aorta?
   - A. Brachiocephalic
   - B. Left subclavian
   - C. Left common carotid
   - D. Right common carotid

3. Each common carotid artery bifurcates into the internal and external arteries at the level of the:
   - A. C4 vertebra
   - B. C6 vertebra
   - C. C2 vertebra
   - D. C2 vertebra

4. Which of the following arteries arises from the brachiocephalic artery rather than the aortic arch?
   - A. Right vertebral
   - B. Left vertebral
   - C. Right common carotid
   - D. Left common carotid

5. The external carotid does not supply blood to the:
   - A. Anterior portion of brain
   - B. Facial area
   - C. Anterior neck
   - D. Greater part of the scalp and meninges

6. Two branches of each internal carotid artery, which are well visualized with an internal carotid arteriogram, are the:
   - A. Posterior and middle cerebral arteries
   - B. Anterior and middle cerebral arteries
   - C. Right and left vertebral arteries
   - D. Facial and maxillary arteries

7. The two vertebral arteries enter the cranium through the foramen magnum and unite to form the:
   - A. Brachiocephalic artery
   - B. Vertebrobasilar artery
   - C. Arterial circle
   - D. Basilar artery

8. The basilar artery rests upon the clivus of the _____ bone.
   - A. Ethmoid
   - B. Parietal
   - C. Temporal
   - D. Sphenoid

9. Which of the following veins do not drain blood from the head, face, and neck regions?

    A. Right and left internal jugular veins   C. Internal and external cerebral veins

    B. Right and left vertebral veins   D. Right and left external jugular veins

10. The superior and inferior sagittal sinuses join certain other sinuses, such as the transverse sinus, at the base of the brain to become the:

    A. External jugular vein   C. Subclavian vein

    B. Internal jugular vein   D. Vertebral vein

11. Which vein receives blood from the intercostal, esophageal, and phrenic veins?

    A. Superior vena cava   C. Azygos vein

    B. Inferior vena cava   D. Brachiocephalic vein

12. Which vessels carry oxygenated blood from the lungs back to the heart?

    A. Pulmonary veins   C. Coronary arteries

    B. Pulmonary arteries   D. Aorta

13. Match the following abdominal arteries with the labeled parts on Fig. 17-15:

    _____ 1. Inferior mesenteric

    _____ 2. Superior mesenteric

    _____ 3. Left renal

    _____ 4. Right renal

    _____ 5. Common hepatic

    _____ 6. Celiac (trunk) artery

    _____ 7. Left common iliac

    _____ 8. Left internal iliac

    _____ 9. Left external iliac

    _____ 10. Left gastric

    _____ 11. Abdominal aorta

    _____ 12. Splenic

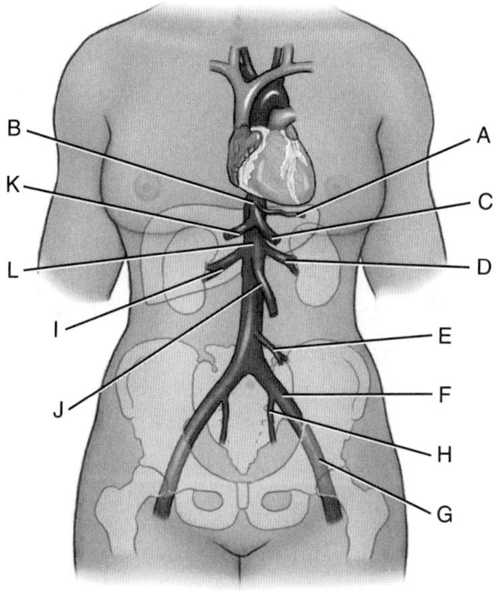

Fig. 17-15. Abdominal arteries.

14. True/False: The right subclavian artery arises directly from the aortic arch.

15. What is another term for the aortic bulb?

    A. Aortic stem   C. Aortic root

    B. Aortic confluence   D. Aortic sphincter

16. How many segments make up the thoracic aorta?

    A. Three   C. Five

    B. Four   D. Two

17. A condition in which the aortic arch is located in the right side of the thorax is a variation termed:

   A. Left circumflex aorta

   B. Inverse aorta

   C. Pseudocoarctation

   D. Situs inversus

18. Which of the following vessels carries blood from the intestine to the liver for filtration?

   A. Portal vein

   B. Hepatic veins

   C. Superior mesenteric vein

   D. Inferior vena cava

19. True/False: The cephalic vein is most commonly used for venipuncture.

20. True/False: The great (long) saphenous vein is the longest vein in the body.

21. True/False: The thoracic duct is the largest lymph vessel in the body.

22. Which one of the following functions is *not* performed by the lymphatic system?

   A. Produce lymphocytes and microphages

   B. Synthesize simple carbohydrates

   C. Filter the lymph

   D. Return proteins and other substances to the blood

23. Solid food should be withheld for approximately _____ hours before an angiographic procedure.

   A. 1

   B. 4

   C. 8

   D. 24

24. Which of the following vessels is most often punctured for the Seldinger technique?

   A. Abdominal aorta

   B. Femoral vein

   C. Femoral artery

   D. Axillary artery

25. Match each of the following terms with its definition or description:

_____ 1. Also known as red blood cells

_____ 2. Component of blood that helps repair tears in blood vessel walls and promotes blood clotting

_____ 3. Carries deoxygenated blood from the right ventricle of the heart to the lungs

_____ 4. Heart valve found between the left atrium and left ventricle

_____ 5. Heart valve found between the right atrium and right ventricle

_____ 6. The vessels that provide blood to the heart muscle

_____ 7. The artery that bifurcates to form the right common carotid and right subclavian artery

_____ 8. The artery that primarily supplies blood to the anterior neck, scalp, and meninges

_____ 9. The artery that bifurcates into the anterior and middle cerebral artery

_____ 10. The aspect of the sphenoid bone on which the basilar artery rests

_____ 11. The membranous portion of the dura mater containing the superior sagittal sinus

_____ 12. The artery that forms the left gastric, hepatic, and splenic arteries

_____ 13. The vein created by the splenic and superior mesenteric veins

_____ 14. The vessel that carries oxygenated blood from the lungs to the left atrium of the heart

A. Brachiocephalic artery

B. Pulmonary veins

C. Celiac artery

D. Coronary arteries

E. Superior vena cava

F. Portal vein

G. Falx cerebri

H. Inferior mesenteric artery

I. Coronary sinus

J. External carotid artery

K. Tricuspid (right atrioventricular) valve

L. Clivus

M. Mitral (left atrioventricular or bicuspid) valve

N. Erythrocytes

O. Pulmonary artery

P. Platelets

Q. Internal carotid artery

26. Injection flow rate in angiography is *not* affected by:

A. Viscosity of contrast media
B. Length and diameter of catheter
C. Body temperature
D. Injection pressure

27. Which one of the following imaging modalities will best demonstrate velocity of blood flow within a vessel?

A. Computed tomography angiography
B. Color duplex ultrasound
C. Magnetic resonance imaging
D. CO_2 angiography

28. What is the minimum amount of time a patient should remain on bed rest following an angiographic procedure?

A. 1 hour
B. 4 hours
C. 8 hours
D. 24 hours

29. What type of angiographic imaging system does not require the use of an image intensifier or video camera?

    A. C-arm conventional fluoroscopy   C. Pulsed generator fluoroscopy

    B. Analog-to-digital conversion fluoroscopy   D. Flat panel detector fluoroscopy

30. True/False: Digital subtraction demonstrates only the bony anatomy during an angiographic study.

31. True/False: Multislice CT scanning does not require arterial puncture and catheter insertion to demonstrate vascular structures.

32. True/False: Contrast media must be used during magnetic resonance angiography.

33. True/False: CO_2 angiography requires the use of a special injector.

34. Which of the following is *not* a clinical indicator for cerebral angiography?

    A. Vascular lesions   C. Coarctation

    B. Aneurysm   D. Arteriovenous malformation

35. True/False: The three vascular phases visualized during cerebral angiography should be arterial, capillary, and venous.

36. Pulmonary arteriography is most often performed to diagnose:

    A. Heart valve disease   C. Arteriovenous malformation

    B. Pulmonary emboli   D. Coarctation of the aorta

37. The most common vascular approach during pulmonary arteriography is the:

    A. Femoral vein   C. Superior vena cava

    B. Femoral artery   D. Axillary artery

38. Which one of the following positions prevents superimposition of the proximal aorta and aortic arch during a thoracic aortogram?

    A. 45° RPO   C. 45° LAO

    B. 45° LPO   D. Lateral

39. During angiocardiography, the catheter is advanced from the aorta into the:

    A. Superior vena cava   C. Left ventricle

    B. Right ventricle   D. Brachiocephalic artery

40. The imaging rate during angiocardiography is:

    A. 1 to 3 frames per second   C. 10 to 12 frames per second

    B. 4 to 8 frames per second   D. 15 to 30 frames per second

41. Which of the following would not be a common pathologic indicator for abdominal angiography?

    A. Aneurysm   C. Trauma

    B. Stenosis or occlusions of aorta   D. Bowel obstruction

42. A peripherally inserted central catheter (PICC line) can remain in the patient up to:

    A. 7 days   C. 180 days

    B. 30 days   D. 6 months

43. The tip of a central line is placed near the _____.

    A. Left ventricle   C. Brachiocephalic vein

    B. Right atrium   D. Inferior vena cava

44. For upper limb angiograms, the catheter is advanced along the _____.

    A. Right carotid artery   C. Iliac vein of the affected side

    B. Inferior vena cava   D. Abdominal and thoracic aorta

45. True/False: Angiographic lower limb imaging can only be conducted unilaterally.

46. True/False: A clinical indication for a transcatheter embolization includes stopping active bleeding at a specific site.

47. The most common pathologic indication for chemoembolization is to treat:

    A. Brain aneurysm   C. AV malformation

    B. Stenosed vessels   D. Malignancies

48. Match the following descriptions to the correct term or interventional procedure. (Use each choice only once.)

    _____ A. Intravascular administration of drugs   1. Embolization

    _____ B. Device to extract urethral stones   2. Nephrostomy

    _____ C. Procedure to dissolve blood clots   3. Infusion therapy

    _____ D. Technique to restrict uncontrolled hemorrhage snare catheter   4. Basket or loop

    _____ E. Technique to decompress obstructed bile duct gastrostomy   5. Percutaneous

    _____ F. Direct puncture and catheterization of the renal pelvis   6. Thrombolysis

    _____ G. Placement of an extended feeding tube into the stomach   7. Percutaneous into biliary drainage

49. True/False: A vena cava filter is placed superior to the renal veins to prevent renal vein thrombosis.

50. True/False: Radiofrequency ablation (RFA) is ideal for treating tumors in the liver and lung.

18 Computed Tomography

This chapter presents the general principles of computed tomography (CT) and the various equipment systems in use today. A study of soft tissue anatomy of the central nervous system (CNS) as viewed in axial sections is included. An introduction into the purpose, pathologic indications, and procedure of cranial, thoracic, abdominal, and pelvic computed tomography is also covered in this chapter. Selected sectional images of these three regions are presented.

CHAPTER OBJECTIVES

After you have successfully completed the activities of this chapter, you will be able to:

_____ 1. List the two general divisions of the CNS.

_____ 2. Identify the specialized cells (neurons) of the nervous system and describe their specific parts and functions.

_____ 3. List the specific membranes or coverings of the CNS and identify the meningeal spaces or potential spaces associated with them.

_____ 4. List the three primary divisions of the brain.

_____ 5. List the four major cavities of the ventricular system and identify specific structures and passageways of the ventricular system.

_____ 6. Identify select gray and white matter structures in the brain.

_____ 7. Describe the concept of the blood-brain barrier.

_____ 8. List the 12 cranial nerves.

_____ 9. List three advantages of computed tomography over conventional radiography.

_____ 10. Identify the generational changes and advances in computed tomography (CT) systems.

_____ 11. List the major components of a CT system.

_____ 12. Explain the basic operating principles of CT imaging, including x-ray transmission, data acquisition, image reconstruction, window width, window level, and slice thickness.

_____ 13. Define and calculate the pitch ratio for a volume CT scan using different variables.

_____ 14. Identify the scan parameters for cranial CT studies.

_____ 15. Identify specific structures of the brain, seen on axial drawings, photographs, and CT sectional images.

_____ 16. Describe various specialized CT procedures to include purpose, procedure, and scan parameters.

LEARNING EXERCISES

Complete the following review exercises after reading the associated pages in the textbook as indicated by each exercise. Answers to each review exercise are given at the end of this workbook.

REVIEW EXERCISE A: Brain and Spinal Cord Anatomy (see textbook pp. 719-727)

1. The central nervous system can be divided into the following two main divisions:

   A. _____

   B. _____

2. A. The solid spinal cord terminates at the level of the lower border of which vertebra?

   _____

   B. This tapered terminal area of the spinal cord is called the _____.

3. A. The specialized cells of the nervous system that conduct electrical impulses are called

   _____.

   B. The parts of these cells that receive the electrical impulse and conduct them toward the cell body are called

   _____.

4. Three membranes or layers of coverings called meninges enclose both the brain and the spinal cord. Certain important spaces or potential spaces are associated with these meninges. List these three meninges and three associated spaces as described in the following:

   Meninges   *Spaces*

   Skull or cranium

   A. _____   D. _____
      (Outer "hard" or "tough" layer)   (Space or potential space)

   B. _____   E. _____
      (Spiderlike avascular membrane)   (Narrow space containing thin layer of fluid)

   C. _____   F. _____
      (Inner "tender" layer)   (Wider space filled with cerebrospinal fluid)

5. The outer "hard" or "tough" membrane described in the preceding has an inner and outer layer tightly fused except for certain larger spaces between folds or creases of the brain and skull, which provide for large venous

   blood channels called _____.

6. The large cerebrum is divided into right and left hemispheres. Each hemisphere of the cerebrum is further divided into five lobes, with four of the lobes lying under the cranial bone of the same name. List these five lobes:

   A. _____   D. _____

   B. _____   E. _____

   C. _____

7. The brain (encephalon) can be divided into three general divisions: the (1) forebrain, (2) midbrain, and (3) hindbrain. The forebrain and hindbrain are both divided into three divisions. List the three divisions of the forebrain and the hindbrain as labeled on Fig. 18-1. (Note: Secondary terms for these divisions as found in the textbook are included in parentheses.)

1. Forebrain   A. _____

   (Prosencephalon)   (Telencephalon)—largest division

   (Diencephalon)   B. _____

                        C. _____

2. Midbrain   (Mesencephalon)

3. Hindbrain   D. _____

   (Rhombencephalon)   E. _____

                        F. _____

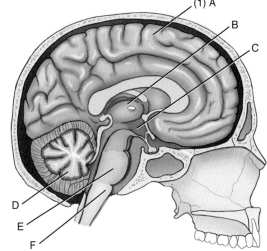

Fig. 18-1. Divisions of the forebrain and hindbrain, midsagittal view.

8. Identify the three lobes of the right cerebral hemisphere, as labeled A through C in Fig. 18-2. The deep fissure separating the two cerebral hemispheres is labeled D. (Note: There is a fold of dura mater, called the falx cerebri, that extends deep within this fissure, separating the two hemispheres that is visualized on CT scans.)

A. _____ lobe

B. _____ lobe

C. _____ lobe

D. _____ fissure

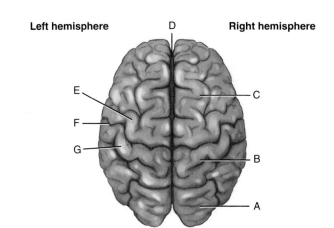

Fig. 18-2. Structures of the cerebral hemispheres.

9. The surface of each cerebral hemisphere contains numerous grooves and convolutions or raised areas. Identify labeled parts E through G in Fig. 18-2. Two of these raised areas, E and G, have specific names and are frequently demonstrated and identified on cranial CT scans. Part F is a shallow groove with a specific name.

E. _____

F. _____

G. _____

10. What is the name of the arched mass of transverse fibers (white matter) that connects the two cerebral hemispheres?

    A. Falx cerebri   C. Central sulcus

    B. Anterior central gyrus   D. Corpus callosum

11. What is the name of the large groove that separates the cerebral hemispheres?

    A. Anterior central gyrus   C. Central sulcus

    B. Longitudinal fissure   D. Posterior central gyrus

12. The fluid manufactured and stored in the ventricular system is called (A) _____,

    abbreviated as (B) _____. This fluid completely surrounds the brain and spinal cord

    by filling the space called the (C) _____ space. A blockage within this system may
    result in excessive accumulation of this fluid within the ventricles, creating a condition known as (D)

    _____.

13. The cerebrospinal fluid–filled space and ventricular system are important in CT because these areas can be
    differentiated from tissue structures by their density differences.

    A. The larger spaces or areas within the CSF-filled space are called _____.

    B. The largest of these is the _____, located just posterior and inferior to the
    fourth ventricle.

14. The central midline portion of the brain connecting the midbrain, pons, and medulla to the spinal cord is called the

    _____.

15. A. The optic chiasma, the site at which some of the optic nerves cross to the opposite side, is located in the

    _____, a division of the forebrain.

    B. An important gland that is located just inferior to this division of the forebrain is the

    _____.

16. A second important midline structure gland is the _____.

17. The CNS can be divided by appearance into white matter and gray matter, which can be differentiated by CT. The
    difference in appearance between these two results from their makeup. Describe this difference by indicating what
    each consists of:

    A. White matter: _____

    B. Gray matter: _____

18. In general, the thin, outer cerebral cortex is (A) _____ matter, whereas the more

    centrally located brain tissue is (B) _____ matter.

19. List the three significant structures associated with the hypothalamus:

    A. _____   B. _____   C. _____

20. List the three primary structures of the brainstem:

   A. _____   B. _____   C. _____

21. Which aspect of the brain serves as an interpretation center for certain sensory impulses?
   A. Midbrain   C. Thalamus
   B. Pituitary gland   D. Hypothalamus

22. Which aspect of the brain coordinates important motor functions such as coordination, posture, and balance?
   A. Pons   C. Midbrain
   B. Cerebellum   D. Cerebrum

23. Which aspect of the brain controls important body activities related to homeostasis?
   A. Pons   C. Thalamus
   B. Cerebellum   D. Hypothalamus

24. Which structure of the brain controls a wide range of body functions, including growth and reproductive functions?
   A. Pineal gland   C. Thalamus
   B. Pituitary gland   D. Hypothalamus

25. List the four groupings of cerebral nuclei (basal ganglia):

   A. _____   C. _____

   B. _____   D. _____

26. Ventricles: There are four major cavities in the ventricular system. These are labeled in Fig. 18-3 and demonstrate the four ventricles in relationship to other brain structures. Two of the ventricles are located within the right and left cerebral hemispheres (A); the remaining two are midline structures (B and C).

   The larger two ventricles (A) have four significant parts labeled 1, 2, 3, and 6 in Fig. 18-4. The small ductlike structure (4) provides communication between ventricles, and number 5 indicates a connection between the third and fourth ventricles. An important gland (8) is also shown. Number 7 represents an important communication with the subarachnoid space on each side of the fourth ventricle.

   Identify the ventricles and their parts as labeled on these two drawings:

   Fig. 18-3

   A. Right and left _____ ventricles

   B. _____ ventricle

   C. _____ ventricle

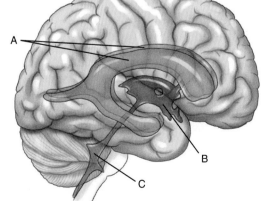

Fig. 18-3. Cavities in the ventricular system.

Fig. 18-4

1. _____ (occipital)

2. _____

3. _____ (frontal)

4. _____ (foramen)

5. _____

6. _____ (temporal)

7. _____

8. _____ (gland)

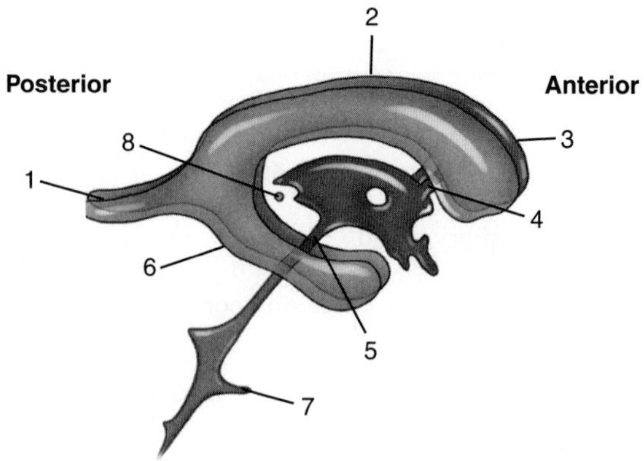

Fig. 18-4. Anatomy of the ventricles.

27. There are 12 pairs of cranial nerves, most of which originate from the brainstem and travel to various parts of the brain, controlling both sensory and motor functions. List these 12 pairs of cranial nerves:

A. _____	E. _____	I. _____
B. _____	F. _____	J. _____
C. _____	G. _____	K. _____
D. _____	H. _____	L. _____

REVIEW EXERCISE B: Basic Principles of Computed Tomography (see textbook pp. 728-732)

1. Match the following characteristics with the correct generation of CT scanner. (Answers may be used more than once, and some blanks have more than one answer.)

_____ 1. First scanner with fan-shaped beam and 30 or more detectors

_____ 2. 1- to 2-detector system

_____ 3. 8 times faster than a 1-second, single-slice scanner

_____ 4. First scanner to rotate a full 360° around patient

_____ 5. Capable of volume scanning (multiple answers)

_____ 6. 1 minute scan time for entire exam (multiple answers)

_____ 7. Contains a bank of up to 960 detectors

_____ 8. Scan times of 4½ minutes per slice

_____ 9. 4800 or more detectors on a fixed ring

_____ 10. Continuous volume scanning (CVS) (multiple answers)

_____ 11. The first type with fixed detectors rather than detectors rotating with an x-ray tube

_____ 12. Capable of acquiring four or more slices simultaneously

_____ 13. First scanner with larger aperture, which permitted full body scanning

A. First-generation

B. Second-generation

C. Third-generation

D. Fourth-generation

E. Multislice scanner

2. True/False: The primary difference between each generation of CT scanners was the speed of the system.

3. True/False: Noninvasive studies of the heart are possible with multislice CT.

4. True/False: Volume CT scanners are limited to one 360° rotation per slice in the same direction.

5. Which of the following devices replaced high-tension cables in helical CT scanners?

A. Microswitches
B. Variable diodes
C. Slip rings
D. Optic fiber lines

6. True/False: Terms such as "helical" and "spiral" are vendor-specific terms for volume CT scanners.

7. Which of the following is not an advantage of multislice CT scanners?

A. Fast imaging speed
B. Acquires large number of slices rapidly
C. Minimizes patient motion
D. Low-cost system to operate

8. Reconstruction of patient data into alternative planes (coronal, sagittal, three-dimensional) is termed:

A. Algorithmic reconstruction
B. 3-D reconstruction
C. Multiplanar reconstruction
D. Modulated reconstruction

9. List the three primary components of a computed tomographic system:

A. _____   B. _____   C. _____

10. Which part of the CT system houses the x-ray tube, detector array, and collimators?

_____

11. The central opening in the CT support structure at which the patient is scanned is called the

_____.

12. List the scintillation materials that make up the solid-state detector array: _____

13. With multidetector CT systems, actual thickness of a tomographic slice is determined by:

A. Size of detector row   C. Effective focal spot

B. Prepatient collimator   D. Postpatient collimator

14. With a 512- × 512-image matrix, the CT computer must perform _____ mathematical calculations per slice.

A. 128   C. 187,818

B. 1280   D. 262,144

15. Image archiving for most modern CT systems is performed through a(n):

A. PACS   C. Optical disk

B. Magnetic disk or tape   D. Laser printer

16. What do the detectors measure in a CT system? _____

17. What is the basic definition of the term *voxel*? _____

18. A voxel is a _____-dimensional image of the tissue, whereas a pixel is a

_____-dimensional representation of the reconstructed image.

19. The depth of the voxels is determined by:

A. Slice thickness   C. Actual scan time

B. Speed of computer   D. Size of the pixel

20. Data sets from image voxels are referred to as:

A. Bytes   C. Dimensions

B. Isotropic   D. Spatial differences

21. Pixels represent varying degrees of:

A. Resolution   C. Attenuation

B. Contrast   D. Scatter radiation

22. Air would have a _____ (higher or lower) differential absorption as compared with soft tissue.

23. CT numbers are a numerical scale that represents tissue _____.

24. List the general CT number or range for the following tissue types:

   A. Cortical bone _____

   B. White brain matter _____

   C. Blood _____

   D. Fat _____

   E. Lung tissue _____

   F. Air _____

   G. Water _____

25. Which medium serves as the baseline for CT numbers? _____

26. Match the most common appearance of the following tissue types as displayed on a CT image:

   _____ A. Bone   1. White

   _____ B. Gray brain matter   2. Gray

   _____ C. CSF   3. Black

   _____ D. Iodinated contrast media

27. Window width (WW) controls:

   A. Displayed image density   C. Slice thickness

   B. Displayed image contrast   D. Total number of slices

28. Window level (WL) controls:

   A. Image brightness   C. Slice thickness

   B. Image contrast   D. Total number of slices

29. Pitch is defined as: _____

30. Pitch is a relationship between _____ and _____.

31. Calculate the pitch ratio using the following parameters: Couch movement at a rate of 20 mm per second with a

   slice collimation of 10 mm _____.

32. The pitch ratio calculated in question 31 is an example of:

   A. Undersampling   C. Perfect pitch

   B. Oversampling   D. Intermittent pitch

33. Which of the following parameters would produce a 0.5:1.0 pitch ratio?

   A. 10-mm couch movement and 10-mm slice thickness

   B. 15-mm couch movement and 10-mm slice thickness

   C. 10-mm couch movement and 20-mm slice thickness

   D. 30-mm couch movement and 10-mm slice thickness

34. True/False: Hard-copy images of axial CT scans are viewed as though the viewer were facing the patient.

35. How must the intravenous contrast media be administered during a multislice CT scan?

A. Hand, bolus injection   C. Slow drip infusion

B. Electromechanical injector   D. Fast drip infusion

36. What is commonly injected following the administration of intravenous contrast media during a multislice CT scan?

A. Saline   C. Lasix

B. Heparin   D. Sterile water

37. CT can detect tissue density differences as low as:

A. 1% or less   C. 15%

B. 10%   D. 20%

38. What is the name of the technology that uses the optimal mAs per slice to minimize the patient dose during a CT scan?

A. Modulation transfer function   C. Detector calibration

B. Scan-dose calibration   D. Dose modulation

39. What type of shields can be used to minimize dose to radiosensitive organs (eye, breasts, pelvis, and thyroid)?

A. Lead   C. Plastic acrylic

B. Bismuth   D. Copper

40. What is the primary goal of the Image Gently campaign?

_____

REVIEW EXERCISE C: Clinical Applications of Computed Tomography and Imaging of the Brain (see textbook pp. 733-737)

1. List the four advantages of CT over conventional radiography:

A. _____

B. _____

C. _____

D. _____

2. A scanogram or topogram is another term for:

A. CT scan of the head   C. Warm up procedure for scanner

B. Scout view   D. Calibration procedure for scanner

3. Approximately _____% to _____% of all cranial CTs require contrast media.

4. True/False: Oxygen deprivation of *2 minutes* will lead to permanent brain cell injury.

5. True/False: Iodinated contrast media are able to pass through the blood-brain barrier in the normal individual.

6. True/False: Iodinated contrast media are often required to visualize neoplasms during a head CT scan.

7. Which one of the following substances will not pass through the blood-brain barrier?

   A. Proteins   C. Oxygen

   B. Glucose   D. Select ions found in the blood

8. True/False: Patient dose is higher for a CT scan of the head as compared with a routine skull series.

9. True/False: The higher the pitch ratio during a volume CT scan, the greater is the patient dose.

10. Head CT images are viewed in what two window settings?

    A. _____

    B. _____

11. The most important aspect of positioning the head for cranial CT is to ensure there is no

    _____ and no _____ of the head.

12. Trauma to the skull may lead to a collection of blood accumulating under the dura mater called

    _____.

13. Identify the labeled parts on this axial section through the region of the midventricular level (Figs. 18-5 and 18-6):

    A. _____

    B. _____

    C. _____

    D. _____

    E. _____

    F. _____

    G. _____

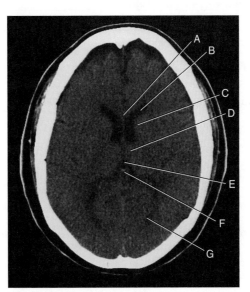

Fig. 18-5. Structure identification on an axial CT scan at midventricular level.

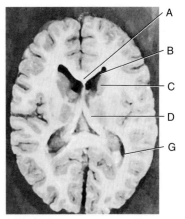

Fig. 18-6. Brain tissue specimen, midventricular level.

14. Identify the labeled parts on this axial section through the level of the middle third ventricle (Figs. 18-7 and 18-8):

A. _____

B. _____

C. _____

D. _____

E. _____

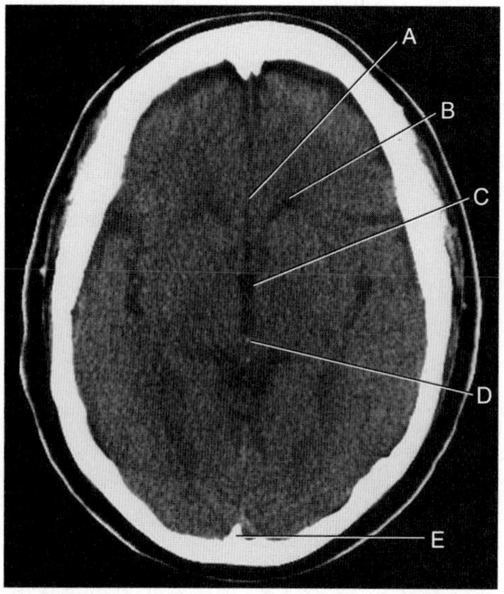

Fig. 18-7. Structure identification on an axial CT scan at mid third ventricle level.

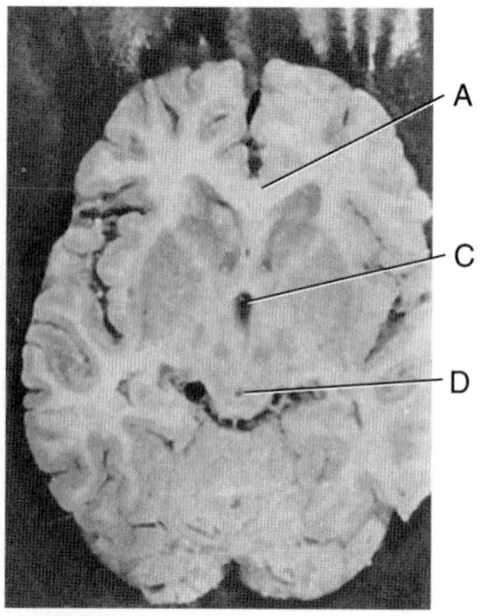

Fig. 18-8. Brain tissue specimen, mid third ventricle level.

REVIEW EXERCISE D: Additional and Specialized Computed Tomography Procedures and Computed Tomography Terminology (see textbook pp. 738-742)

1. CT scan of the neck for a possible tumor of the nasopharynx requires slice thicknesses of no greater than:

   A. 2-3 mm   C. 7-10 mm

   B. 5 mm   D. 1 cm

2. True/False: Air may be injected into the joint for a CT scan of synovial joints.

3. Common pathologic indications for a CT study of the spine include the following *except*:

   A. Infection   C. Spinal cord deformity

   B. Spinal stenosis D. Fracture of the vertebrae

4. True/False: Different CT scans can be combined and reformatted to create a three-dimensional image.

5. True/False: Three-dimensional imaging requires a data set created during a volume acquisition.

6. What is the contrast medium of choice for most CT virtual endoscopic procedures?

   _____

7. What two positions must the patient assume during a CT colonography? _____

8. Other than air, what other contrast media is often used for a CT colonography?

   _____

9. True/False: CT angiography (CTA) does not require the use of iodinated contrast media.

10. How much oral contrast media is instilled for a CT enteroclysis?

    A. Up to 100 mL   C. Up to 1000 mL

    B. Up to 500 mL   D. Up to 2000 mL

11. What is the purpose of ECG gating during a cardiac CT scan? _____

12. True/False: Traditional coronary angiography remains the gold standard for evaluation of the coronary arteries over cardiac CT.

13. True/False: The patient/table is stationary during CT fluoroscopy.

14. During CT fluoroscopy, partially reconstructed images are obtained and displayed at a rate of:

    A. 1 to 3 images per second   C. 8 to 12 images per second

    B. 6 to 8 images per second   D. 20 to 25 images per second

15. One of the most common applications for CT fluoroscopy is:

    A. CT myelography   C. Virtual colonoscopy

    B. GI motility studies   D. Biopsies

16. What is used to minimize exposure to the hands of the radiologist during a CT fluoroscopic biopsy?

    A. Lead gloves   C. Special filters

    B. Low kV   D. Special needle holders

17. True/False: CT percutaneous biopsies have an equal accuracy rate as compared with surgical biopsies.

18. The success rate for CT percutaneous abscess drainage is approximately:

    A. 10% to 15%   C. 50% to 60%

    B. 20% to 25%   D. 85%

19. Identify the name of the device that houses the CT x-ray tube, detectors, and collimators.

    _____

20. What is the term for a series of rows and columns of pixels that give form to the digital image?

    _____

21. What are the terms (more than one answer) for a preliminary image taken before a CT procedure?

    _____

22. A device that transmits electrical energy and allows continuous rotation of the CT x-ray tube for volumetric

    acquisition is called _____.

23. _____ controls the brightness of a CT reconstructed image within a certain range.

24. _____ controls the gray level or contrast of a CT image.

25. _____ is a technique used to view vessels demonstrated during a CTA.

LABORATORY EXERCISES

Part A of this learning activity needs to be carried out in a special procedures room equipped for whole-body CT. A supervising technologist or instructor should be present for this activity. Part B can be carried out in a classroom or any room in which illuminators and other CT viewing facilities are available.

Laboratory Exercise A: Positioning

Complete the following steps and place a check mark by each when completed.

_____ 1. Review the equipment in the room, noting the location of patient support equipment, such as oxygen, suction, the IV pole, and the emergency cart.

_____ 2. Role-play using another student as the patient. Prepare the "patient" by explaining the procedure, the breathing instructions that will be given, the sounds that will be experienced, and what he or she will see and experience as the patient is placed into the gantry aperture for the examination.

_____ 3. Place your patient on the table (couch) in a supine position with the arms above the head. Raise the patient and table to the correct height and slowly move into the gantry aperture until the x-ray beam trajectory coincides with the starting scan position for the part being examined. Using the intercom device, talk to the patient from the control console. Finally, remove your patient when the procedure is completed.

_____ 4. Review the controls and monitors at the operator console. Have someone demonstrate the image parameters and the other variables controlled by the technologist and explain how whole-body scanning is different from head CT scanning.

Directions: This self-test should be taken only after completing all of the readings, review exercises, and laboratory activities for a particular section. The purpose of this test is not only to provide a good learning exercise, but also to serve as a strong indicator of what your final evaluation exam will be. It is strongly suggested that if you do not receive at least a 90% to 95% grade on this self-test, you should review those areas in which you missed questions before going to your instructor for the final evaluation exam for this chapter.

1. A. The parts of the neuron that conduct impulses toward the cell body are called

   _____.

   B. The part that conducts impulses away from the cell body is the _____.

2. Three protective membranes that cover or enclose the entire central nervous system are collectively called:

   _____

3. The three specific membranes from question 2 are called (starting externally):

   A. _____   B. _____   C. _____

4. The various layers of the membranes just discussed have specific spaces of various sizes between these layers. Each has a specific name. Identify these various membrane layers and their associated spaces on Fig. 18-9:

   A. _____

   B. _____

   C. _____

   D. _____

   E. _____

   F. _____

   G. _____

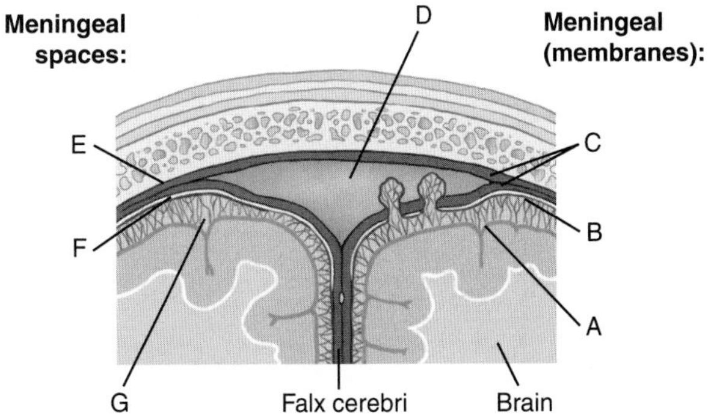

Fig. 18-9. Meninges and meningeal spaces.

5. Which of the spaces in question is normally filled with cerebrospinal fluid? _____

6. Match the following structures to the correct division of the brain:

_____ A. Pons   1. Forebrain

_____ B. Cerebellum   2. Midbrain

_____ C. Cerebrum   3. Hindbrain

_____ D. Thalamus

_____ E. Cerebral aqueduct

7. The largest division of the brain is the _____.

8. The right and left cerebral hemispheres are separated by a deep fissure called the

_____.

9. The fibrous band of white tissue deep within this fissure connecting the right and left cerebral hemispheres is

called the _____.

10. The inner layers of dura mater within the longitudinal fissure join to form the

_____.

11. Which of the following ventricles are located in the upper aspect of the cerebral hemispheres?

A. Lateral ventricles   C. Third ventricle

B. Fourth ventricle   D. Cisterna magna

12. The diamond-shaped fourth ventricle connects inferiorly with a wide portion of the subarachnoid space called the:

A. Interventricular foramen   C. Cisterna cerebellomedullaris

B. Lateral recesses   D. Cisterna pontis

13. Identify the ventricles, their parts, and their associated structures as labeled on both the lateral and top-view drawings (Figs. 18-10 and 18-11):

Ventricles

A. _____

B. _____

C. _____

Connecting passageways for CSF

a. _____

b. _____

c. _____

Parts of lateral ventricles

1. _____

2. _____

3. _____

4. _____

Small gland (only in Fig. 18-10)

5. _____

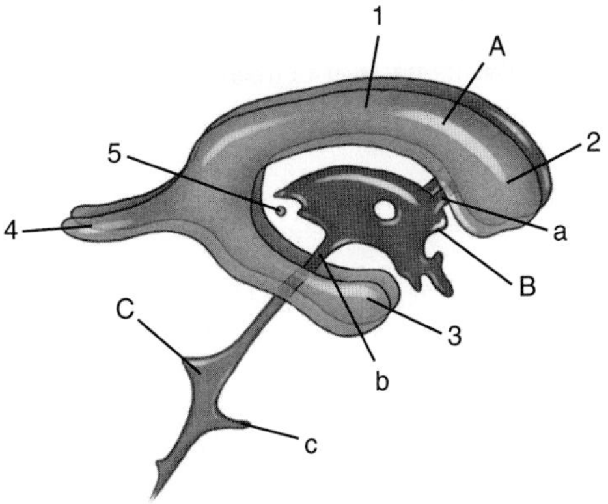

Fig. 18-10. Ventricles, lateral view.

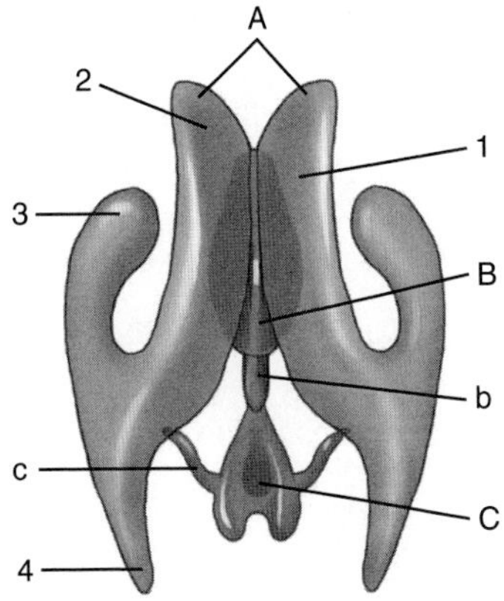

Fig. 18-11. Ventricles, superior view.

14. The condition known as _____ results from abnormal accumulation of cerebrospinal

fluid within the _____.

15. Enlarged regions of the subarachnoid space are called _____.

16. Identify the four lobes of the cerebrum as labeled in Fig. 18-12:

A. _____

B. _____

C. _____

D. _____

E. The fifth lobe, which is more centrally located and not shown on this drawing,

   is called the _____.

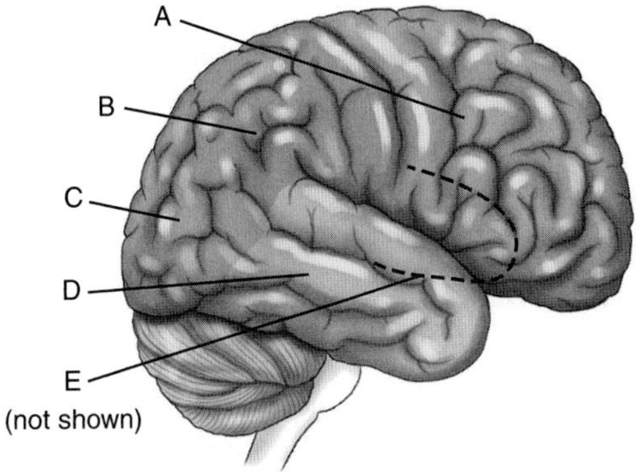

Fig. 18-12. Four lobes of the cerebrum.

17. Identify each of the following terms as either gray matter or white matter brain structures:

_____ A. Cerebral cortex   1. Gray matter

_____ B. Axons (fibrous parts of neuron)   2. White matter

_____ C. Corpus callosum

_____ D. Thalamus

_____ E. Centrum semiovale

_____ F. Cerebral nuclei

18. Which generation of CT scanner uses a pencil-thin x-ray beam and a single detector?
   A. First-generation   C. Third-generation
   B. Second-generation   D. Fourth-generation

19. Which generation of CT scanner allows continuous volume type of scanning?
   A. First-generation   C. Third-generation
   B. Second-generation   D. Fourth-generation

20. Which devices in the volume CT scanners allow continual tube rotation in the same direction?

_____

21. CT can detect tissue density differences as low as:
   A. 1%   C. 10%
   B. 5%   D. 20%

22. Which device shapes and limits the x-ray beam in the CT tube? _____

23. What must be done to the numeric data (CT numbers) to create the displayed CT image?

_____

24. The three major components of the scan unit are:

   A. _____   B. _____   C. _____

25. Each tiny picture element in the display matrix is called a(n) _____.

26. Which of the following parameters *cannot* be varied by appropriate manipulation at the operator console?
   A. kV   D. Vertical adjustment of table height
   B. Scan time   E. Thickness of slice
   C. Pitch ratio

27. What is the name of the three-dimensional element that provides height, width, and depth to the display matrix of the digital image?
   A. Pixel   C. Image volume
   B. Voxel   D. Isotropic data set

28. True/False: Submillimeter slice thicknesses are possible with multislice CT scanners.

29. A 64-slice CT scanner can acquire up to _____ images per second.
    - A. 64
    - B. 160
    - C. 525
    - D. 1048

30. What does the detector actually measure in a CT system? _____

31. What substance serves as the baseline for CT numbers? _____

32. What is the CT number for the substance described in question 31? _____

33. What is the CT number for fat?
    - A. −100
    - B. −200
    - C. +100
    - D. +250

34. Pitch is defined as a ratio between table speed and:
    - A. Number of tube rotations
    - B. Size of total tissue acquisition
    - C. Slice thickness
    - D. Tissue attenuation

35. Which one of the following pitch ratios represents "undersampling"?
    - A. 1:1
    - B. 2:1
    - C. 0.5:1
    - D. 0.7:1

36. True/False: CT exceeds the contrast resolution seen on a conventional radiograph.

37. Contrast media does not ordinarily cross the _____ barrier.

38. Which one of the following pathologic indications does *not* apply to head CT?
    - A. Brain neoplasm
    - B. Brain atrophy
    - C. Multiple sclerosis
    - D. Trauma
    - E. All of the above apply

39. True/False: An intravenous injection of iodinated contrast media is often given during a CT enteroclysis study.

40. Images produced during CT angiography (CTA) are viewed with a technique termed

_____.

41. What type of technical factors are employed with CT fluoroscopy?
    - A. High kV; high mA
    - B. Low kV; high mA
    - C. High kV; low mA
    - D. Low kV; low mA

42. The typical slice thickness for a spine CT ranges between:
    - A. 3 mm
    - B. 7 mm
    - C. 10 mm
    - D. 15 mm

43. A CT colonography requires the use of _____ as a contrast medium.

    A. Barium sulfate

    B. Iodinated rectal contrast

    C. Air

    D. All of the above

44. What is the chief disadvantage of CT colonography over conventional endoscopy?

    A. Cost

    B. Cannot biopsy or remove polyps

    C. Bowel prep required

    D. Time-consuming procedure

45. True/False: Special filters can be used during CT fluoroscopy to reduce patient skin dose during biopsies.

46. How long is the catheter left in place following a percutaneous abscess drainage (PAD) procedure?

    A. 1 hour

    B. 6 hours

    C. 12 hours

    D. 24 to 48 hours

47. _____ is a method by which images acquired in the axial plane may be reconstructed in the coronal or sagittal plane.

48. _____ controls the gray level of an image (the contrast).

49. _____ is a computer that serves as a digital postprocessing station and/or an image review station.

50. Devices that transmit electrical energy and allow continuous rotation of the x-ray tube for volumetric acquisition are called _____.

19 | Special Radiographic Procedures

This chapter discusses those additional diagnostic imaging procedures that are less common in most radiology departments. Arthrograms, biliary duct procedures, myelograms, orthoroentgenograms, and conventional tomograms are largely being replaced with other imaging modalities such as computed tomography (CT) or magnetic resonance imaging (MRI). However, in some departments, these procedures are still being performed in sufficient numbers that technologists must be familiar with them so that they can perform them when requested.

The anatomy for these procedures has been studied in previous chapters; therefore this chapter covers only the procedures themselves and the related positioning. The exception to this is the anatomy of the female reproductive organs as described in the section on hysterosalpingography.

CHAPTER OBJECTIVES

After you have successfully completed the activities of this chapter, you will be able to:

ARTHROGRAPHY

_____ 1. Identify the purpose, clinical indications, patient preparation, equipment, general procedure, and positioning routines related to knee arthrography.

_____ 2. Identify the purpose, clinical indications, patient preparation, equipment, general procedure, and positioning and imaging sequence related to shoulder arthrography.

BILIARY PROCEDURES

_____ 1. Describe the purpose, clinical indications, patient preparation, equipment, general procedure, and positioning and imaging sequence for the postoperative (T-tube or delayed) cholangiography.

_____ 2. Describe the purpose, clinical indications, patient preparation, equipment, general procedure, and the positioning and imaging sequence for an endoscopic retrograde cholangiopancreatography (ERCP).

HYSTEROSALPINGOGRAPHY

_____ 1. Identify specific aspects of the female reproductive system.

_____ 2. Identify the purpose, clinical indications, patient preparation, equipment, general procedure, and the positioning routines related to hysterosalpingography.

MYELOGRAPHY

_____ 1. Identify the purpose, clinical indications, contraindications, equipment, and general procedure related to myelography.

_____ 2. Identify positioning routines performed for lumbar, thoracic, and cervical myelography.

ORTHOROENTGENOGRAPHY

_____ 1. Define orthoroentgenography and the purpose of this procedure.

_____ 2. Identify the specific positioning and procedure for lower and upper limb orthoroentgenography.

CONVENTIONAL TOMOGRAPHY

_____ 1. Define the specific terms associated with conventional tomography.

_____ 2. Identify the controls and variables that are common features on conventional tomographic units.

_____ 3. Identify the three influencing and controlling factors related to tomographic blur.

_____ 4. Demonstrate the principles and controlling factors of conventional tomography in laboratory exercises.

LEARNING EXERCISES

The following review exercises should be completed only after careful study of the associated pages in the textbook as indicated by each exercise. Answers to each review exercise are given at the end of this workbook.

REVIEW EXERCISE A: Arthrography (see textbook pp. 716-719)

1. What classifications of joints are studied with arthrography? _____

2. Other than conventional radiography of synovial joints (e.g., arthrography), what imaging procedure is preferred

   by physicians for studying synovial joints? _____

3. List the three common forms of knee injury that require arthrography:

   A. _____

   B. _____

   C. _____

4. Give an example of nontraumatic pathology of the knee joint indicating arthrography.

   _____

5. What are the two primary contraindications for arthrography of any joint? _____

6. True/False: An arthrogram must be approached as a sterile procedure. Proper skin prep and sterility must be maintained.

7. True/False: Once the contrast medium is introduced into the knee joint, the knee must *not* be flexed or exercised.

8. What is the normal appearance of synovial fluid?

9. List the two types of contrast media used for a knee arthrogram:

   A. _____

   B. _____

10. List the two projections for conventional radiographic projections used for knee arthrography:

A. _____

B. _____

11. A. On average, how many exposures are taken of each meniscus during horizontal beam arthrography of the knee?

_____

B. How many degrees of rotation of the leg are used between exposures? _____

12. What four aspects of shoulder anatomy are demonstrated with shoulder arthrography?

A. _____   C. _____

B. _____   D. _____

13. What is the general name for the conjoined tendons of the four major shoulder muscles?

_____

14. What type of needle is commonly used for shoulder arthrograms? _____

15. List three clinical indications for a shoulder arthrogram:

A. _____

B. _____

C. _____

16. List the six projections frequently taken during a shoulder arthrogram:

A. _____   D. _____

B. _____   E. _____

C. _____   F. _____

REVIEW EXERCISE B: Biliary Procedures (see textbook pp. 720-721)

1. Postoperative (T-tube) cholangiograms are usually performed to detect:

A. Pancreatitis   C. Liver cyst

B. Biliary stones   D. Infected gallbladder

2. True/False: T-tube cholangiography is usually performed by a surgeon during a colectomy.

3. Which two blood values must be checked before a postoperative (T-tube) cholangiogram?

A. _____

B. _____

4. Why is the contrast media for a T-tube cholangiogram occasionally diluted before injection?

_____

5. True/False: Bile is sterile and standard precautions do not apply when handling it.

6. **Situation:** A T-tube cholangiogram image demonstrates the biliary ducts superimposed over the spine. The patient is in an AP position. Which position would remove the ducts from the spine?

_____

7. Postoperative (T-tube) cholangiograms are generally performed _____.

8. Which one of the following procedures may be performed during a postoperative (T-tube) cholangiogram?

   A. Remove the gallbladder   C. Remove a biliary stone

   B. Remove a liver cyst   D. Catheterize the hepatic portal vein

9. A. A radiographic procedure of examining the biliary and main pancreatic ducts is called a(n)

   _____. (Write out the full term.)

   B. What initials are commonly used as an abbreviation for this procedure? _____

   C. What type of special endoscope is commonly used for this procedure? _____

   D. Which member of the health care team usually performs this procedure? _____

   E. Why should a patient remain NPO at least 1 hour after this procedure? _____

10. Which condition of the pancreas may contraindicate a direct injection into the biliary ducts?

   _____

REVIEW EXERCISE C: Hysterosalpingography (see textbook pp. 722-724)

1. The hysterosalpingogram is a radiographic study of the _____ and

   _____.

2. The uterus is situated between the _____ posteriorly and the

   _____ anteriorly.

3. List the four divisions of the uterus:

   A. _____

   B. _____

   C. _____

   D. _____

4. The largest division of the uterus is the _____.

5. The distal aspect of the uterus extending to the vagina is the _____.

6. List the three layers of tissue that form the uterus (from the innermost to the outermost layer):

    A. _____

    B. _____

    C. _____

7. Which of the following terms is not an aspect of the uterine tube?

    A. Cornu   C. Isthmus

    B. Ampulla   D. Infundibulum

8. True/False: Fertilization of the ovum occurs in the uterine tube.

9. True/False: The distal portion of the uterine tube opens into the peritoneal cavity.

10. Which of the following terms is used to describe the "degree of openness" of the uterine tube?

    A. Stenosis   C. Atresia

    B. Patency   D. Gauge

11. The most common pathologic indication for the hysterosalpingogram (HSG) is:

    _____.

12. In addition to the answer for question 11, what are two other clinical indications for HSG?

    A. _____

    B. _____

13. List the three common types of lesions that can be demonstrated during a hysterosalpingogram:

    A. _____

    B. _____

    C. _____

14. The contrast medium preferred by most radiologists for a hysterosalpingogram is:

    A. Water-soluble, iodinated   C. Oxygen

    B. Oil-based, iodinated   D. Nitrogen

15. What device may be needed to aid the insertion and fixation of the cannula or catheter during the

    hysterosalpingogram? _____

16. To help facilitate the flow of contrast media into the uterine cavity, which position is the patient placed into

    following the injection of contrast media? _____

17. In addition to the supine position, what two other positions may be imaged to adequately visualize pertinent anatomy for an HSG?

A. _____

B. _____

18. Where is the CR centered for radiographic projections taken during an HSG using a 24- × 30-cm (10- × 12-inch) image receptor?

A. At level of ASIS   C. Iliac crest

B. Symphysis pubis   D. 2 inches (5 cm) superior to symphysis pubis

REVIEW EXERCISE D: Myelography (see textbook pp. 726-728)

1. Myelography is a radiographic study of the:

A. _____

B. _____

2. List the four common lesions or clinical indications demonstrated during myelography:

A. _____   C. _____

B. _____   D. _____

3. Of the four clinical indications just mentioned, which is the most common for myelography?

_____

4. True/False: Myelography of the cervical and thoracic spinal regions is most common.

5. List the four common contraindications for myelography:

A. _____   C. _____

B. _____   D. _____

6. To reduce patient anxiety, a sedative is usually administered _____ hour(s) before the procedure.

7. What type of radiographic table must be used for myelography? _____

8. Into which spinal space is the contrast medium introduced during myelography?

_____

9. List the two common puncture sites for contrast media injection during myelography:

A. _____

B. _____

10. Which one of the puncture sites from question 9 is preferred? _____

11. What is the patient's general body position for each of the following punctures? (Note: There may be more than one acceptable answer for each.)

A. Lumbar _____

B. Cervical _____

12. Why is a large positioning block placed under the abdomen for a lumbar puncture in the prone position?

_____

13. Which type of contrast medium is most commonly used for myelography? _____

14. The contrast medium in question 13 provides good radiopacity up to _____ after injection.

A. 20 minutes   C. 1 hour

B. 30 minutes   D. 8 hours

15. What dosage range of contrast medium is usually injected for myelography?

A. 8 to 10 mL   C. 9 to 15 mL

B. 20 to 30 mL   D. Approximately 1 mL

16. Indicate the correct sequence of events for a myelogram by numbering the following steps in order (from 1 through 8):

_____ A. Introduce needle into subarachnoid space

_____ B. Collect CSF and send to laboratory

_____ C. Take overhead radiographic images

_____ D. Explain procedure to the patient

_____ E. Introduce contrast medium

_____ F. Have patient sign informed consent form

_____ G. Take fluoroscopic spot images

_____ H. Prepare patient's skin for puncture

17. Which position is performed to demonstrate the region of C7 during a cervical myelogram?

_____

18. Why should the patient's head and neck remain hyperextended during cervical myelography?

_____

19. True/False: Generally, AP supine, PA prone, or horizontal beam lateral projections are not taken during thoracic spine myelography.

20. Complete the following for suggested routine projections (following fluoroscopy and spot filming) for the different levels of the spine:

Projection/Position   **Level of CR**

1. Cervical region   A. _____

                            B. _____

2. Thoracic region   A. _____

                            B. _____

                            C. _____

3. Lumbar region   A. _____

21. True/False: Myelography is largely being replaced by MRI and CT.

22. How is the contrast medium removed from the body after myelography?

_____

REVIEW EXERCISE E: Orthoroentgenography (see textbook pp. 760-763)

1. What are the chief disadvantages of using CT over orthoroentgenography for long bone measurements?

_____

2. What is the literal meaning of the term orthoroentgenogram? _____

3. Why should separate projections be taken of limb joints rather than including the entire extremity on a single

projection? _____

4. When performing an orthoroentgenographic procedure, what device must be placed on top of the table next to the

affected limb? _____

5. What is the name of the surgical procedure that shortens a limb by fusing the epiphyses?

_____

6. Which three joints are included on one image receptor for a long bone study of the lower limb?

_____

7. True/False: Both right and left lower limbs can be placed on the same radiograph for a long bone study.

8. True/False: For a bilateral study, all three joints of both lower limbs can be placed on the same 35- × 43-cm (14- × 17-inch) IR.

9. If both lower limbs are radiographed together on one image receptor, why should two rulers be used with one under each limb rather than placing one midway between the two limbs?

_____

10. True/False: For a long bone study of the upper limb, all three projections must be taken with the IR placed in the Bucky tray.

11. True/False: The wrist is examined in the pronated position (PA) for a long bone study of the upper limb.

12. True/False: The proximal humerus must be rotated internally for the shoulder projection taken during upper limb orthoroentgenography.

REVIEW EXERCISE F: Conventional Tomography (see textbook pp. 764-765)

1. Define each of the following terms in short, concise answers:

   A. Tomograph _____

   B. Fulcrum _____

   C. Fulcrum level _____

   D. Objective (focal) plane _____

   E. Sectional thickness _____

   F. Exposure angle (exposure amplitude) _____

   G. Amplitude _____

   H. Blur _____

2. Which locks on the x-ray tube must be opened or unlocked during linear tomography?

   _____

3. True/False: The Bucky tray lock must be securely locked before a tomographic exposure.

4. True/False: Anatomy at the fulcrum level becomes blurred and difficult to see on a radiograph.

5. List four common adjustments or features found on the tomographic control panel:

   A. _____

   B. _____

   C. _____

   D. _____

6. True/False: Objects closer to the objective plane will experience maximum blurring.

7. Briefly describe the tomographic blurring principle. (Why, or how, does blurring of some objects occur while others remain in sharp focus?)

   _____

8. List the four factors that determine the amount of blurring:

   A. _____

   B. _____

   C. _____

   D. _____

9. True/False: As the exposure angle decreases, slice thickness also decreases (becomes thinner).

10. True/False: As the distance from the image receptor increases, object blurring increases.

11. To gain maximum blurring of the body of the sternum during tomography, it should be placed to tube movement.

   A. Parallel   C. Diagonally

   B. Perpendicular   D. 5° angle

12. Which of the following exposure angles would produce the least amount of blurring outside of the objective plane?

   A. 10°   C. 5°

   B. 20°   D. 40°

13. Which of the following exposure angles would produce the greatest amount of blurring outside of the objective plane?

   A. 10°   C. 5°

   B. 8°   D. 20°

14. What exposure angle is required with the tomographic process described in question 14?

   _____

15. True/False: Blurring is a desired outcome of tomography.

16. A tomographic principle in which the anatomic structure moves but the image receptor/tube remain stationary is

   called _____. (Hint: Found in Chapter 8 in text.)

17. What is the *minimum* exposure time required to produce a breathing lateral projection of the thoracic spine? (Review Chapter 8 in text.)

   A. 1 second   C. 4 seconds

   B. 2 seconds   D. 6 seconds

LABORATORY EXERCISES

The following exercises involve two procedures for which supplies and equipment are most commonly available to students.

Exercise A: Orthoroentgenography Long Bone Measurement

1. Using an upper and lower limb radiographic phantom (if available), produce long bone measurement radiographs of the following:

_____ Unilateral lower limb (AP projection of hip, knee, and ankle on one image receptor with a correctly placed Bell-Thompson ruler)

_____ Bilateral lower limbs (AP projections of hips, knees, and ankles on one image receptor with correctly placed Bell-Thompson ruler)

_____ Unilateral upper limb (AP projections of shoulder, elbow, and wrist on one image receptor with correctly placed ruler)

Exercise B: Conventional Tomography

This part of the learning exercise needs to be carried out in an energized radiographic room equipped with a linear type tomographic unit. Check off the following steps as they are completed:

_____ **Step 1. Equipment setup:** Set up the necessary tomographic equipment, including the adjustable fulcrum level attachment connected to the tube and to the Bucky. Ensure that the Bucky tray locks are released (as well as the tube angle and tube distance locks), allowing the tube and Bucky tray to move freely.

_____ **Step 2. Preparation of "phantom" for experiments:** Design a series of experiments to demonstrate the tomographic blurring principle and the effect of the four controlling and influencing factors on blurring. Commercial tomographic phantoms are available with various lead numbers or other metallic devices placed at specific levels within the phantom. If these are not readily available, one can easily be made with paper clips in combination with a wire mesh or other flat metallic objects placed in horizontal layers in three different books or in three different layers within the same book. The shape or the configuration of the metallic objects can be varied in each layer so that the various levels can be differentiated on the radiograph.

_____ **Step 3. Determine exposure factors:** Determine approximate exposure factors to visualize the metallic objects as placed in the books and stacked on the radiographic table. Start with an approximate upper limb exposure technique. Make a test exposure. Set the factors on the control panel of the tomographic unit as needed.

OPTIONAL EXPERIMENTS TO DEMONSTRATE TOMOGRAPHIC PRINCIPLES AND VARIABLES

Using your knowledge and understanding of tomographic blurring principles as studied in this chapter, design and carry out exercises as needed to demonstrate the following:

Experiment A: Orientation of Body Part to Tube Travel—Demonstrate that those objects parallel to the direction of tube movement create "streaks" and are not as effectively blurred as when they are perpendicular to the tube movement. This can be readily shown by changing the longitudinal direction of the metallic objects (e.g., paper clips) so that the levels above and below the focal plane will be at some angle or completely perpendicular to the direction of the tube travel. This should demonstrate increased blurring of the objects above and below the focal plane.

Experiment B: Influencing and Controlling Factors for Tomographic Blurring—Design experiments to demonstrate how each of the four factors or variables listed in the following influences or controls the amount of blurring. On these types of experiments, remember to change only one factor at a time, keeping all other factors constant.

_____ **Factor 1—Object-focal plane distance**

Demonstrate that those objects farther from the focal plane have greater movement on the image receptor and therefore increased blurring as compared with those closer to the focal plane.

This can be done by first taking tomographs with the objects above and below those in the focal plane. Compare these with tomographs taken when the objects above and below are placed at increased distances from the focal plane. You should be able to demonstrate markedly increased blurring on the second set of tomographs.

_____ **Factor 2—Exposure angle or amplitude**

By changing the exposure angle, demonstrate that an increase in exposure angle with greater tube travel will increase the blurring, resulting in a thinner focal plane. Likewise, a decrease in exposure angle with less tube travel will decrease the movement of the objects above and below the focal plane, creating less blurring and a thicker section remaining in focus.

Remember that the amplitude or speed of tube movement must also increase as the exposure angle is increased so that the exposure continues throughout the full arc of tube travel.

_____ **Factor 3—Object image receptor distance (OID)**

Demonstrate that as the distance of the objects from the IR is increased, greater blurring will occur.

Sponge blocks can be placed between objects (e.g., books or phantom) and the table to increase the object-IR distance. (This will demonstrate why the upside or side away from the IR on a tomogram of a lateral TMJ or of a lateral of inner ear structures should be examined rather than the downside.)

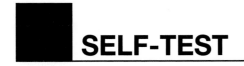

SELF-TEST

MY SCORE = _____%

Directions: This self-test should be taken only after completing all of the readings, review exercises, and laboratory activities for a particular section. The purpose of this test is not only to provide a good learning exercise but also to serve as a strong indicator of what your final evaluation exam will be. It is strongly suggested that if you do not receive at least a 90% to 95% grade on this self-test that you review those areas in which you missed questions before going to your instructor for the final evaluation exam for this chapter.

1. List the two synovial type of joints most commonly examined with an arthrogram:

   A. _____   B. _____

2. List the two contraindications for an arthrogram:

   A. _____   B. _____

3. An indication of a possible "Baker's cyst" suggests the need for an arthrogram procedure for the

   _____.

4. List the two types of contrast media commonly used for a knee arthrogram:

   A. _____

   B. _____

5. What is the purpose of flexing the knee gently after the contrast medium has been injected for an arthrogram

   procedure? _____

6. How many exposures are made, and how much is the leg rotated, between each exposure for horizontal beam knee arthrograms?

   A. Number of exposures: _____

   B. Degrees of rotation between exposures: _____

7. The term *rotator cuff* refers to what structures of the shoulder? _____

8. What type of needle is most often used to introduce contrast media during a shoulder arthrogram?

   _____

9. List the overhead projections that may be requested for a shoulder arthrogram:

Scout

A. _____

Postinjection

B. _____

C. _____

D. _____

E. _____

F. _____

10. How is the contrast medium instilled into the biliary ducts during an ERCP? _____

11. Other than a radiologist, what type of physician often performs ERCP? _____

12. What is the most common clinical reason for performing a T-tube cholangiogram?

_____

13. Which one of the following conditions may contraindicate an ERCP?
   A. Biliary obstruction   C. Jaundice
   B. Stone in main pancreatic duct   D. Pseudocyst

14. List the four divisions of the uterus:

   A. _____   C. _____

   B. _____   D. _____

15. Which of the following is *not* a tissue layer of the uterus?
   A. Osseometrium   C. Endometrium
   B. Myometrium   D. Serosa

16. True/False: The uterine tubes are connected directly to the ovaries.

17. List the three contraindications for a hysterosalpingogram:

   A. _____

   B. _____

   C. _____

18. True/False: An oil-based contrast medium is preferred for the majority of hysterosalpingograms.

19. True/False: Hysterosalpingography can be a therapeutic procedure in correcting certain obstructions within the uterine tube.

20. List the four common lesions or conditions diagnosed through a myelogram:

    A. _____   C. _____

    B. _____   D. _____

21. List the four contraindications for a myelogram:

    A. _____   C. _____

    B. _____   D. _____

22. The most common clinical indication for a myelogram is:

    A. Benign tumors   C. HNP

    B. Spinal cysts   D. Bony injury to the spine

23. Where is the contrast medium injected during a myelogram? _____

24. Which position will move the contrast media column from the lumbar to the cervical region during a myelogram?

    A. Fowler's   C. Trendelenburg

    B. Left lateral decubitus   D. Prone

25. What is the most common spinal puncture site for a lumbar myelogram?

    A. L3-L4   C. L4-L5

    B. L1-L2   D. L5-S1

26. A cervical puncture is indicated for an upper spinal region myelogram if:

    A. The patient has severe lordosis   C. The patient has HNP of the L4-L5 level

    B. The patient has mild scoliosis   D. The patient has complete blockage at T-spine level

27. The absorption of the water-soluble contrast media into the vascular system of the body begins approximately

    _____ minutes after injection and is totally undetectable radiographically after

    _____ hours.

28. Which position is performed during a cervical myelogram to demonstrate the C7-T1 region?

    _____

29 The formal term for a radiographic long bone measurement study is _____.

30. True/False: To properly measure the length of a long bone, the entire lower limb should be included on a single projection.

31. True/False: Epiphysiodesis is an operation to lengthen bone by widening the epiphyseal plate.

32. True/False: Movement of the body part between exposures will compromise the long bone study.

33. True/False: If a long bone study of both lower limbs is ordered, the use of two metal rulers is recommended with both limbs exposed at the same time on the same image receptor.

34. What is the proper name for the special metal ruler used for long bone measurement?

_____

35. What size of image receptor and how many exposures are recommended for a long bone study of the upper limbs for an adult? (More than one answer is possible.)

_____

36. Another term for tomography is _____.

37. Match each of the following tomographic terms with its correct definition:

_____ A. Objective plane   1. Distortion of objects outside the objective plane

_____ B. Exposure angle   2. The total distance the x-ray tube travels

_____ C. Tomogram   3. Radiograph produced by a tomographic unit

_____ D. Blur   4. The plane where the target anatomy is clear

_____ E. Fulcrum   5. The pivot point between tube and image receptor

_____ F. Amplitude   6. The factor that determines slice thickness

38. True/False: Maximum blurring of anatomy is achieved when it is perpendicular to tube travel.

39. True/False: The primary factor affecting the sectional thickness, as controlled by the operator, is exposure angle.

40. True/False: Increased blurring occurs when the object is farther from the image receptor.

41. True/False: More blurring occurs with a shorter exposure angle.

20 | Diagnostic and Therapeutic Modalities

This chapter introduces select alternative diagnostic and therapeutic imaging modalities, including nuclear medicine (NM), positron emission tomography (PET), radiation oncology (therapy), ultrasound imaging (sonography), mammography, bone densitometry, and magnetic resonance imaging (MRI). The information and review exercises contained in Chapter 20 are intended to introduce students to basic concepts related to each of these modalities. Basic definitions, physical principles, clinical applications, and technologist responsibilities will be covered.

A more extensive presentation is provided in the MRI section, which introduces MRI terminology and the basics of MRI physics and instrumentation. The important clinical aspects related to personnel and patient safety are discussed. An introduction to the imaging parameters that affect the quality of the images and clinical applications of MRI is included.

CHAPTER OBJECTIVES

Nuclear Medicine

_____ 1. Identify basic operating principles related to nuclear medicine imaging.

_____ 2. List the purpose, radionuclide used, and pathologic indications demonstrated with select nuclear medicine procedures.

_____ 3. List specific responsibilities for members of the nuclear medicine team.

Positron Emission Tomography (PET)

_____ 1. Describe the PET imaging process.

_____ 2. Identify the different types of radionuclides used in PET imaging.

_____ 3. Describe the basic operating principles of PET imaging.

_____ 4. Identify the pathologic conditions best demonstrated with PET imaging.

_____ 5. Define terms and concepts specific to nuclear medicine technology.

Radiation Oncology (Therapy)

_____ 1. Distinguish between internal and external types of radiation therapy.

_____ 2. Identify the energy level, characteristics, and advantages of the major types of radiation therapy units.

_____ 3. List the specific responsibilities of radiation oncology team members.

Ultrasound Imaging (Sonography)

_____ 1. Identify basic operating principles related to ultrasound.

_____ 2. List the characteristics, advantages, and disadvantages of specific types of ultrasound systems.

_____ 3. List the purpose, transducer used, and pathologic indications demonstrated with select ultrasound procedures.

Mammography

_____ 1. List statistics for breast cancer in the United States and worldwide.

_____ 2. Describe the recommendations from the American Cancer Society and American College of Radiology (ACR) in regard to mammography.

_____ 3. Describe the impact of the Mammography Quality Standards Act (MQSA) on mammography facilities and mammographers.

_____ 4. On drawings and radiographs, identify specific anatomy of the female breast.

_____ 5. Identify specific regions of the breast using the quadrant and the clock systems.

_____ 6. List the three general categories of breast tissue according to their tissue composition, age of the patient, and radiographic density (brightness).

_____ 7. Identify the three classifications of the breast.

_____ 8. Describe the general patient preparation concerns before a mammogram.

_____ 9. Identify key questions that should be asked as part of the clinical history taking before a mammogram.

_____ 10. List the technical considerations and equipment essential for quality images of the breast.

_____ 11. Identify the diagnostic benefits of breast compression and the precautions when applying compression.

_____ 12. Identify the principal way patient dose can be decreased or controlled during mammography.

_____ 13. Compare and contrast the advantages and disadvantages of film-screen and digital mammography.

_____ 14. List the benefits of using computer-aided detection (CAD) in mammographic interpretation.

_____ 15. Identify alternative imaging modalities available to study the breast, including advantages and disadvantages of each system.

_____ 16. Describe the basic and special projections most commonly performed in mammography; include patient positioning, CR placement, and anatomy demonstrated.

_____ 17. Describe the Eklund method for imaging breasts with implants.

_____ 18. List the average skin dose and mean glandular dose (MGD) range for each projection of the breast as described in the textbook.

_____ 19. Define specific types of breast pathology.

_____ 20. List the American College of Radiology nomenclature of terms and abbreviations for mammographic positioning.

_____ 21. Given mammographic images, identify specific positioning and exposure factor errors.

Mammography Positioning and Image Critique

_____ 1. Using a peer in a simulated setting, position for basic and special mammographic projections.

_____ 2. Using appropriate radiographic phantoms, produce satisfactory radiographs of specific positions (if equipment is available).

_____ 3. Critique and evaluate mammographic images based on the five divisions of radiographic criteria: (1) anatomy demonstrated, (2) position, (3) collimation and CR, (4) exposure and (5) anatomic image markers.

_____ 4. Distinguish between acceptable and unacceptable mammographic images based on exposure factors, motion, collimation, positioning, or other errors.

Bone Densitometry

_____ 1. List the major components of bone and their function.

_____ 2. List common clinical and pathologic indicators for osteoporosis.

_____ 3. Define and list the risk factors for fracture risk and osteoporosis.

_____ 4. List the World Health Organization (WHO) criteria for the diagnosis of osteoporosis.

_____ 5. List and describe the general types of agents approved by the FDA for the treatment and prevention of osteoporosis and the specific drugs approved under each type.

_____ 6. Identify the most common types of equipment, methods, and techniques for determining bone mineral density.

_____ 7. Define and describe the meaning of the two terms _DXA precision_ and _DXA accuracy_ as used in the performance of bone densitometry procedures.

Magnetic Resonance Imaging

_____ 1. Explain how MRI produces an image.

_____ 2. Compare the process of MRI image production with that of other imaging modalities.

_____ 3. Explain how a tissue signal is generated and received from body tissues.

_____ 4. Explain how image contrast is produced in the MR image.

_____ 5. Identify basic MRI safety considerations.

_____ 6. Identify information to be included when preparing a patient for an MRI exam.

_____ 7. Identify the type of contrast agent used in MRI.

_____ 8. State the appearance of specific tissue types on both T1- and T2-weighted images.

_____ 9. Define the terms and pathologic indications related to MRI.

_____ 10. Explain the purpose and applications of functional MRI (fMRI).

LEARNING EXERCISES

The following review exercises should be completed only after careful study of the associated pages in the textbook as indicated by each exercise. Answers to each review exercise are given at the end of this workbook. The review exercises are separated by imaging modality.

REVIEW EXERCISE A: Nuclear Medicine and PET (see textbook pp. 771-776)

1. A group of radioactive drugs used in the diagnosis and treatment of disease is termed

_____.

2. True/False: Nuclear medicine examines physiologic functions of an organ on the molecular level.

3. How are the materials identified in question 1 introduced into the body?

   A. Inhalation   C. Instilled

   B. Ingested   D. All of the above

4. The most common nuclide used in nuclear medicine procedures is:

   A. Sulfur colloid   C. Technetium 99m

   B. Iodine 123 (^{123}I)   D. Thallium

5. The nuclide identified in question 4 has a physical half-life of _____.

6. SPECT is an abbreviation for _____.

7. The typical patient dose for most diagnostic nuclear medicine procedures ranges between

   _____ to _____.

8. A bone scan can detect a fracture up to _____ post injury.

9. A common genitourinary nuclear medicine study is performed for:

   A. Kidney transplants   C. Pyelonephritis

   B. Renal cyst   D. All of the above

10. Nuclear medicine procedure to evaluate the motility of both solids and liquids through the GI tract is termed

    _____ study.

    A. HIDA   C. Gastroesophageal reflux

    B. Gastric emptying   D. GI flow

11. Which one of the following radiopharmaceuticals is given for a nuclear thyroid uptake scan?

    A. Technetium 99m   C. Sodium iodide 123 (^{123}I)

    B. Thallium   D. Neo Tect

12. Match the following responsibilities to the correct nuclear medicine team member:

    _____ A. Properly disposes of contaminated materials   1. Nuclear medicine technologist

    _____ B. Calibrates nuclear medicine imaging equipment   2. Nuclear medicine physician

    _____ C. Performs statistical analysis of study data   3. Health physicist

    _____ D. Administers radionuclide to patient   4. Radiation safety officer

    _____ E. Interprets procedure

    _____ F. Often serves as department radiation safety officer

    _____ G. Licensed to acquire and use radioactive materials

    _____ H. Reviews all dosimetry records

    _____ I. Performs audits on the record keeping

    _____ J. Digitally processes the images

13. Match each of the following nuclear medicine terms to its correct definition (use each choice only once):

_____ A. Synonym for a product of decay

_____ B. Time required for disintegration of half of the original activity of a nuclide

_____ C. Type of atom whose nucleus disintegrates spontaneously

_____ D. External indication of a device designed to enumerate ionizing events

_____ E. SI unit of radioactivity

_____ F. Stage in a reaction in which the concentration of the reactive species is no longer changing

_____ G. Traditional or standard unit of radioactivity

_____ H. Spontaneous nuclear transmutation characterized by the emission of energy and/or mass from the nucleus

1. Becquerel

2. Radionuclide

3. Daughter

4. Curie

5. Equilibrium

6. Half-life

7. Disintegration

8. Count

14. Technetium 99m will allow target tissue to return to background radiation levels within:

   A. 6 hours
   B. 12 hours
   C. 24 hours
   D. 48 hours

15. Technetium 99m has an energy level of:

   A. 70 keV
   B. 140 keV
   C. 5.11 MeV
   D. 5.11 keV

16. PET is an acronym for _____.

17. PET is a process that demonstrates:

   A. Anatomic appearance of tissues and organs

   B. Molecular makeup of tissues

   C. Biochemical function of the body's organs and tissue

   D. Pathologic processes of brain tissue only

18. True/False: The PET scanner produces radiation with an intensity of 5.11 MeV.

19. PET uses radioactive compounds that emit _____ during the radioactive decay process.

   A. Electrons
   B. Positrons
   C. Two gamma rays
   D. Neutrinos

20. The disappearance of the electron-positron pair and, in their place, two 511 keV photons that travel out in opposite directions is termed _____.

21. The PET scanner detector array measures:

   A. Emitted photons   C. Positrons

   B. Electrons   D. Neutrons

22. The energy detection process used with PET is termed _____ imaging.

23. PET uses radioactive compounds, which include oxygen and nitrogen, as well as:

   A. Selenium and iron   C. Carbon and argon

   B. Hydrogen and iodine   D. Carbon and fluorine

24. PET radioactive compounds measure all of the following vital cellular biochemical processes except:

   A. Oxygen use   C. Cellular reproduction

   B. Tissue perfusion   D. Glucose metabolism

25. Match each of the following PET tracer compounds to the cellular function that it measures (different compounds may measure the same biologic process):

   _____ A. Glucose metabolism   1. ^{13}N-ammonia

   _____ B. Blood flow/perfusion   2. ^{18}F-FDG

   _____ C. Amino acid metabolism   3. ^{15}O-water

   _____ D. Blood flow, blood volume, and oxygen consumption   4. ^{11}C-methionine

26. What is the name of the device required to produce the PET radioactive compounds?

   _____

27. Most PET tracers have a half-life of:

   A. 120 seconds to 110 minutes   C. 15 minutes to 8 hours

   B. 10 to 60 seconds   D. 8 to 12 hours

28. True/False: PET is superior to MRI in demonstrating anatomic structures of the brain.

29. True/False: PET can be used to investigate the location of seizure sites in patients with epilepsy who are not responding to drug therapy.

30. PET plays an important role in the initial diagnosis and _____ of malignancy.

   A. Destruction   C. Staging

   B. Prevention   D. Cure

31. True/False: Active tumor growth will lead to a decreased uptake of FDG.

32. True/False: Decreased uptake of an ammonia tracer in the heart tissue may indicate that coronary artery disease (CAD) is present.

33. Two common radionuclides used for PET perfusion coronary artery disease studies include ^{13}N-ammonia and

   A. ^{82}Rbn chloride   C. ^{18}F-FDG

   B. ^{15}O-water   D. ^{11}C-methionine

34. True/False: PET/CT scanners can determine the location of an atherosclerotic lesion and its impact on cardiac perfusion.

35. True/False: Generally, malignant cells have an accelerated glucose metabolism.

36. PET brain mapping is performed to:

    A. Identify possible tumors in the brain

    B. Distinguish between the gray and white matter of the brain

    C. Identify the transmission or impulse patterns of the brain

    D. Identify the location of key motor and sensory regions of the brain

37. In patients with Alzheimer's disease, glucose metabolism is dramatically _____ (increased or decreased) in several key areas of the brain.

38. Coregistration is another term for:

    A. PET image manipulation

    B. Increased tracer uptake in the brain

    C. Artifact seen on certain PET images

    D. Fusion technology

39. PET may be combined with an _____ study to determine if any epileptic activity is present.

40. True/False: It is possible to acquire functional PET and anatomic CT images in the same scanning session when the correct technology is employed.

REVIEW EXERCISE B: Radiation Oncology (Therapy) (see textbook p. 777)

1. True/False: Cancer is the second leading cause of death in the United States and Canada.

2. The use of radiation therapy to relieve symptoms of cancer only is termed _____ therapy.

3. Identify the two primary mechanisms for delivering therapeutic or palliative radiation:

    A. _____

    B. _____

4. Prostate cancer is a common candidate for which of the two types of radiation therapy treatment from

    question 3? _____

5. List the two sources of external beam radiation:

    A. _____

    B. _____

6. Cobalt-60 units emit gamma rays at the average intensity of _____ MeV.

    A. 1.25   C. 10.4

    B. 5.25   D. 15.25

7. What is the source of the high-energy x-rays produced with a linear accelerator therapy unit?

   A. Cobalt-60

   B. High-speed neutrons striking an anode

   C. Uranium 235

   D. High-speed electrons striking tungsten target

8. 4D imaging takes into account movement of the tumor caused by _____ functions.

9. SBRT is the abbreviation for _____.

10. _____ is a technique to administer radiation directly to an organ or area at the time of surgery.

11. Match the following responsibilities to the correct radiation oncology team member:

   _____ A. Plans the treatment as prescribed

   _____ B. Administers radiation treatments

   _____ C. Responsible for patient education

   _____ D. Serves as a conduit for patient referrals

   _____ E. Prescribes treatment plan

   _____ F. Advises oncologists on dosage calculations

   _____ G. Maintains daily treatment documentation

   1. Radiation therapist

   2. Radiation oncologist

   3. Medical dosimetrist

   4. Radiation oncology nurse

12. Another term for brachytherapy is _____.

REVIEW EXERCISE C: Ultrasound Imaging (Sonography) (see textbook pp. 778-781)

1. List three additional terms for medical ultrasound:

   A. _____

   B. _____

   C. _____

   D. Which of those listed above is the preferred term? _____

2. Sonography uses high-frequency sound waves in the range between _____ to

   _____ MHz.

3. True/False: Sonography is an ideal imaging modality for diagnosing an ileus.

4. True/False: Sonography is often used to locate a bone cyst in the femur.

5. True/False: Current research studies conclude that there are no adverse biologic effects associated with the use of medical sonography.

6. What is the fundamental purpose or function of the transducer? _____

   _____.

7. What type of material comprises the functional aspect of the transducer, which produces the high-frequency sound waves?

   A. Tungsten alloy   C. Silver/chromium alloy

   B. Ceramic   D. Ferrous alloy

8. True/False: A diagnostic medical transducer serves as both a transmitter and receiver of sound waves.

9. True/False: Lower frequency transducers permit greater penetration for imaging organs within the abdominal cavity.

10. List the three major imaging specialty areas that are within diagnostic sonography:

    A. _____

    B. _____

    C. _____

11. What is the chief advantage in using sonography for obstetric and pediatric patients?

    _____

12. What animal uses echo location in nature? _____ .

13. Which generation of sonographic equipment introduced grayscale imaging?

    A. A-mode   C. Real-time dynamic

    B. B-mode   D. Doppler

14. Which type of ultrasound system is used to examine the structure and behavior of flowing blood?

    A. A-mode   C. Real-time dynamic

    B. B-mode   D. Doppler

15. True/False: Advances in digital sonographic technology have eliminated film as an image storage medium.

16. True/False: Advances in digital sonographic technology have greatly reduced musculoskeletal injuries to the sonographer.

17. True/False: ALARA principles apply to sonography.

18. True/False: Thermal index or TI refers to heating of the face of transducer.

19. True/False: Mechanical index or MI refers to changes in cell structure.

20. The safety goal for each sonographic procedure performed is to use the least amount of scan time with the

    _____.

21. True/False: Contrast media is widely used for abdominal ultrasound studies in the United States.

22. Match the following procedures and/or situations to the correct frequency transducer (use each choice only once):

    _____ A. For an average or small abdomen   1. 3.5 MHz

    _____ B. For a larger abdomen   2. 5.0 to 7.0 MHz

    _____ C. For a study of breast   3. 17 MHz

23. True/False: Sonographers must provide technical or preliminary report based on their findings of an examination.

24. Sonography is highly diagnostic for studies of all of the following structures except the:
    A. Liver
    B. Stomach
    C. Gallbladder
    D. Uterus

25. What is the name of the ultrasound procedure in which the breast is scanned to distinguish between a cystic and solid mass? _____

26. Sonography is very effective in evaluating the Achilles tendon for tears.

27. What is placed between the transducer and the anatomy to prevent air distortion of the ultrasound signal?
    A. Water bath
    B. Nitrogen gas
    C. Gel
    D. Saline disk

28. True/False: The bones in the growing fetus are not well seen during a sonographic procedure.

29. Match each of the following sonographic terms to its correct definition (use each choice only once):

    _____ A. Uses heat to destroy tissues

    _____ B. Alteration in sound frequency or wavelength

    _____ C. Acoustic energy that travels through a medium

    _____ D. An anatomic object that does not produce any echoes

    _____ E. Ultrasound images that demonstrate dynamic motion

    _____ F. Highly reflective (echogenic) structures as compared with the surrounding structures

    _____ G. Acoustic energy that is reflected from a structure back towards the transducer

    _____ H. An anatomic structure or region of the body that highly reflects sound energy

    _____ I. An aspect of acoustic energy reflected back toward the source or origin

    _____ J. An anatomic object that produces fewer echoes than normal

    1. Anechoic
    2. Backscatter reflected by moving structures
    3. Doppler effect
    4. Echogenic
    5. Hyperechoic
    6. Hypoechoic
    7. Real-time imaging
    8. High-intensity focused ultrasound
    9. Wave
    10. Reflection

30. Sonoelastography is performed for the detection of:
    A. Muscular injuries
    B. Arterial wall calcification
    C. Meniscal tears in the knee joint
    D. Normal from abnormal breast tissue

MAMMOGRAPHY
REVIEW EXERCISE A: Breast Cancer, Anatomy of the Breast, and Mammography Quality Standards Act (see textbook pp. 782-786)

1. Radiographic examination of the mammary gland or breast is called _____.

2. The American Cancer Society recommends that women over the age of _____ should have a screening mammogram performed.

   A. 35   C. 45

   B. 40   D. 50

3. The Mammography Quality Standards Act (MQSA), which went into effect on October 1, _____, was passed to ensure high-quality mammography service requiring certification by the secretary of the Department of Health and Human Services (DHHS).

   A. 1992   C. 1994

   B. 1993   D. 1995

4. There are more than _____ documented cases of breast cancer worldwide.

5. Men have _____ % chance of developing breast cancer as compared with women.

6. Research indicates that once a breast cancer tumor has reached a size of _____ cm, it has often metastasized.

7. Breast cancer accounts for _____ of all new cancers detected in women.

   A. 12%   C. 32%

   B. 15%   D. 50%

8. In Canada, mammography guidelines are set by the _____.

9. Which of the following mammography facilities are exempt from MQSA standards?

   A. Medicare facilities   C. Not-for-profit facilities

   B. VA facilities   D. No facilities are exempt

10. The junction of the inferior part of the breast with the anterior chest wall is called the _____.

11. The pigmented area surrounding the nipple is the _____.

12. Breast tissue extending into the axilla is called the tail of the breast or the _____.

13. In the average female breast, the _____ (craniocaudad or mediolateral) diameter is usually greater.

14. Using the clock localization system, five o'clock on the right breast would be in what quadrant?
_____

15. Based on the clock system method, a suspicious mass at two o'clock on the right breast would be at _____ o'clock if it were in a similar position on the left breast.

16. What is the large muscle commonly seen on a mammogram that is located between the bony thorax and the mammary gland? _____

17. Two fibrous sheets of tissue join together just posterior to the breast to form _____ the space.

18. What is the function of the mammary gland? _____

19. List the three tissue types found in the female breast:

    A. _____   B. _____   C. _____

20. Various small blood vessels, fibrous connective tissues, ducts, and other small structures seen on finished mammograms are collectively called _____.

21. Bands of fibrous tissue passing through the breast tissue are known as _____.

22. Classify the following types of breasts into one of the three general categories: fibroglandular (FG), fibrofatty (FF), or fatty (F).

    _____ 1. 20 years, no children   _____ 5. 50 years, two children

    _____ 2. 35 years, no children   _____ 6. Male

    _____ 3. 35 years, three children   _____ 7. 35 years, lactating

    _____ 4. 25 years, pregnant   _____ 8. 10 years

23. Which is the least dense of the following tissues: fibrous, glandular, or adipose?

    _____

24. Identify the labeled parts on this sagittal section drawing (Fig. 20-1):

    A. _____

    B. _____

    C. _____

    D. _____

    E. _____

    F. _____

    G. _____

    H. _____

    I. _____

    J. _____

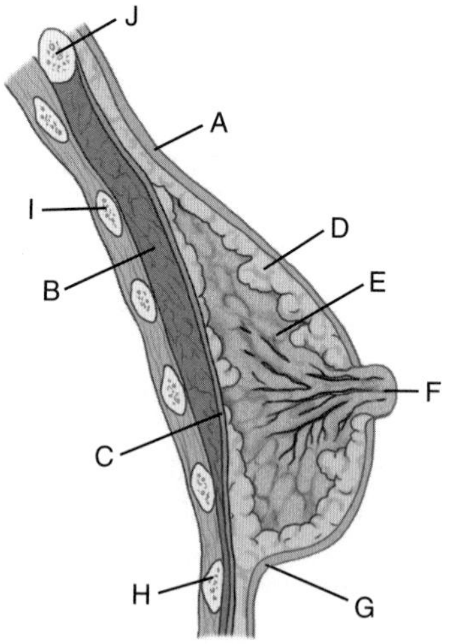

Fig. 20-1. Sagittal section of the breast.

25. Identify the labeled parts on Fig. 20-2:

A. _____

B. _____

C. _____

D. _____

E. _____

F. _____

G. _____

H. _____

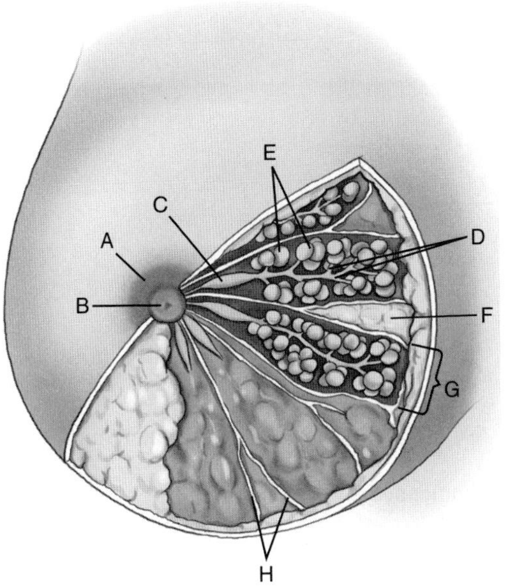

Fig. 20-2. Cutaway anterior view of the breast.

26. The glandular tissue of the breast is divided into _____lobes.

27. Which portion of the breast is nearest to the chest wall (apex or base)? _____

28. Which portion of the breast is nearest to the nipple (apex or base)? _____

29. The central ray is usually directed through the _____ of the breast.

30. What is the typical skin dose for a mammographic projection?

    A. 100 to 200 mrad   C. 800 to 900 mrad

    B. 400 to 600 mrad   D. 1200 to 1500 mrad

31. To minimize patient dose, the ACR recommends a repeat rate of less than:

    A. 2%   C. 10%

    B. 5%   D. 15%

32. True/False: MGD, as used in patient dose measurements in mammography, refers to mean gonadal dose.

33. True/False: A thyroid shield should be worn by the patient during mammography.

REVIEW EXERCISE B: Patient Preparation, Technical Considerations, Alternative Modalities, and Radiographic Positioning (see textbook pp. 787-798)

1. Other than jewelry and clothing, what substances must be removed from the patient's body before mammography

    to prevent artifacts? _____

2. True/False: Certain lotions with glitter may produce artifacts on the mammographic image.

3. List the six questions that should be included in the patient history taking before a mammogram:

   A. _____

   B. _____

   C. _____

   D. _____

   E. _____

   F. _____

4. True/False: Skin tattoos on the breast may produce an artifact on the image.

5. True/False: The apex of the breast is much thicker and contains denser tissues than at the base.

6. The recommended kV for analog (film-based) mammography is between _____and _____ kV.

7. Name the target material commonly used in mammography x-ray tubes: _____

8. The focal spot size on a dedicated mammography unit is usually between _____ and _____mm.

9. Typically, compression applied to the breast is _____ to _____ pounds of pressure.

10. List the six benefits of applying breast compression during mammography:

    A. _____

    B. _____

    C. _____

    D. _____

    E. _____

    F. _____

11. How does breast compression improve image quality or resolution?

    A. _____

    B. _____

12. The average required mAs range in mammography when using 25 to 28 kV is:

    A. 10 to 15   C. 40 to 60

    B. 20 to 30   D. 75 to 85

13. What is the three-part hallmark of good analog (film-screen) mammography (i.e., what are the three image qualities that need to be present on a diagnostic mammogram)?

   A. _____   B. _____   C. _____

14. True/False: Grids and AEC are used for most mammograms.

15. True/False: Breast compression cannot be applied for a patient with breast implants.

16. Magnification is performed during mammography primarily to:

   A. Increase signal-to-noise ratio   C. Reduce dose per projection

   B. Magnify specific regions of interest   D. Demonstrate the deep chest wall

17. What is the average mean glandular dose (MGD) for projections of the breast?

   A. 130 to 150 mrad   C. 500 to 700 mrad

   B. 200 to 400 mrad   D. 900 to 1000 mrad

18. List the four advantages of computed radiographic mammography over conventional film-screen mammography:

   A. _____

   B. _____

   C. _____

   D. _____

19. What is the name of the device that captures the image with direct digital mammography?

   _____

20. True/False: Digital mammography can almost match the overall spatial resolution produced with film-screen systems.

21. Studies have shown that using computer-aided detection (CAD) as a second reader to interpret screening mammograms improves the cancer detection rate by as much as _____.

   A. 10%   C. 20%

   B. 15%   D. 30%

22. The major benefit of sonography (sonomammography) of the breast is _____.

23. True/False: Functional imaging utilizes a radiopharmaceutical.

24. True/False: Scintimammography is considered unreliable for any lesion smaller than 1 cm.

25. Scintimammography uses which radionuclide?

   A. Cardiolyte   C. Thallium

   B. Iodine 131   D. Technetium-99m-sestamibi

26. A second type of nuclear medicine procedure called sentinel node studies is performed to:

    A. Determine whether a malignant lesion is present in the breast

    B. Detect metastasis to a lymph node surrounding the breast

    C. Distinguish between a benign and a malignant tumor of the breast

    D. Diagnose a lymphoma

27. What type of radionuclide is often used with sentinel node studies?

    A. Sulfur colloid   C. Sestamibi

    B. Technetium   D. FDG

28. PET studies of the breast can detect early cancerous cells by measuring the rate of:

    A. Oxygen metabolism   C. Glucose (sugar) metabolism

    B. Phosphorus metabolism   D. Osmosis through the cell membrane

29. The primary difference between breast-specific gamma imaging (BSGI) and scintimammography is

    _____.

30. List the two major disadvantages of using positron emission mammography (PEM) as a breast screening tool:

    A. _____

    B. _____

31. True/False: Patients with the BRCA1 and BRCA2 genes have reduced risk of developing breast cancer.

32. List the three disadvantages in using MRI to study the breast:

    A. _____

    B. _____

    C. _____

33. Which of the following technologies will produce a 3D image of the breast tissue?

    A. DDR   C. Sentinel node study

    B. DBT   D. Sonomammography

34. The most common form of benign tumor of the breast is:

    A. Fibroadenoma   C. Fibrocystic lesion

    B. Adenocarcinoma   D. Adenosarcoma

35. The most common form of breast cancer is:

    A. Fibroadenoma   C. Infiltrating (invasive) ductal carcinoma

    B. Intraductal papilloma   D. Lobular carcinoma

36. Which of the following breast lesions has well-defined margins?

    A. Gynecomastia   C. Fibroadenoma

    B. Lobular carcinoma   D. Infiltrating ductal carcinoma

37. True/False: Gynecomastia involves primarily the male breast.

38. What are the two routine projections performed for screening mammograms?

  A. _____   B. _____

39. What surface landmark determines the correct height for placement of the image receptor for the craniocaudad

  projection? _____

40. Anatomic side markers and patient identification information need to be placed near the

  _____ side of the breast.

41. In the craniocaudad projection, what structure must be in profile? _____

42. In the craniocaudad projection, the head should be turned _____ (toward or away
  from) the side being radiographed.

43. Which routine projection taken during a screening mammogram will demonstrate more of the pectoral muscle?

  _____

44. How much CR/IR angulation is used for an average-size breast for the mediolateral oblique projection?

  _____

45. True/False: The desired patient position for the mediolateral oblique projection is seated.

46. For the mediolateral oblique projection, the arm of the side being examined should be placed:
  A. On the hip   C. Resting on top of the head
  B. Forward, toward the front of the body   D. Behind the back, palm out

47. Which special projection is usually requested when a lesion is seen on the mediolateral oblique but not on the

  craniocaudad projection? _____

48. In both the craniocaudad and the mediolateral projections, the central ray is generally directed to the

  _____ of the breast.

49. What is the most frequently requested special projection of the breast? _____

50. Which projection will most effectively show the axillary aspect of the breast? _____

51. How much is the CR/IR angled from vertical for the mediolateral, true lateral projection?

  _____

52. True/False: Mark each of the following statements either T for true or F for false.

_____ A. It is important for all skinfolds to be smoothed out and all wrinkles and pockets of air removed on each projection for the breast.

_____ B. Since the base of the breast is well shown on the craniocaudad projection, this area does not need to be shown on the mediolateral oblique projection.

_____ C. The axillary aspect of the breast is usually well visualized on the craniocaudad projection.

_____ D. Mammography is usually done in the standing position.

_____ E. Because of a short exposure time, the patient does not need to be completely motionless during the exposure.

_____ F. Use of AEC often results in an underexposed image with breast implants.

_____ G. In the craniocaudad projection, the chest wall must be pushed firmly against the image receptor.

_____ H. Standard CC and MLO projections should be performed on patients who have breast implants.

_____ I. Compression should not be used on patients with breast implants.

_____ J. The mediolateral projection is recommended to demonstrate air/fluid structures in the breast.

53. Which technique (method) is commonly used for the breast with an implant? _____

54. During the procedure identified in question 53, what must be done to allow the anterior aspect of the breast to be compressed and properly visualized? _____

55. If a lesion is too deep toward the chest wall and cannot be visualized with a laterally exaggerated craniocaudal projection, a(n) _____ projection should be performed.

    A. Mediolateral oblique   C. Mediolateral

    B. Craniocaudal   D. Axillary tail

56. Identify the correct positioning term or description for each of the following ACR abbreviations:

    A. MLO _____   F. LM _____

    B. SIO _____   G. XCCL _____

    C. AT _____   H. LMO _____

    D. CC _____   I. ID _____

    E. RL _____

These questions relate to the radiographs found in Chapter 20 of the textbook. Evaluate these radiographs for the radiographic criteria categories (1 through 5) that follow. Describe the corrections needed to improve the overall image. The major, or "repeatable," errors are specific errors that indicate the need for a repeat exposure, regardless of the nature of the other errors.

A. CC projection (Fig. C20-79)

Description of possible error:

1. Anatomy demonstrated: _____

2. Part positioning: _____

3. Collimation and central ray: _____

4. Exposure: _____

5. Markers: _____

Repeatable error(s): _____

B. MLO projection (Fig. C 20-80)

Description of possible error:

1. Anatomy demonstrated: _____

2. Part positioning: _____

3. Collimation and central ray: _____

4. Exposure: _____

5. Markers: _____

Repeatable error(s): _____

C. CC projection (Fig. C 20-81)

Description of possible error:

1. Anatomy demonstrated: _____

2. Part positioning: _____

3. Collimation and central ray: _____

4. Exposure: _____

5. Markers: _____

Repeatable error(s): _____

D. MLO projection (Fig. C 20-82)

Description of possible error:

1. Anatomy demonstrated: _____

2. Part positioning: _____

3. Collimation and central ray: _____

4. Exposure: _____

5. Markers: _____

Repeatable error(s): _____

E. CC projection (Fig. C 20-83)

Description of possible error:

1. Anatomy demonstrated: _____

2. Part positioning: _____

3. Collimation and central ray: _____

4. Exposure: _____

5. Markers: _____

Repeatable error(s): _____

F. CC projection (Fig. C 20-84)

Description of possible error:

1. Anatomy demonstrated: _____

2. Part positioning: _____

3. Collimation and central ray: _____

4. Exposure: _____

5. Markers: _____

Repeatable error(s): _____

LABORATORY EXERCISES

Exercise A below needs to be carried out in the radiology department where the mammography machine is located. Part B can be carried out in a classroom or any room where illuminators are available.

Laboratory Exercise A: Positioning

For this section you need another person to act as your "patient." Male and female students should be separated for this exercise, and students can be fully clothed for the simulated positioning. A clinical instructor must be present. Include each of the following during this exercise (check off when completed):

_____ Manipulate the x-ray machine into all the positions and become familiar with the locks and devices.

_____ Place or exchange the compression cone on the x-ray machine.

_____ Place an IR into the cassette holder.

_____ Place a fist on the IR tray and compress it by using the compression device. (This should be performed so that the student can sense the pressure of the device.)

_____ Place another student in position and simulate the CC, MLO, XCCL, and ML positions.

_____ Optional: If the department or school has a breast phantom, perform the basic and special mammogram positions.

Laboratory Exercise B: Image Critique and Evaluation

Your instructor will provide various breast radiographs for these exercises. Some will be optimal-quality radiographs that meet all or most of the evaluation criteria described for each projection in the textbook. Others will be of less than optimal quality, and others will be unacceptable, requiring a repeat exam. Evaluate each radiograph as specified below.

Radiographs

1	2	3	4	5	6	
_____	_____	_____	_____	_____	_____	a. Correct alignment and centering of part
_____	_____	_____	_____	_____	_____	b. Pectoral muscle included
_____	_____	_____	_____	_____	_____	c. Tissue thickness distributed evenly
_____	_____	_____	_____	_____	_____	d. Optimal compression noted
_____	_____	_____	_____	_____	_____	e. Dense areas adequately penetrated
_____	_____	_____	_____	_____	_____	f. High tissue contrast and optimal resolution noted
_____	_____	_____	_____	_____	_____	g. Absence of artifacts
_____	_____	_____	_____	_____	_____	h. Markers in proper position; accurate patient identification, including date
_____	_____	_____	_____	_____	_____	i. Based on acceptable variances to criteria factors, determine which of these radiographs are acceptable and which are unacceptable and should have been repeated. (Place a check mark if the radiograph needs to be repeated.)

REVIEW EXERCISE: Bone Densitometry (see textbook pp. 800-806)

1. Each year in the United States, approximately _____ million people have, or are at risk for developing, osteoporosis.

2. Bone strength is determined by two factors:

    A. _____

    B. _____

3. For osteoporosis to be visible on conventional radiographs, a loss of _____ % to

    _____ % of the trabecular bone must occur.

4. Cells responsible for new bone formation are called _____, and cells that help to

    break down and remove old bone are _____.

5. Approximately by the age of _____ years, more bone is being removed than is being replaced by new bone formation.

6. Bone matrix is _____% collagen and _____% other proteins.

7. The quantity or mass of bone measured in grams is the definition for _____.

8. The purpose of bone densitometry is to:

    A. Establish the diagnosis of osteoporosis

    B. Assess the response to osteoporosis therapy

    C. Measure bone mineral density

    D. All of the above

9. Clinical indications for bone densitometry include all of the following except:

    A. Estrogen deficiency in women

    B. Hyperparathyroidism

    C. Vertebral abnormalities

    D. Polycystic kidney disease

10. True/False: A sedentary lifestyle can lead to osteoporosis.

11. Place a check mark by each of the following that are *not* risk factors for low bone mass as identified in the textbook:

    _____ A. Family history of osteoporosis

    _____ B. Excessive physical activity

    _____ C. Low sodium and niacin intake

    _____ D. Smoking

    _____ E. Low body weight

    _____ F. Alcohol consumption

    _____ G. High-fat diet

    _____ H. Low calcium intake

    _____ I. Height greater than 6 feet (183 cm)

    _____ J. Previous fractures

12. True/False: Women on estrogen replacement therapy (ERT) are at greater risk for acquiring osteoporotic fractures.

13. True/False: Bone strength and bone density are directly proportional.

14. True/False: Patients who had intestinal bypass surgery are at greater risk of acquiring an osteoporotic fracture.

15. Osteoporosis in postmenopausal, Caucasian women is defined by the World Health Organization (WHO) as a bone mineral density (BMD) value of:

    A. 1.0 standard deviation below the average for the young normal population

    B. 1.5 standard deviations below the average for the same age and sex population

    C. 2.0 standard deviations below the average for the same age and sex population

    D. 2.5 standard deviations below the average for the young normal population

16. A T-score is defined as _____.

17. A T-score of no lower than −1.0 indicates:

    A. Normal bone   C. Osteopenia

    B. Osteoporosis   D. Severe osteoporosis

18. BMD reporting for premenopausal females or males younger than 50 should be reported in

    _____ rather than T-scores.

19. Which of the following drugs is given as a stimulator for new bone growth and reduces the risk for vertebral fracture?

    A. Estrogen   C. Calcitonin

    B. Parathyroid hormone D. Alendronate

20. True/False: Estrogen replacement therapy (ERT) is classified as an antiresorptive agent.

21. List the three most common diagnostic systems utilized for bone densitometry:

    A. _____

    B. _____

    C. _____

22. Which of the following is the preferred modality for evaluating both trabecular and cortical bone?

    A. Quantitative computed tomography (QCT)

    B. Dual-energy x-ray absorptiometry (DXA)

    C. Quantitative ultrasound (QUS)

    D. Dual-energy photon absorptiometry

23. True/False: Current DXA systems use a pencil x-ray beam to reduce dose to the patient.

24. Patient dose delivered during bone densitometry procedures using an x-ray source is measured in what units of

    measurement? _____

25. Effective dose delivered during a bone density exam of both spine and hip is _____.

26. A Z-score produced during a DXA scan compares the patient's bone density with that of:

    A. An average young, healthy individual with peak bone mass

    B. An average individual of the same sex and age

    C. A person with a slight degree of osteoporosis

    D. A person with a severe degree of osteoporosis

27. QCT involves a scan taken between the vertebral levels of:

    A. C4 to T5

    B. T7 to T12

    C. T12 to L5

    D. L5 to S1

28. True/False: QCT permits three-dimensional analysis of the scanned region of the spine.

29. True/False: QCT produces less patient dose as compared with DXA.

30. Quantitative computed tomography (QCT) provides bone mineral density measurements of

    _____ and _____ bone.

31. Average patient dose with QCT is approximately _____.

32. The most common anatomic site selected for QUS is the:

    A. Spine   C. Os calcis (calcaneus)

    B. Femur   D. Pelvis

33. Which of the following bone densitometry methods results in no radiation to the patient?

    A. DXA   C. QUS

    B. QCT   D. None of the above

34. Central or axial analysis using DXA or QCT includes bone density measurements of the:

    A. _____

    B. _____

35. True/False: Severe scoliosis or kyphosis may result in less accurate results for bone densitometry procedures.

36. True/False: New DXA technology allows for bilateral hips to be scanned at the same time; therefore a hip prosthesis should not compromise the quality of the study.

37. True/False: If a patient has severe scoliosis, DXA can be performed on the forearm to gain a true measurement of BMD.

38. True/False: DXA of the hip requires the lower limb to be rotated 45° internally.

39. True/False: A patient history of hyperparathyroidism is considered as a contraindication for a DXA scan.

40. Another term for *precision* in regard to the ability of a DXA system to obtain repeated measurements on the same patient is:

    A. Reliability   C. Validity

    B. Reproducibility   D. Duplicity

41. Which of the following factors has the greatest impact of precision during a DXA scan?

    A. Patient positioning   C. Post-processing algorithm

    B. Exposure factors   D. Quality of x-ray beam

42. Typically, the accuracy of a DXA system is better than _____ %.

43. Vertebral fractures are most common in patients over the age of _____.

44. Which region of the body is scanned during a vertebral fracture assessment (VFA) study?

    A. Thoracolumbar spine   C. Bilateral hips

    B. Pelvis   D. Ribs and sternum

45. _____ of vertebral fractures diagnosed on x-ray examination are asymptomatic.

    A. 10%   C. 50%

    B. 23%   D. 66%

MAGNETIC RESONANCE IMAGING (MRI)
REVIEW EXERCISE A: Physical Principles of MRI (see textbook pp. 807-812)

1. MRI uses _____ and _____ to obtain a mathematically reconstructed image.

2. The MRI image represents differences in the patient's tissues in the number of _____ and the rate at which they recover from radiofrequency stimulation.

3. To compare the energy of x-rays and MRI radio waves and the relative effect on irradiated tissue, fill in the blanks in the following:

	Wavelength	*Frequency*	*Energy*
1. Typical x-rays	A. 10^{-11} M	B. 10^{19} Hz cycles/sec	C. 60,000 electron volts
2. MRI radio waves	A. _____	B. _____	C. _____

4. A. Which nucleus is most suitable for MRI? _____

    B. Why? _____

5. Which component of the nucleus is affected by radio waves and static magnetic fields?

    _____

6. A typical cubic centimeter of the human body contains approximately _____ hydrogen atoms.

    A. 1022   C. 1010

    B. 10,020   D. 10^{20}

7. Define *precession* by comparing it to another, more well-known phenomenon. _____

8. The rate of precession of a proton in a magnetic field _____ (increases or decreases) as the strength of the magnetic field increases.

9. Precession occurs as a result of _____ acting on a spinning nuclei.

10. The angle of precession of protons can be altered by the introduction of _____.

11. How does an increase in the length of application time of the radio wave affect the angle of precession of the exposed nuclei? _____

12. Timing of the radio wave frequency to the rate of the precessing nuclei is an example of the concept of

_____.

13. The signal that is received by the antenna or the receiving coil comes from which part of the atoms in the body tissues? _____

14. The nucleus emits _____ waves because it is a tiny magnet that is also

_____.

15. Relaxation of the nuclei as soon as the radiofrequency pulse is turned off can be divided into two categories:

_____ and _____.

16. T1 relaxation is known as _____ (transverse or longitudinal), or spin-lattice, relaxation.

17. T2 relaxation is known as _____ (transverse or longitudinal), or spin-spin, relaxation.

18. The quantity of hydrogen nuclei per given volume of tissue is referred to as the _____,

which is a _____ (major or minor) contributor to the appearance of the MR image.

19. Describe the main purpose of the gradient magnetic fields (the magnetic field strengths through only specific regions or slices of body tissue). _____

20. What are three primary factors that determine the signal strength?

A. _____

B. _____

C. _____

REVIEW EXERCISE B: Clinical Applications, Safety Considerations, and Appearance of Anatomy (see textbook pp. 813-816)

1. Complete the following list of MRI safety concerns:

A. _____

B. _____

C. _____

D. Local heating of tissues and metallic objects

E. Electrical interference with normal functions of nerve cells and muscle fibers

2. The danger of projectiles becomes _____ (greater or lesser) as ferromagnetic objects are moved toward the scanner because the field strength is _____ (directly or inversely) proportional to the cube of the distance from the bore of the magnet.

3. In an emergency situation, the patient is removed from the scan room because of the danger of

_____.

4. Pacemakers are not allowed inside the _____ -gauss line.

5. As a general rule, O_2 tanks, IV pumps, and wheelchairs are not allowed inside the

_____ -gauss line.

6. Patients with internal drug infusion pumps and cochlear implants are not allowed inside the

_____ -gauss line.

7. The most important contraindication to MRI of the brain involves torquing of _____.

8. What unit of measurement is used to calculate local heating of tissues? _____

9. Which term is used to describe the amount of tissue heating delivered during an MRI procedure?

_____

10. What is the whole-body averaged SAR permitted for a 15-minute MRI procedure with a 1.5 Tesla system?

_____

11. True/False: MR should be avoided in the first 6 months of pregnancy unless diagnosis is crucial for conditions.

12. True/False: Before giving gadolinium-DTPA (Gd-DTPA), creatinine levels should be checked.

13. MRI has excellent _____, which allows visualization of soft tissue structures.

14. Diagnosis of diseases such as those involving the CNS can be made with MRI by comparing the signals produced

in _____ (normal or abnormal) tissues with those produced in (normal or abnormal) tissues.

15. List three types of histories that should be obtained from patients before an MRI exam.

A. _____

B. _____

C. _____

16. The _____ rate is a measurement of normal of kidney function.

17. In addition to tumor detection, what other pathology may indicate the use of contrast media during an MRI scan?

_____

18. The average amount of contrast media given during an MRI examination is _____ mL/kg;

the injection rate should not exceed _____ mL/min.

19. List the ten absolute contraindications to patient MRI scanning as listed in the textbook.

A. _____

B. _____

C. _____

D. _____

E. _____

F. _____

G. _____

H. _____

I. _____

J. _____

20. Match the following pulse sequence descriptions with the correct designation.

_____ A. Pulse sequences using a combination
of short TR and short TE

_____ B. Pulse sequences using a combination
of long TR and long TE

1. T1 relaxation

2. T2 relaxation

21. For each tissue listed below, identify the T1- and T2-weighted appearances: dark, bright, light gray, or dark gray:
(Note: The first tissue has been completed as an example.)

	T1	*T2*
A. Cortical bone	Dark	Dark
B. Red bone marrow	_____	_____
C. Fat	_____	_____
D. White brain matter	_____	_____
E. CSF	_____	_____
F. Muscle	_____	_____
G. Vessels	_____	_____

22. True/False: Flowing blood is not visualized with a conventional spin-echo pulse sequence.

23. True/False: Tissues filled with air do not produce a T1 or T2 signal and therefore appear as bright.

1. Complete the list of six structures or tissue types best demonstrated by MRI of the brain:

   A. Gray matter

   B. _____

   C. _____

   D. _____

   E. Basal ganglia

   F. Brainstem

2. Complete the list of six possible pathologies best demonstrated by MRI of the brain:

   A. _____

   B. _____

   C. _____

   D. _____

   E. Hemorrhagic disorders

   F. CVA

3. MRI of the brain is considered superior to the CT in visualizing the following three regions of the brain or changes in tissues:

   A. _____

   B. _____

   C. _____

4. Which of the following technical factors may be used in spine imaging?

   A. T1-weighted sequence   C. Gradient echo

   B. T2-weighted sequence   D. All of the above

5. T1-weighted MRI of the spine is effective in evaluating:

   A. _____

   B. _____

   C. _____

6. List two major advantages of MRI over CT imaging of the spine:

   A. _____

   B. _____

7. True/False: CT is superior to MRI for evaluation of a vertebral arch fracture.

8. List the four conditions or diseases best demonstrated with MRI of the joints:

   A. _____

   B. _____

   C. _____

   D. _____

9. T1-weighted images of the abdomen are helpful in identifying tumors containing _____

and _____.

10. T2-weighted images of the abdomen are useful to demonstrate changes in _____.

11. True/False: As magnet or field strength increases, quality and resolution of the MRI image increases.

12. True/False: Cardiac gating during an MRI procedure is a process in which heart wall motion is studied.

13. True/False: During the cardiac-gated MRI procedure, signal collection occurs at the same point during the cardiac cycle.

14. Which one of the following devices/equipment is required during a cardiac-gated MRI procedure?
    A. CT   C. PET
    B. ECG   D. Pulse oximeter

15. True/False: Functional MRI (fMRI) provides both an anatomic and functional assessment of the brain.

16. Neural activity is measured by _____ during a functional MRI procedure.
    A. Decreased RF signal   C. Blood oxygen level-dependent (BOLD) signal
    B. Increased RF signal   D. Water shift signal

17. True/False: fMRI does not require the injection of radiopharmaceuticals.

18. True/False: fMRI scan times are typically longer than similar PET studies of the brain.

19. True/False: Spatial image resolution with fMRI is less than with PET or SPECT.

20. Match the following MRI terms with the correct definition.

    _____ A. MRI technique to minimize involuntary
              motion artifacts

    _____ B. False features on an image caused by patient
              instability or equipment deficiencies

    _____ C. Slow gyration of an axis of a spinning body
              caused by an application of torque

    _____ D. Method of improving SNR by averaging
              several FIDs or spin echoes

    _____ E. Spin lattice or longitudinal relaxation time

    _____ F. SI unit of magnetic field intensity

    _____ G. Stray magnetic field that exists outside the
              imager

    _____ H. A new growth of the white substance of the
              nerve sheath

    _____ I. A tumor growing from nerve cells affecting
              the sense of hearing

    _____ J. Spin-spin or transverse relaxation time

    1. T2

    2. Tesla

    3. Signal averaging

    4. Acoustic neuroma

    5. Fringe field

    6. Schwannoma

    7. Artifacts

    8. Physiologic gating

    9. Precession

    10. T1

21. Match the following MRI terms with the correct definition:

_____ A. Measure of the geometric relationship between the RF coil and the body

_____ B. Atmospheric gases such as nitrogen and helium used for cooling

_____ C. Reappearance of MR signal after the FID has disappeared

_____ D. Amount of rotation of the net magnetization vector produced by an RF pulse

_____ E. Force that causes or tends to cause a body to rotate

_____ F. Repetition time

_____ G. In flowing fluid, velocity component that fluctuates randomly

_____ H. A malignant tumor arising from the embryonic remains of the notochord

_____ I. A hard, slow-growing vascular tumor

_____ J. Ability of an imaging process to distinguish adjacent soft tissue from one another

1. Contrast resolution

2. Chordoma

3. Turbulence

4. Spin echo

5. Filling factor

6. Meningioma

7. Cryogen

8. Torque

9. TR

10. Flip angle structures

Directions: This self-test should be taken only after completing all of the readings, review exercises, and laboratory activities for a particular section. **Please note:** Self-test is divided into sections specific to each imaging modality described in the chapter. The purpose of this test is not only to provide a good learning exercise but also to serve as a good indicator of what your final evaluation exam will be. It is strongly suggested that if you do not get at least a 90% to 95% grade on this self-test, you should review those areas in which you missed questions before going to your instructor for the final evaluation exam for this chapter.

NUCLEAR MEDICINE AND PET

1. One of the most common radionuclides used in nuclear medicine is:

    A. Thallium

    B. Technetium 99m

    C. Cardiolite

    D. Sulfur colloid

2. What type of imaging device used in nuclear medicine provides a three-dimensional image of anatomic structures?

    A. SPECT camera

    B. B-mode unit

    C. Linear accelerator

    D. Real-time scanner

3. An abnormal region detected during a nuclear medicine bone scan is often described as a(n):

    A. Signal void

    B. Hot spot

    C. Acoustic shadow

    D. Region of high attenuation

4. Which one of the following is a common clinical indicator for a nuclear medicine gastrointestinal study?

    A. Duodenal ulcer

    B. Bezoar

    C. Hepatobiliary disease

    D. Ileus

5. How is the heart stressed during a nuclear cardiac perfusion study?

    A. Giving the patient a radiopharmaceutical

    B. Giving the patient Valium

    C. Giving the patient Lasix

    D. Having patient run on treadmill

6. Which radiopharmaceutical is given during a thyroid uptake study?

    A. Technetium 99m

    B. Sodium iodide (^{123}I)

    C. Sulfur colloid

    D. Thallium

7. Which one of the following duties is *not* a typical responsibility of the nuclear medicine technologist?

    A. Calibrates imaging equipment

    B. Processes images

    C. Administers radionuclides

    D. Decontaminates area after spills

8. A device for accelerating charged particles in a circular orbit to high energies by means of an alternating electric field is a:

   A. Cyclotron
   C. Linear accelerator
   B. Particle accelerator
   D. Pulsed accelerator

9. A helium nucleus, consisting of 2 protons and 2 neutrons, is a(n):

   A. Alpha particle
   C. Beta particle
   B. Neutrino
   D. Radionuclide

10. A type of atom whose nucleus disintegrates spontaneously is a(n):

    A. Alpha particle
    C. Radiopharmaceutical
    B. Beta particle
    D. Radionuclide

11. PET demonstrates the _____ of the body's organs and tissues.

    A. Anatomy
    C. Physiology
    B. Biochemical function
    D. Chemical structure

12. What is produced when a positron and electron join and then undergo annihilation?

    A. X-ray
    C. Radionuclide
    B. Alpha particle
    D. Two 511-keV photons

13. Which of the following elements is *not* used in the PET imaging process?

    A. Hydrogen
    C. Fluorine
    B. Carbon
    D. Oxygen

14. Which of the following biochemical compounds is used to gauge glucose metabolism in tissues during PET scan?

    A. ^{15}O-water
    C. ^{18}F-FDG
    B. ^{13}N-ammonia
    D. ^{11}C-methionine

15. Most PET tracers have a half-life of:

    A. 1 to 13 seconds
    C. 150 to 320 seconds
    B. 120 seconds to 110 minutes
    D. 8 to 12 hours

16. True/False: Malignant cells have a high rate of glucose metabolism.

17. True/False: During an epileptic seizure, there is a decrease in sugar (glucose) use at the seizure site in the brain.

18. Brain mapping is a PET procedure used to identify:

    A. Primary tumors
    C. Critical motor or sensory regions
    B. Metastatic spread
    D. Regions of brain responsible for dementia

19. True/False: CNS tumors examined with PET will demonstrate decreased glucose metabolism.

20. True/False: Dementia, when studied with PET, is demonstrated by decreased glucose metabolism in aspects of the brain.

21. The most common form of coregistration, or fusion technology is the use of:

   A. PET/MRI   C. PET/X-ray

   B. CT/MRI   D. PET/CT

Radiation Oncology

22. Which one of the following is *not* an example of a teletherapy unit?

   A. Linear accelerator   C. Intraoperative radiation therapy (IORT)

   B. Interstitial irradiation   D. Cobalt-60 unit

23. Palliative radiation therapy is intended to:

   A. Treat deep tumors   C. Treat tumors during surgery

   B. Treat superficial tumors   D. Help relieve a patient's symptoms caused by a cancer

24. True/False: Brachytherapy employs the use of sealed radioactive isotopes.

25. Which one of the following is *not* a responsibility of the certified radiation therapist?

   A. Uses fluoroscopy for treatment planning   C. Prescribes the treatment

   B. Interacts directly with the patient   D. Maintains therapy records

Ultrasound Imaging (Sonography)

26. Which of the following is *not* an alternative term for medical ultrasound?

   A. Echosonography   C. Piezosonography

   B. Sonography   D. Ultrasonography

27. Medical sonography operates at a frequency range between:

   A. 1 to 5 KHz   C. 1 to 17 KHz

   B. 25 to 50 KHz   D. 1 to 20 MHz

28. Which generation of ultrasound equipment first introduced grayscale imaging?

   A. A-mode   C. Real-time dynamic

   B. B-mode (patient-mode)   D. Doppler

29. An ultrasound transducer converts _____ energy to ultrasonic energy.

   A. Electrical   C. Light

   B. Heat   D. Magnetic

30. Which of the following transducer frequencies would most likely be used on a large abdomen?

   A. 3.5 MHz   C. 10 MHz

   B. 5.0 to 7.0 MHz   D. 17 MHz

31. True/False: A higher-frequency transducer will increase penetration through the anatomy but will produce lower image resolution.

32. True/False: A normal gallbladder is an example of a *hyperechoic* structure.

33. True/False: Breast sonography is used primarily to distinguish between solid and cystic masses.

34. True/False: High-intensity focused ultrasound (HIFU) utilizes heat to destroy tissues.

Mammography

35. What does the acronym MQSA represent, and what year did it go into effect? _____

36. Which health facilities (if any) are exempt from the MQSA requirements? _____

37. In 1992 the American Cancer Society recommended that all women over the age of

_____ undergo annual screening mammography.

38. Currently, 1 in _____ American women will develop breast cancer sometime during her life.

39. The junction between the inferior aspect of the breast and chest wall is called the _____.

40. In which quadrant of the breast is the tail, or axillary prolongation, found? _____

41. Using the clock system, one o'clock in the left breast would correspond to _____ in the right breast.

42. Which large muscle is located directly posterior to the breast? _____

43. What is the function of the mammary gland? _____

44. Name the bands of connective tissue passing through the breast tissue to provide support.

_____

45. Which one of the three breast tissue types is the least dense radiographically? _____

46. What is the term used by radiologists for various small structures (blood vessels, etc.) seen on the mammogram?

_____

47. Which term describes the thickest portion of the breast near the chest wall? _____

48. Which one of the following tissue types would be found in the breasts of a 25-year-old pregnant female?

   A. Fibroglandular   C. Fatty

   B. Fibrofatty   D. Cystic

49. Which one of the following tissue types would be found in the breasts of a 35-year-old female who has borne two children?

   A. Fibroglandular   C. Fatty

   B. Fibrofatty   D. Cystic

50. The male breast would be classified as:

   A. Fibroglandular   C. Fatty

   B. Fibrofatty   D. Cystic

51. Which one of the following tissue types requires more compression during mammography as compared with the others?

   A. Fibroglandular   C. Fatty

   B. Fibrofatty   D. Cystic

52. Identify the anatomy labeled on Fig. 20-3:

A. _____

B. _____

C. _____

D. _____

E. Which basic mammogram projection is demonstrated in

Fig. 20-3? _____

F. The right side marker on this mammogram is correctly

placed on the _____ side of the breast.

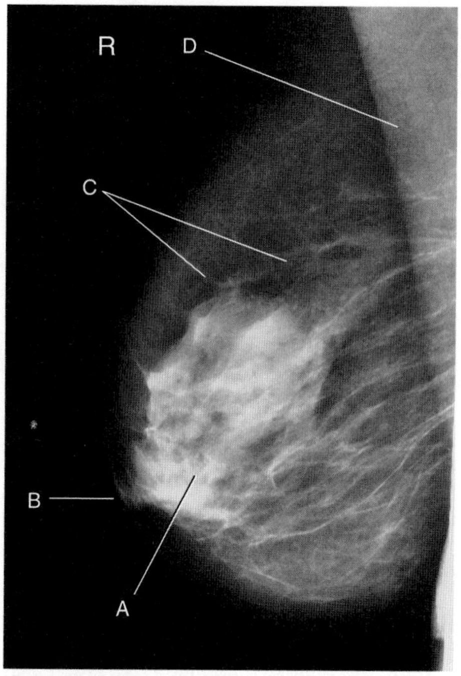

Fig. 20-3. Breast anatomy on a mammogram.

53. The target material commonly used in most mammographic x-ray tubes is _____.

54. To use the maximum advantage of the anode-heel effect, the anode side of the x-ray tube should be over the

_____ (base or apex) of the breast.

55. True/False: Automatic exposure control (AEC) can be used for most mammographic projections.

56. True/False: Compression of the breast will improve image quality by reducing scatter radiation.

57. True/False: A grid is generally not used for mammography.

58. What size focal spot should be used for magnification of small breast nodules or tissue samples?

_____

59. What is the magnification factor for an exposure with a source object distance (SOD) of 20 inches and a source

image receptor distance (SID) of 40 inches? _____

60. The average mean glandular dose received by the patient during a basic two-projection mammogram examination
is in the range of:

A. 50 to 150 mrad   C. 400 to 600 mrad

B. 200 to 300 mrad   D. 800 to 1100 mrad

61. Which imaging modality is best suited to distinguish a cyst from a solid mass within the breast?

_____

62. Which imaging modality is best suited to diagnose an extracapsular rupture of a breast implant?

_____

63. True/False: Breast imaging using sonography has been performed since the mid-1970s.

64. True/False: The primary way to reduce patient dose during analog mammography is to use higher mAs.

65. True/False: One reason that mammoscintigraphy is not ordered more frequently is the high number of false positives reported with this procedure.

66. Which one of the following radionuclides is used during a BSGI study?
   A. Sulfur colloid   C. Technetium
   B. Sestamibi   D. Iodine 131

67. Carcinoma of the breast is divided into two categories: _____ and

_____.

68. Which one of the following ACR abbreviations refers to the exaggerated craniocaudal (lateral) projection?
   A. LECC   C. LCC
   B. LXCC   D. XCCL

69. What is the ACR abbreviation for a mediolateral oblique projection?

70. List the two routine projections taken during a screening mammogram:

   A. _____   B. _____

71. Which of the routine projections taken during a mammogram will best demonstrate the pectoral muscle?

_____

72. The typical kV range for analog mammography is _____.

73. Which projection best demonstrates the axillary aspect of the breast?

74. What is the ACR abbreviation for the special projection, lateromedial oblique, often used with pacemaker

patients? _____

75. The use of AEC when performing a projection with a breast implant in place can lead to

_____ (overexposure or underexposure) of the breast.

76. A. The technique of "pinching" the breast to push an implant posteriorly to the chest wall is known as the

_____ method.

   B. What is the correct ACR term and abbreviation for this method? _____

77. What other special projection can be taken if a lesion is too deep into the axillary tail aspect of the chest wall to be seen with an exaggerated craniocaudal projection? (Include the correct ACR term and abbreviation.)

_____

78. Identification markers should always be placed near the _____.

79. How is the opposite breast prevented from superimposing the breast being examined on the MLO projection?

_____

80. With a large breast, which of the two routine projections is most likely to require two images to include all the breast tissue? _____

81. Which projection is usually requested when a lesion is seen on the MLO (mediolateral oblique) but not on the CC (craniocaudad) projection? _____

82. What soft-tissue landmark determines the correct height for placement of the image receptor for the CC (craniocaudad) projection? _____

83. Which one of the following projections is recommended for demonstrating evaluating air-fluid levels in structures of the breast?
   A. Craniocaudal   C. Mediolateral (true lateral)
   B. Mediolateral oblique   D. Exaggerated craniocaudal (lateral)

84. **Situation:** A mammogram is performed for a patient with breast implants. The resultant images are overexposed. The following factors were used: 28 kV, AEC, grid, and gentle compression. Which one of the following modifications would produce more diagnostic images during the repeat study?
   A. Lower the kV.   C. Use manual exposure factors.
   B. Do not use a grid.   D. Do not use breast compression.

85. What device or system is part of direct digital mammography?
   A. Imaging plate   C. Bucky tray
   B. Image intensifier   D. Flat panel detector

86. True/False: The spatial resolution of digital mammography nearly equals that of film-screen imaging.

87. CAD is an acronym for _____.

88. It is reported that CAD can improve breast cancer detection rate as much as _____%.

89. What type of radionuclide is used with mammoscintigraphy?
   A. Technetium-99m-sestamibi   C. Sulfur colloid
   B. Iodine 131   D. Gadolinium

90. Which imaging modality will produce sectional images of the breast with a 3D appearance?
   A. Mammoscintigraphy   C. Sonomammography
   B. DBT   D. BSGI

91. True/False: Patient dose from a PEM scan of the breast is comparable to that of a film-screen mammogram.

92. Which of the following imaging modalities is most effective in studying the breast with implants?
   A. Ultrasound   C. MRI
   B. PEM (PET)   D. IR-screen mammography

93. One of the major disadvantages of using MRI as a breast screening tool is:

   A. Higher patient dose   C. Patient discomfort

   B. High false-positive rate   D. Length of the exam

94. The most common form of breast cancer is:

   A. Fibroadenoma   C. Lobular carcinoma

   B. Infiltrating sarcoma   D. Infiltrating ductal carcinoma

Bone Densitometry

95. Which of the following is not a risk factor for osteoporosis?

   A. Excessive physical activity   C. Low body weight

   B. Alcohol consumption   D. Low calcium intake

96. Newer dual-energy x-ray absorptiometry (DXA) use:

   A. Fan-beam x-ray source   C. Pencil-thin x-ray source

   B. Positron-emission source   D. Super voltage x-ray source

97. A T-score obtained with the DXA system compares the patient with a(n):

   A. Average patient of the same age, sex, and ethnic background

   B. Young healthy individual with peak bone mass

   C. Young healthy individual of the same sex and ethnic background

   D. Patient with severe osteoporosis

98. The two disadvantages of quantitative computed tomography (QCT) are:

   A. _____

   B. _____

99. The anatomic area most commonly scanned with quantitative ultrasound (QUS) is the

   _____.

100. What specific cells are responsible for bone resorption? _____

101. Which of the following factors often leads to advanced bone loss?

   A. Being a female over the age of 21 years   C. Undergoing glucocorticoid therapy

   B. Undergoing hormone replacement therapy   D. Undergoing cardiac rehab

102. True/False: African-American women are at greater risk for developing osteoporosis than are Caucasian women.

103. A T-score acquired during a DXA scan of lower than −1.0 but higher than −2.5 indicates:

   A. Normal BMD   C. Osteoporosis

   B. Osteopenia   D. Severe osteoporosis

104. True/False: Estrogen replacement therapy (ERT) often stimulates new bone formation.

105. What is the average effective dose delivered to a patient during a bone density scan of the spine and hip?

A. 5 μSv

C. 1 to 30 Seiverts

B. 10 to 30 μSv

D. 1 to 3 mSv

106. True/False: As the technology is refined, QUS may replace existing peripheral techniques.

107. Which vertebral region(s) is (are) analyzed during a DXA scan?

A. T12

C. L1 to L4

B. Between T7 and L1

D. L4 to S1

108. The ability of a DXA system to obtain consistent BMD values of repeated measurements of the same patient is

called _____.

109. True/False: If trabecular and cortical bone is being evaluated, QCT is the method of choice.

110. True/False: QCT of the hip is most valuable to predict future hip fracture.

111. The presence of _____ prevents accurate measurement of the BMD of an extremity.

A. Cancer

C. Metallic prosthesis

B. Paget's disease

D. Osteoporosis

112. True/False: Single-energy photon absorptiometry (SPA) is no longer used in clinical practice.

113. Parathyroid hormone 1-34 analog (teriparatide, brand name Forteo) is given to patients with osteoporosis to:

A. Heal hip fractures

C. Relieve pain

B. Stimulate bone formation

D. Reduce bone loss

114. Boniva belongs to a group of drugs termed:

A. Calcitonin

C. Teriparatide

B. Selective estrogen receptor modulators

D. Bisphosphonates

Magnetic Resonance Imaging (MRI)

115. The MRI image represents differences in the number of:

A. X-rays attenuated

C. Frequencies of nuclei

B. Nuclei and the rate of their recovery

D. Radio waves

116. The MRI process excites the nuclei in the body with:

A. X-rays

C. Sound waves

B. Radio waves

D. Visible light

117. The most common nuclei in the body used to receive and reemit radio waves are:

A. Hydrogen

C. Oxygen

B. Carbon

D. Phosphorus

118. The nuclei that receive and reemit radio waves are under the influence of:

A. Gravitational force

C. X-ray energy

B. The sun and the planets

D. A static magnetic field

119. Which of the following properties results in a nucleus behaving like a small magnet?

    A. An even number of neutrons and protons   C. An even number of electrons

    B. An odd number of neutrons or protons   D. The presence of a magnet

120. Precession of the magnetic nuclei occurs because of:

    A. Oscillation in the presence of other atoms   C. The influence of a static magnetic field

    B. Regression under the influence of a magnet   D. Ionization exposed atoms

121. A precessing nucleus produces _____ in a nearby loop of wire.

    A. An alternating current   C. A direct current

    B. A dipole   D. Magnetic regression

122. Precession of magnetic nuclei can be altered by the application of:

    A. X-rays   C. Microwaves

    B. Radio frequency waves   D. Visible light

123. Resonance occurs when radio waves are:

    A. Of the same frequency as the precessing nuclei   C. At the same rate as T2 relaxation

    B. At the same rate as T1 relaxation   D. Received by an antenna

124. The angle of precession of the nuclei is altered because the:

    A. Nuclei must be vertical   C. Electrostatic properties of the nuclei dominate

    B. Magnetic force dominates   D. MR signal is strongest when nuclei are in horizontal or transverse plane

125. Emitted signals from the exposed nuclei are _____ and sent to the computer.

    A. Evaluated   C. In resonance

    B. Received by an RF antenna   D. Precessing

126. The _____ among T1, T2, and spin density signals of tissues produce(s) contrast in the MRI image.

    A. Similarities   C. Differences

    B. Phase   D. Frequency

127. In T2 relaxation, the spins of the exposed nuclei:

    A. Are vertical in orientation   C. Are reduced in density

    B. Move to the north   D. Become out of phase with one another

128. In T1 relaxation, the spins of the exposed nuclei:

    A. Are relaxing back to a vertical orientation   C. Are reduced in density

    B. Stay in a horizontal position   D. Become out of phase with one another

129. Spin density refers to the _____ of hydrogen nuclei.

    A. Quality   C. Phase

    B. Quantity   D. Wavelength

130. The signal strength and thus the brightness of points in the image are primarily determined by:

    A. Differences in T1 and T2 relaxation rates of tissues   C. The longitudinal component of nuclei

    B. Differences in spin density of tissues   D. Exposure of the nuclei to the static magnetic field

131. Common strengths of magnets used in MRI range from:

    A. 1 to 3 tesla   C. 12 to 15 tesla

    B. 5 to 7 tesla   D. 15 to 20 tesla

132. Which one of the following types of MRI magnets requires the use of cryogens?

    A. Permanent   C. Resistive

    B. Superconducting magnets   D. Open magnets

133. TR can be defined simply as:

    A. Time reversal   C. Timing range

    B. Repetition time   D. Time of resonance

134. TE can be defined simply as:

    A. Echo phase   C. Temporary echo

    B. Time net   D. Echo time

135. TR and TE have a profound influence on:

    A. Image noise deletion   C. Signal averaging

    B. Image contrast   D. Image density

136. One tesla equals:

    A. 10,000 times the earth's magnetic field   C. 10 gauss

    B. 0.00005 gauss   D. 10,000 gauss

137. Which one of the following is *not* a similarity between MRI and CT?

    A. The outward appearance of the unit   C. The use of ionizing radiation

    B. The use of a computer to analyze information   D. Images viewed as a slice of tissue

138. Primary safety concerns for the technologist, patient, and medical personnel are due to:

    A. Fringe field strengths less than 1 gauss

    B. Gravitational pull on metallic objects

    C. Magnetic fields and heat production

    D. Interaction of magnetic fields with ferrometallic objects and tissues

139. Projectiles are a concern because of:

    A. Force of ferromagnetic objects being pulled to the magnet   C. Nerve cell function

    B. Fringe fields less than 10 gauss   D. Local heating of tissues and metallic objects

140. Pacemakers are not allowed inside the:

    A. 5-gauss line   C. 1.0-gauss line

    B. 2.5-gauss line   D. 0.5-gauss line

141. IV pumps, wheelchairs, and O_2 tanks are not allowed inside the:

    A. 150-gauss line   C. 5-gauss line

    B. 50-gauss line   D. 1-gauss line

142. The most important MRI safety contraindication in regard to torquing of metallic objects is:

    A. Intraabdominal surgical staples   C. Ferromagnetic intracranial aneurysm clips

    B. Stainless steel femoral rods   D. Titanium hip prosthesis

143. Local heating of tissues (referred to as *SAR*, or *specific absorption ratio*) is measured in:

    A. W/kg   C. RF frequency

    B. Joules/kg   D. W/cm^2

144. The contrast agent commonly used for MR examinations is:

    A. Iodine 131   C. Gadolinium oxysulfide

    B. Lanthanum oxybromide   D. Gadolinium-diethylene triamine pentaacetic acid

145. Contrast agents are generally used in conjunction with:

    A. T1-weighted pulse sequences   C. Spin-density weighted pulse sequences

    B. T2-weighted pulse sequences   D. All of the above

146. True/False: Contrast media used in MRI carry a higher risk for allergic reaction as compared with iodinated contrast agents.

147. Which of these pathologic indications would indicate the use of contrast media during an MRI procedure?

    A. Cerebral bleed   C. HNP

    B. C-spine fracture   D. Spinal cord abscess

148. True/False: T1-weighted images will demonstrate free air within the abdominal cavity.

149. On T1-weighted images, CSF will appear:

    A. Dark   C. Same as white matter

    B. Bright   D. Same as gray matter

150. On T2-weighted images, CSF will appear:

    A. Dark   C. Same as white matter

    B. Bright   D. Same as gray matter

151. MRI of the brain allows visualization of:

    A. White matter disease   C. Small calcifications

    B. Acute cerebral bleeds   D. Skull anomalies

152. MRI of the brain includes the use of a standard head coil and:

    A. Prone position   C. Sedation

    B. Cardiac gating   D. T1- and T2-weighted pulse sequences

153. Which of the following is not best evaluated by MRI of the spine?

    A. Bone marrow changes   C. Disk herniation

    B. Cord abnormalities   D. Degree of scoliosis present in spine

154. MRI of the joints or limbs demonstrates all of the following except:

   A. Ligaments   C. Muscle

   B. Tendons   D. Cortical bone

155. The largest drawback to MRI of the abdomen is:

   A. Motion artifacts   C. Coil selection

   B. Metallic implants   D. Sequence times

156. True/False: High-field strength MRI magnets can produce up to 7 tesla.

157. True/False: A titanium hip prosthesis is an example of an MRI safe device.

158. A stray magnetic field that exists outside the MRI gantry is the definition for:

   A. RF field   C. Magnetic field

   B. Fringe field   D. Field of influence

159. Functional MRI is performed to study:

   A. Anatomy of the brain

   B. Specific functions of the brain

   C. Processes such as language, vision, movement, hearing, and memory

   D. All of the above

160. True/False: Functional MRI of the brain exceeds the spatial resolution seen with PET and SPECT images.

Answers to Review Exercises

CHAPTER 1

Review Exercise A: General, Systemic, and Skeletal Anatomy and Arthrology

1. Chemical level
2. A. Epithelial
   B. Connective
   C. Muscular
   D. Nervous
3. A. Skeletal
   B. Circulatory
   C. Digestive
   D. Respiratory
   E. Urinary
   F. Reproductive
   G. Nervous
   H. Muscular
   I. Endocrine
   J. Integumentary
4. 1. C
   2. E
   3. H
   4. G
   5. I
   6. D
   7. J
   8. F
   9. B
   10. A
5. True
6. B. Integumentary
7. C. Integumentary
8. A. Axial skeleton
   B. Appendicular skeleton
9. False (206)
10. False (part of appendicular)
11. True
12. True
13. A. Long bones
    B. Short bones
    C. Flat bones
    D. Irregular bones
14. D. Periosteum
15. C. Medullary aspect
16. C. Periosteum

17. A. Body (diaphysis)
    B. Epiphyses
18. False (25 years)
19. C. Metaphysis
20. A. Synarthrosis
    B. Amphiarthrosis
    C. Diarthrosis
21. A. Fibrous
    B. Cartilaginous
    C. Synovial
22. 1. C
    2. A
    3. C
    4. A
    5. B
    6. C
    7. A
    8. B
    9. B
    10. C
23. A. Plane (gliding)
    B. Ginglymus (hinge)
    C. Trochoid (pivot)
    D. Ellipsoid (condylar)
    E. Sellar (saddle)
    F. Spheroidal (ball and socket)
    G. Bicondylar
24. 1. E
    2. B
    3. F
    4. A
    5. D
    6. G
    7. C
    8. B
    9. C
    10. E
    11. G
    12. D

Review Exercise B: Positioning Terminology

1. Radiograph
2. Central ray
3. Anatomic
4. Median or midsagittal

5. Midcoronal
6. Transverse or axial
7. True
8. False
9. A. Projection
10. C. Position
11. True
12. True
13. Lateral position
14. Left posterior oblique (LPO)
15. Right anterior oblique (RAO)
16. Dorsal decubitus (left lateral)
17. Right lateral
18. Left lateral decubitus (PA)
19. 1. H
    2. G
    3. F
    4. I
    5. B
    6. D
    7. J
    8. C
    9. E
    10. A
20. Anteroposterior (AP)
21. Axial
22. (Apical) lordotic position
23. True
24. False (inward, toward midline)
25. 1. B
    2. A
    3. A
    4. A
    5. A
    6. B
    7. B
    8. A
    9. B
    10. A
26. A. Extension
    B. Radial deviation
    C. Plantar flexion
    D. Inversion
    E. Medial (internal) rotation
    F. Adduction
    G. Pronation

H. Protraction

I. Elevation

27. 1. F
    2. D
    3. G
    4. E
    5. C
    6. J
    7. I
    8. H
    9. A
    10. B
28. Protraction
29. Radial deviation
30. A. Patient identification and date
    B. Anatomic side markers

Review Exercise C: Positioning Principles

1. False
2. True
3. True
4. False
5. False
6. A. A minimum of two projections 90° from each other
   B. A minimum of three projections when joints are in the prime interest area
7. A. 3
   B. 2
   C. 3
   D. 2
   E. 2
   F. 3
   G. 2
   H. 2
   I. 3
   J. 1 (see text)
8. A. (d) Two
   B. (c) Rather than move the forearm for additional projections, place the image receptor and x-ray tube as needed.
9. Palpation
10. A. Ischial tuberosity
    B. Symphysis pubis
11. False (Place as if technologist were facing the patient; the patient's right to the technologist's left.)
12. True

Review Exercise D: Image Quality in Analog (Film-Screen) Imaging

1. Silver
2. A. Density
   B. Contrast
   C. Spatial resolution
   D. Distortion
3. C. Exposure latitude
4. Kilovoltage (kV)
5. Milliseconds
6. Density
7. Milliampere seconds (mAs)
8. B. Decrease density to 25%
9. Underexposed
10. Doubling
11. False
12. C. 25% to 30%
13. Anode
14. Cathode
15. Compensating filters
16. A. Wedge filter
    B. Trough filter
    C. Boomerang filter
17. Wedge filter
18. Boomerang filter
19. D. 10 mAs
20. Radiographic contrast
21. Kilovoltage (kV)
22. A. Long-scale contrast (low contrast)
    B. Short-scale contrast (high contrast)
23. Long-scale contrast (low)
24. True
25. True
26. D. 110 kV, 10 mAs
27. B. 8 to 10 kV increase
28. 10 cm
29. A. 2. Off-level grid cutoff
    B. 3. Off-focus grid cutoff
    C. 4. Upside down grid cutoff
30. *Spatial* resolution or definition
31. Blur or unsharpness
32. A. Focal spot size
    B. Source image receptor distance (SID)
    C. Object image receptor distance (OID)
33. Penumbra
34. False
35. Motion
36. D. Shorten exposure time
37. A. Decrease OID
38. D. 0.3-mm focal spot and 40-inch SID
39. Distortion

40. False (There is always some magnification and distortion caused by OID and divergence of the x-ray beam.)
41. A. Source image receptor distance (SID)
    B. Object image receptor distance (OID)
    C. Object IR alignment
    D. Central ray placement
42. False (increase distortion)
43. False (increase distortion)
44. True
45. C. 44 inches (112 cm)
46. B. 72 inches (183 cm)
47. True
48. False
49. True
50. True

Review Exercise E: Image Quality in Digital Radiography

1. False
2. True
3. False
4. D. Algorithms
5. C. Digital processing
6. Wide
7. A. Brightness
   B. Contrast
   C. Spatial resolution
   D. Distortion
   E. Exposure indicator
   F. Noise
8. A. Brightness
9. True
10. False
11. D. Contrast resolution
12. C. Application of processing algorithms
13. B. Contrast resolution
14. A. Acquisition pixel size
    B. Display pixel size
15. Acquisition pixel size
16. False
17. D. 2.5 lp/mm to 5.0 lp/mm
18. B. Display matrix
19. False
20. Exposure indicator
21. A. mAs
    B. kV
    C. Total detector area irradiated
    D. Objects exposed
22. Underexposure
23. Underexposure
24. Least possible dose to the patient

25. Noise
26. Signal-to-noise ratio
27. Low-SNR
28. C. Mottle
29. Post-processing
30. A. Annotation
    B. Edge enhancement
    C. Image reversal
    D. Magnification
    E. Smoothing
    F. Subtraction

Review Exercise F: Applications of Digital Technology

1. A. Image plates (IP)
   B. IP reader
   C. Technologist QC workstation
2. True
3. A. Image archiving
4. A. Bar code reader
5. False
6. True
7. True
8. A. Bright light
9. Archiving
10. D. A minimum of 72" (183 cm) required for all projections
11. False
12. False
13. D. Both A and B
14. True
15. False
16. False
17. C. CCD-based systems
18. 1. D
    2. E
    3. A
    4. C
    5. F
    6. B
19. True
20. Picture Archiving Communication System
21. False
22. A. Digital Imaging Communications Medicine
    B. Radiology Information System
    C. Hospital Information System
    D. Health care Level 7
23. Teleradiography
24. FPD-TFT
25. A. Display matrix
    B. Exposure latitude
    C. Windowing

D. Penumbra
E. Exposure indicator
F. Bit depth
G. Distortion
H. Kilovoltage
I. Noise
J. Spatial resolution (detail, sharpness, or definition)
K. Post-processing
26. A. Radiology Information System
    B. Image Receptor
    C. Object Image Distance
    D. Digital Radiography
    E. Automatic Exposure Control
    F. Hospital Information System
27. A. 5
    B. 7
    C. 3
    D. 2
    E. 1
    F. 4
    G. 6

Review Exercise G: Radiation Protection

1. Roentgen or Coulombs per kilogram (C/kg)
2. Gray (rad)
3. Effective dose
4. 50 mSv (5 rem) per year
5. 350 mSv (35 rem)
6. A. Coulombs per kilogram (C/kg) of air
   B. Gray (Gy)
   C. Sievert (Sv)
7. A. 0.03 Gy
   B. 4.48 mGy
   C. 0.38 Sv
   D. 150 mSv
8. A. 0.5 mSv (50 mrem)
   B. 5 mSv (500 mrem)
9. 1 mSv (0.1 rem) per year
10. B. 10%
11. A. Thermoluminescent dosimeter
    B. Optically stimulated luminescence (dosimeter)
12. As Low As Reasonably Achievable
13. A. Family member (if not pregnant)
14. False (still need to be used)
15. True
16. True

17. False (considers dose risk to all organs)
18. C. Poor communication between technologist and patient
19. A. Carelessness in positioning
    B. Selection of incorrect exposure factors
20. A. Inherent
    B. Added
21. Aluminum or copper or combination of both
22. A. Reduces the volume of tissue irradiated
    B. Reduces the accompanying scatter radiation, which adds to patient dose
23. False (2%, not 10%)
24. True
25. True
26. A. Shadow shields
    B. Contact shields
27. C. 1-mm lead equivalent
28. A. 95% to 99%
29. 2 inches; 5 cm
30. Shadow shield
31. True
32. D. Do not use shielding (for initial pelvis projection)
33. Results in reduction in spatial resolution
34. False (only if it does not cover pertinent anatomic parts for that exam)
35. 0.5-mm lead (Pb) equivalent
36. A. Distance
    B. Time
    C. Shielding
37. True
38. False
39. Keep the image intensifier tower as close as possible to the patient. (Also some experts recommend wearing a thyroid shield along with a protective apron.)
40. C. Behind the radiologist
41. D. 10 R/min (air kerma rate of 88 mGy/min)
42. Must not exceed 20 R/min (air kerma rate of 176 mGy/min)
43. C. 1 to 3 R/min (air kerma rate of 8.8 to 26 mGy/min)
44. C. AP abdomen
45. C. Retrograde pyelogram
46. A. Dose Area Product (DAP)
    B. Cumulative total dose

47. B. 3 Gy (300 rad)
48. True
49. True
50. False (Image Gently is intended to reduce unnecessary dose to children.)

CHAPTER 2

Review Exercise A: Radiographic Anatomy of the Chest

1. A. Sternum
   B. Clavicles
   C. Scapulae
   D. Ribs
   E. Thoracic vertebrae
2. A. Vertebra prominens
   B. Jugular notch
3. A. Pharynx
   B. Trachea
   C. Bronchi
   D. Lungs
4. A. Thyroid cartilage
   B. Larynx
   C. Sternum
   D. Scapula
   E. Clavicle
5. A. Nasopharynx
   B. Oropharynx
   C. Laryngopharynx
6. Epiglottis
7. Anteriorly
8. Hyoid
9. A. Right
   B. It is larger in diameter and more vertical.
10. A. Carina
    B. T5
11. Alveoli
12. A. Pleura
    B. Parietal pleura
    C. Pulmonary or visceral pleura
    D. Pleural cavity
    E. Pneumothorax
13. A. Base
    B. Hilum (hilus)
    C. Apex (apices)
    D. Costophrenic angle
14. Presence of liver on right
15. A. Thymus gland
    B. Heart and great vessels
    C. Trachea
    D. Esophagus
16. A. Thymus
    B. Arch of aorta
    C. Heart

D. Inferior vena cava
   E. Superior vena cava
   F. Thyroid
   G. Trachea
   H. Esophagus
17. Pericardial sac or pericardium
18. Ascending, arch, and descending aorta
19. A. Apex of left lung
    B. Trachea
    C. Carina
    D. Heart
    E. Left costophrenic angle
    F. Right hemidiaphragm (or base)
    G. Hilum
    H. Apex of lungs
    I. Hilum
    J. Heart
    K. Right and left hemidiaphragm
    L. Right and left costophrenic angles (superimposed)
20. A. Left main stem bronchus
    B. Descending aorta
    C. T5 (fifth thoracic vertebra)
    D. Esophagus
    E. Region of carina
    F. Right main stem bronchus
    G. Superior vena cava
    H. Ascending aorta
    I. Sternum

Review Exercise B: Technical Considerations

1. Hypersthenic
2. D. Hyposthenic and asthenic
3. 10 ribs
4. A. Necklace
   B. Bra
   C. Religious medallion around neck
   D. Hair fasteners
   E. Oxygen lines
5. True
6. 110 to 125 kV
7. False
8. E. All of the above
9. Should be able to see faint outlines of at least middle and upper vertebrae and ribs through heart and other mediastinal structures
10. False (Situs inversus may be present.)
11. C. Pigg-O-Stat
12. A. 70 to 85 kV, short exposure time
13. True

14. Second
15. 1. Small pneumothorax
    2. Fixation or lack of normal diaphragm movement
    3. Presence of a foreign body
    4. Distinguishing between opacity in rib or lung
16. A. To allow diaphragm to move down farther
    B. To show possible air and fluid levels in the chest
    C. To prevent engorgement and hyperemia of the pulmonary vessels
17. Erect position causes abdominal organs to drop, allowing the diaphragm to move farther down and the lungs to more fully aerate.
18. Reduces distortion and magnification of the heart and other chest structures
19. D. Air bronchogram sign
20. C. Symmetric appearance of sternoclavicular joints
21. Extend the neck upward
22. A. Left
    B. Right
    C. Left
23. Prevents upper arm soft tissue from being superimposed over upper chest fields
24. 1½ to 2 inches (5 cm)
25. Vertebra prominens, 8 inches (20 cm) for male, 7 inches (18 cm) for female
26. A. Crosswise
    B. Lengthwise
27. B. Jugular notch
28. True
29. False (should be equal)
30. True
31. False (greater width)
32. True
33. False
34. False
35. 1. F
    2. J
    3. E
    4. I
    5. G
    6. L
    7. K
    8. B
    9. D
    10. C
    11. A
    12. H

36. Atelectasis +
Lung neoplasm 0
Pulmonary edema + (severe)
RDS or ARDS (HMD in infants) +
Secondary tuberculosis (slight increase) +
Advanced emphysema −
Large pneumothorax 0
Pulmonary emboli 0
Childhood tuberculosis 0
Asbestosis 0
37. B. Emphysema
38. D. AP lordotic

Review Exercise C: Positioning of the Chest

1. Places the heart closer to the image receptor to reduce magnification of the heart
2. T7
3. Scapulae
4. A left lateral better demonstrates the heart region
5. Greater than 1 cm (½ to ¾ inch)
6. A. Caudad (±5°)
   B. Sternum
7. Pleural effusion
8. Left lateral decubitus
9. Pneumothorax
10. Right lateral decubitus (affected side up)
11. Rule out calcifications or masses beneath the clavicles
12. AP semiaxial projection, central ray 15° to 20° cephalad
13. A. RAO
    B. LPO
14. Left, 60°
15. False (A grid is recommended.)
16. Level of C6-C7, midway between thyroid cartilage and jugular notch
17. Scatter
18. Lift the breasts up and outward and then remove her hands as she leans against the chest board (image receptor) to keep them in the position.
19. False
20. Engorgement, hyperemia

Review Exercise D: Problem Solving for Technical and Positioning Errors

1. Rotation. The patient is rotated into a slight RAO position.
2. The lungs are underinflated. Explain to the patient the need for a deep inspiration, and take the exposure on the second deep inspiration.
3. A. The 75 kV is too low. The ideal kV range is 110 to 125.
   B. Increase the kV and reduce the mAs for the repeat exposure.
4. Center the central ray higher (to the level of T7, which will be found 7 to 8 inches below the vertebra prominens). Make sure the image receptor is centered to the central ray and the top collimation light border is at the vertebra prominens.
5. B. Decrease the kV moderately (− −).
6. C. Increase the kV slightly (+).
7. Ensure placement of the correct right or left anatomic side marker on the image receptor, because the heart and other thoracic structures may be transposed from right to left.
8. Determine which hemidiaphragm (right or left) is more posterior or more anterior. The left hemidiaphragm can frequently be identified by visualization of the gastric air bubble or the inferior heart shadow, both of which are associated with the left hemidiaphragm.
9. Right lateral decubitus; in a patient with hemothorax (fluid), the side of interest should be down.
10. A. AP and lateral upper airway projections
11. AP lordotic
12. Inspiration and expiration PA projections and/or a lateral decubitus AP chest with affected side up
13. C. Erect PA and lateral
14. AP semiaxial projection; CR is angled 15° to 20° cephalad to project the clavicles above the apices and clearly demonstrate the possible tumor.

15. Both the LPO and RAO oblique positions will best demonstrate or elongate the left lung.

CHAPTER 3

Review Exercise A: Abdominopelvic Anatomy

1. Psoas muscles
2. Gastro-
3. A. Duodenum
   B. Jejunum
   C. Ileum
4. Ileum
5. Right lower, cecum
6. Descending colon, rectum
7. B. Spleen
8. A. Pancreas
   B. Liver
   C. Gallbladder
9. Posteriorly
10. B. Spleen
11. Presence of liver on right
12. Suprarenals (adrenal)
13. False (intravenous urogram [IVU])
14. Peritoneum
15. Retroperitoneal
16. D. Mesentery
17. C. Greater omentum
18. 1. A
    2. C
    3. B
    4. A
    5. C
    6. B
    7. A
    8. C
    9. B
    10. A
    11. B
    12. B
19. A. RUQ
    B. LUQ
    C. LLQ
    D. LUQ
    E. LUQ
    F. RLQ
    G. LUQ
20. C. Umbilical
21. A. Pubic
22. A. Ischial tuberosity
    B. Greater trochanter
    C. Iliac crest or crest of ilium
    D. Anterior superior iliac spine (ASIS)
    E. Symphysis pubis

23. Superior border; 1½ (inches), 1 to 4 (cm), distal
24. Symphysis pubis
25. Inferior costal margin
26. Interspace between L4-L5
27. A. Stomach
    B. Jejunum
    C. Ileum
    D. Region of ileocecal
    E. Duodenum
    F. Duodenal bulb
28. A. Stomach
    B. Pancreas
    C. Spleen
    D. Kidney (left)
    E. Liver
    F. Duodenum
    G. Gallbladder

Review Exercise B: Shielding, Pathology, Exposure Factors, and Positioning

1. A. Patient breathing
   B. Patient movement during exposure
2. Careful breathing instructions
3. Peristaltic action of the bowel
4. Use the shortest exposure time possible.
5. False
6. False
7. A. It obscures essential anatomy.
8. B. Female
9. ASISs; Symphysis pubis
10. C. 70 to 80 kV, grid, 40-inch (102-cm) SID
11. D. All of the above
12. True
13. C. Computed tomography (CT)
14. A. Ultrasound
15. A. Ultrasound
16. 1. E
    2. D
    3. F
    4. C
    5. B
    6. A
    7. G
17. 1. F
    2. E
    3. A
    4. C
    5. D
    6. B
18. Iliac crest
19. Expiration
20. A. Iliac wings

B. Obturator foramina (if visible)
C. Ischial spines
D. Outer rib margins
21. Hypersthenic body type
22. True
23. False
24. To increase the room for expansion of the abdominal organs within the abdominal cavity
25. C. Pancreas
26. Increased object image receptor distance (OID) of kidneys on PA
27. Left lateral decubitus (free air best visualized in upper right abdomen in area of liver)
28. To allow intraabdominal air to rise or abnormal fluids to accumulate
29. Dorsal decubitus
30. Lateral position
31. A. AP supine
    B. AP erect or lateral decubitus abdomen
    C. PA erect chest
32. PA chest
33. Two-way abdomen; AP supine abdomen, and left lateral decubitus
34. C. PA, erect chest for free air under diaphragm
35. 2 inches (5 cm) above iliac crest; axilla
36. 3 to 5 cm (1 to 2 inches)
37. B. Long scale

Review Exercise C: Problem Solving for Technical and Positioning Errors

1. No. A KUB must include the symphysis pubis on the radiograph to ensure that the bladder is seen. The positioning error involves centering of the central ray to the iliac crest. The technologist should also palpate the symphysis pubis (if permitted by institutional policy) or greater trochanter to ensure that it is above the bottom of the cassette.
2. The selected kilovoltage (90 kV) was too high. The technologist needs to lower the kilovoltage to between 70 and 80 kV. The milliamperage and exposure time can be altered to maintain the density.

3. The blurriness may be caused by involuntary motion. To control this motion, the technologist needs to increase the milliamperage and decrease the exposure time (e.g., 400 mA at ¹⁄₁₀ second).
4. Patient was rotated into a slight right posterior oblique (RPO) position. (The downside ilium will appear wider.)
5. The three-way acute abdominal series, including the anteroposterior (AP) supine and erect abdomen and posteroanterior (PA) erect chest projections
6. The two-way acute abdomen series: AP supine abdomen and left lateral decubitus
7. A KUB would be performed with the correct exposure factors to visualize the possible stone.
8. A bedside portable left lateral decubitus projection could be performed to demonstrate any fluid levels in the abdomen.
9. A. The erect AP abdomen position best demonstrates air-fluid levels. Ascites produces free fluid in the intraperitoneal cavity.
10. B. Because the patient may have renal calculi in the distal ureters and urinary bladder, gonadal shielding cannot be used.
11. D. Repeat the exposure using two 14- × 17-inch cassettes placed crosswise. The hypersthenic patient often requires this type of IR placement for abdomen studies.
12. B. Decrease the mAs. Because trapped air is easier to penetrate than soft tissue with x-rays, reducing the mAs will prevent overexposing the radiograph.
13. C. KUB and lateral abdomen. With any foreign body study, two projections 90° opposite is recommended to pinpoint the location of the foreign body.

CHAPTER 4

Review Exercise A: Anatomy of Hand and Wrist

1. A. 14
   B. 5
   C. 8
   D. 27
2. A. Proximal phalanx
   B. Distal phalanx
3. A. Proximal phalanx
   B. Middle phalanx
   C. Distal phalanx
4. A. Head
   B. Body (shaft)
   C. Base
5. A. Base
   B. Body (shaft)
   C. Head
6. Interphalangeal joint
7. Metacarpophalangeal (MCP) joints
8. A. Fifth carpometacarpal (CMC) joint
   B. Body of third metacarpal
   C. Head of fifth metacarpal
   D. Fourth metacarpophalangeal (MCP) joint
   E. Head of proximal phalanx of fifth digit
   F. Base of middle phalanx of fourth digit
   G. Distal interphalangeal (DIP) joint of fourth digit
   H. Body of middle phalanx of second digit
   I. Proximal interphalangeal (PIP) joint of second digit
   J. Body of distal phalanx of first digit
   K. Interphalangeal (IP) joint of first digit
   L. Metacarpophalangeal (MCP) joint of first digit
   M. Head of first metacarpal
   N. Second carpometacarpal (CMC) joint
   O. First carpometacarpal (CMC) joint
9. A. 8
   B. 1
   C. 5
   D. 4
   E. 3
   F. 6
   G. 7
   H. 2
10. Capitate
11. Hamulus or hamular process
12. Scaphoid
13. Either of these two mnemonics is acceptable: (1) Send Letter To Peter To Tell'im (to) Come Home, or (2) Steve Left The Party To Take Carol Home
14. A. 3
    B. 9
    C. 2
    D. 5
    E. 1
    F. 8
    G. 6
    H. 7
    I. 4
15. A. Body of first metacarpal (thumb)
    B. Carpometacarpal joint of first digit
    C. Trapezium
    D. Scaphoid
    E. Lunate
    F. Radiocarpal (wrist) joint (between radius and carpals)

Review Exercise B: Anatomy of the Forearm, Elbow, and Distal Humerus

1. A. Radius
   B. Ulna
2. A. U
   B. U
   C. H
   D. H
   E. U
   F. U
   G. U
   H. H
3. Proximal radioulnar joint
4. A. Trochlea
   B. Capitulum
5. Olecranon fossa
6. A. Trochlear sulcus (groove)
   B. (a) Capitulum
      (b) Trochlea
   C. Trochlear notch
7. A. 1
   B. 5
   C. 1
   D. 2
   E. 2
   F. 4
   G. 1
   H. 3
8. Diarthrodial, 4 (four)

9. True
10. Radial collateral ligament
11. A. Ulnar deviation
    B. Radial deviation
12. Ulnar deviation
13. The proximal radius crosses over the ulna.
14. A. Scaphoid fat stripe
    B. Pronator fat stripe
15. A. Elbow flexed 90°
    B. Optimal exposure factors employed
    C. In a true lateral position
16. False (A nonvisible fat pad suggests a negative exam.)
17. True
18. False
19. Posteroanterior (PA) and oblique wrist
20. Lateral wrist
21. A. Radial tuberosity
    B. Radial neck
    C. Capitulum
    D. Lateral epicondyle
    E. Olecranon fossa
    F. Medial epicondyle
    G. Trochlea
    H. Coronoid tubercle
    I. Olecranon process
    J. Superimposed humeral epicondyles
    K. Radial head
    L. Radial neck
    M. Radial tuberosity
    N. Outer ridges of trochlea and capitulum
    O. Trochlear sulcus (groove)
    P. Trochlear notch
22. A. Radial tubercle
    B. Radial neck
    C. Radial head
    D. Capitulum
    E. Lateral epicondyle
    F. Coronoid process
    G. Trochlea
    H. Olecranon process

Review Exercise C: Positioning of the Fingers, Thumb, Hand, and Wrist

1. A. Low to medium (50 to 70 kV for analog and 60 to 80 kV for digital systems)
   B. Short exposure
   C. Small focal spot
   D. 40 inches (102 cm)
   E. 10 cm

F. Detail screens (analog)
G. 5 to 7 kV
H. 8 to 10 kV
I. 3 to 4 kV
J. Soft tissue, trabecular
2. Collimation borders should be visible on all four sides if the image receptor (IR) is large enough to allow this without cutting off essential anatomy.
3. B, D, E, F
4. False. A good practice is to provide shielding for all patients.
5. True (Ensure adults are given a lead apron to wear during exposures)
6. Arthrography
7. PA, PA oblique, and lateral
8. Distal aspect of metacarpals
9. A. Symmetric appearance of both sides of the shafts of phalanges and distal metacarpals
   B. Equal amounts of tissue on each side of the phalanges
10. A. Perform the medial oblique rather than lateral oblique to decrease OID.
    B. Perform a thumb-down lateral (mediolateral projection) to decrease OID.
11. Proximal interphalangeal (PIP) joint
12. D
13. The AP position produces a decrease in OID and increased resolution.
14. PA oblique
15. 18 × 24 cm (8 × 10 inch)
16. Metacarpophalangeal
17. True
18. C
19. A
20. A. Modified Robert's method
    B. 15° proximal
21. A
22. 1 inch (2.5 cm)
23. True
24. Fan lateral
25. Lateral in extension
26. Norgaard method
27. D
28. 90
29. 45°
30. Anteroposterior (AP) projection (with the hand slightly arched)
31. Excessive lateral rotation from PA

32. B
33. 10 to 15, proximally
34. C
35. 25° to 30°
36. PA projection with radial deviation
37. Tangential inferosuperior or Gaynor-Hart projection
38. 45°
39. 90°

Review Exercise D: Pathologic Features of the Fingers, Thumb, Hand, and Wrist

1. A. Barton's fracture
   B. Multiple myeloma
   C. Osteoporosis
   D. Skier's thumb
   E. Achondroplasia
   F. Boxer's fracture
   G. Osteopetrosis
   H. Colles' fracture
2. A. 4
   B. 2
   C. 3
   D. 1
   E. 5
3. Paget's disease (+)
   Joint effusion (0)
   Rheumatoid arthritis (−)
   Osteoporosis (−)
   Osteopetrosis (+)
   Bursitis (0)

Review Exercise E: Positioning of the Forearm, Elbow, and Humerus

1. AP and lateral
2. False
3. Parallel
4. Two AP projections (partially flexed), one with humerus parallel to IR and one with forearm parallel to IR
5. AP oblique with 45° lateral rotation
6. False (because of scatter, divergent rays, or both reaching gonads)
7. AP oblique with 45° medial rotation
8. Lateral, flexed 90°
9. Two projections-central ray perpendicular to humerus and central ray perpendicular to forearm (acute flexion projections)

10. 45° laterally
11. 45° toward shoulder
12. 45° away from shoulder
13. 80° of flexion
14. The rotational position of hand and wrist

Review Exercise F: Problem Solving for Technical and Positioning Errors

1. Use a small focal spot, minimum 40-inch (102-cm) SID, and detail speed screens (analog) to produce a higher-quality study.
2. Rotation
3. Excessive lateral rotation
4. PA forearm projection was performed rather than AP.
5. The central ray needs to be angled 15° proximally, toward the elbow.
6. The elbow is rotated medially.
7. Increase lateral rotation of the elbow to separate the radius from the ulna.
8. The forearm and humerus are not on the same horizontal plane.
9. Coyle method for radial head (lateral elbow, central ray 45° toward shoulder)
10. PA and lateral-in-extension projection
11. AP and lateral forearm projections to include the wrist
12. Two AP projections with acute flexion and a lateral projection
13. Modified Robert's method
14. Carpal canal position (Gaynor-Hart method)
15. Norgaard method—ball catcher's position
16. PA stress (Folio method) projection
17. Tangential projection—carpal bridge projection
18. Trauma axial lateral projection—Coyle method for coronoid process

Review Exercise G: Critique Radiographs of the Upper Limb

A. PA hand (Fig. C4-159)
1. Because of rotation and flexion, anatomy of hand is distorted and joints are not open.
2. Fingers flexed preventing clear assessment of joint spaces. Medial rotation of hand distorts the proximal phalanges and metacarpals.
3. No collimation evident on this printed radiograph; centering satisfactory for hand
4. Exposure factors are acceptable.
5. No anatomic side marker
   Repeatable error(s): 1 (anatomy demonstrated) and 2 (part positioning)

B. Lateral wrist (Fig. C4-160)
1. All pertinent anatomic structures included
2. Upper limb rotated slightly; radius and ulna not directly superimposed; metacarpals not all superimposed
3. No collimation evident on this printed radiograph; centering slightly off; central ray centered to the distal carpal region; includes too much forearm
4. Acceptable selected exposure factors
5. Anatomic side marker evident on this projection
   Repeatable error(s): 2 (rotation) and 3 (centering)

C. AP oblique elbow (Fig. C4-161)
1. All essential anatomic structures included
2. Elbow is rotated laterally evident by slight separation of proximal radius and ulna
3. No collimation borders evident; central ray centering excellent for elbow
4. Optimal exposure factors
5. No anatomic side marker evident on this projection
   Repeatable error(s): 2 (rotation) and 5 (unless markers are visible elsewhere on radiograph)

D. PA wrist (Fig. C4-162)
Note: This demonstrates a radial deviation for the ulnar side carpals (the opposite of the ulnar deviation for scaphoid).
1. Aspect of pisiform cut off laterally
2. Excellent part positioning with good radial deviation
3. Central ray centering error—central ray centered over scaphoid and medial carpals; would have excellent collimation if central ray were centered correctly
4. Excellent exposure factors
5. Evidence of satisfactory anatomic marker
   Repeatable error(s): 1 (anatomy demonstrated) and 3 (centering)

E. PA forearm—pediatric (Fig. C4-163)
1. All pertinent anatomic structures not included because of PA projection being performed over AP
2. Poor part positioning because proximal radius crossing over ulna due to PA projection being performed
3. No collimation evident on this printed radiograph; acceptable central ray centering. Exposure factors are satisfactory.
4. Anatomic side marker evident
   Repeatable error(s): 1 (anatomy demonstrated) and 2 (Note: Individual immobilizing infant's hand should wear lead glove or use mechanical restraint.)

F. Lateral elbow (Fig. C4-164)
1. All pertinent anatomic structures demonstrated
2. Elbow overflexed (beyond 90°) and not true lateral; too much distance between parts of concentric circles 1 and 2; trochlear notch space not open
3. Satisfactory collimation (i.e., collimation that is evident); central ray centering slightly off center to the elbow joint
4. Acceptable exposure factors

5. Anatomic side marker partially off radiograph and unacceptable (unless it is demonstrated on the actual radiograph)
   Repeatable error(s): 2 (part positioning) and 5 (unless marker is more visible on actual radiograph)

CHAPTER 5

Review Exercise A: Anatomy of Proximal Humerus and Shoulder Girdle

1. A. Proximal humerus
   B. Scapula
   C. Clavicle
2. A. Intertubercular groove (bicipital groove)
   B. Greater tubercle (tuberosity)
   C. Head of humerus
   D. Anatomic neck
   E. Lesser tubercle (tuberosity)
   F. Surgical neck
   G. Neutral (Neither the greater nor lesser tubercle is in profile.)
3. A. Sternal extremity
   B. Body (shaft)
   C. Acromial extremity
4. Male
5. A. Lateral angle
   B. Superior angle
   C. Inferior angle
6. Costal
7. Axilla
8. A. Infraspinous fossa
   B. Supraspinous fossa
9. Synovial (diarthrodial)
10. A. Spheroidal
    B. Plane
    C. Plane
11. 1. C
    2. A
    3. A
    4. D
    5. B
    6. C
    7. D
    8. C
12. A. Neck of scapula
    B. Scapulohumeral joint (glenohumeral joint)
    C. Acromion
    D. Coracoid process

E. Scapular notch
F. Superior angle
G. Medial (vertebral)
H. Lateral (axillary)
I. Ventral (costal)
J. Dorsal (posterior)
K. Spine of scapula
L. Acromion
M. Coracoid process
N. Body (blade, wing, or ala)
O. Inferior angle
13. A. Coracoid process
B. Scapulohumeral
C. Acromion
D. Greater tubercle
E. Lesser tubercle
F. Lateral border
G. Internal (lesser tubercle is in profile medially)
H. Lateral perspective
I. Perpendicular
J. Body of scapula
K. Spine of scapula and acromion
L. Coracoid process
M. Body (shaft) of humerus
N. Scapular Y lateral-anterior oblique projection
14. A. Coracoid process
B. Glenoid process
C. Spine of scapula
D. Acromion
E. Inferosuperior axial projection
F. 90°

Review Exercise B: Positioning of Humerus and Shoulder Girdle

1. 1. A
   2. C
   3. B
   4. A
   5. C
   6. A
   7. B
   8. B
   9. A
2. A. Neutral
   B. External
   C. Internal
3. A. True
   B. False
   C. False
   D. False
   E. True
   F. False
   G. True

4. A. 70 to 80 kV
5. A. Parent or guardian
6. True
7. False
8. True
9. False
10. True
11. 1. D
    2. B
    3. G
    4. A
    5. C
    6. F
    7. E
12. 1. G
    2. E
    3. F
    4. H
    5. I
    6. B
    7. D
    8. A
    9. C
13. D. Osteoporosis
14. A. AP, external rotation
    B. AP, internal rotation
15. CR perpendicular to IR, directed to 1 inch (2.5 cm) inferior to coracoid process
16. Transthoracic lateral projection for humerus
17. B. Rotate affected arm externally approximately 45°
18. A. 25° to 30° medially
19. Posterior oblique; Grashey method
20. A. Fisk modification
21. 10° to 15°
22. D. Scapular Y
23. Tangential projection—Supraspinatus Outlet; Neer method
24. C. PA transaxillary projection (Hobbs modification)
25. A. 5° to 15°
26. D. 15° cephalad
27. True
28. True
29. True
30. False
31. False (10° to 15° cephalad)
32. False
33. Superior angle of the scapula and the AC joint articulation
34. AP apical oblique axial projection
35. Superior

36. More (CR angle)
37. Fracture of clavicle
38. 1. C
    2. B
    3. D
    4. A
    5. C
    6. E
39. CR perpendicular to midscapula, 2 inches (5 cm) inferior to coracoid process, or to level of axilla, and approximately 2 inches (5 cm) medial from lateral border of patient
40. None. CR perpendicular to the IR

Review Exercise C: Problem Solving for Technical and Positioning Errors

1. Lower to 75 kV and double milliamperage seconds (to 40 mAs), which increases radiographic contrast
2. Increase central ray cephalad angle.
3. Ensure that the affected arm is abducted 90° and use a breathing technique.
4. Supinate the hand and ensure that the epicondyles are parallel to the IR for a true AP.
5. Palpate the superior angle of the scapula and AC joint articulation and ensure that the imaginary plane between these points is perpendicular to the IR.
6. Increase rotation of affected shoulder toward IR to closer to 45°.
7. Angle the central ray 10° to 15° cephalad to separate the shoulders.
8. The routine includes an anteroposterior (AP) of right shoulder and humerus without rotation (neutral rotation) and a supine, horizontal beam, right transthoracic shoulder. Note: In those cases in which the opposite arm cannot be elevated or extended, a supine posterior oblique scapular Y lateral projection could also be used as a second option for a lateral shoulder position (see Chapter 15).

9. Possible positioning options: Inferosuperior axial projection with exaggerated external rotation, Inferosuperior axial projection (Clements modification) and AP apical oblique axial projection (Garth method)
10. A. AP—internal rotation
    B. Scapular Y lateral
    C. Posterior oblique (Grashey method)
11. B. MRI
12. C. Ultrasound
13. The humeral epicondyles were not placed parallel to the plane of the IR.
14. Use breathing exposure technique to create blurring of ribs and lung markings.
15. Transthoracic lateral projection for humerus
16. Anterior dislocation of the proximal humerus

Review Exercise D: Critique Radiographs of the Humerus and Shoulder Girdle

A. AP clavicle (Fig. C5-96)
   1. All of clavicle demonstrated
   2. Rotation of body toward the patient's right, superimposing sternal end over the spine and creating overall distortion of the clavicle and associated joints
   3. Collimation much too loose and not evident at all; central ray centered too low (inferiorly), which also adds to distorted appearance of clavicle
   4. Acceptable but slightly underexposed exposure factors
   5. Missing (or not visible) anatomic side marker
      Repeatable error(s): 2 (rotation), 3 (incorrect centering), and 5 (missing anatomic side marker)
B. AP shoulder—external rotation (Fig. C5-97)
   1. All pertinent anatomic structures demonstrated
   2. Greater tubercle is not in profile but note fracture of scapular neck. No rotation of the proximal humerus should be employed. Transthoracic

lateral projection should be performed to provide 90° opposite perspective.
   3. No evidence of collimation
   4. Acceptable but slightly overexposed.
   5. Anatomic side marker is present
      Repeatable error(s): None (considering the degree of trauma). Transthoracic lateral or Scapular Y lateral projection should be performed to provide another perspective.
C. AP scapula (Fig. C5-98)
   1. Lower margin of scapula cut off at bottom edge of radiograph
   2. Arm must be abducted at 90° angle to body
   3. Collimation not evident; need to center central ray and cassette to include the entire scapula
   4. Underexposed scapula and blurring of ribs, not evident from breathing technique
   5. Missing (or not visible) anatomic side marker
      Repeatable error(s): 1 (anatomy), 2 (positioning), 3 (centering), 4 (exposure), and 5 (anatomic side marker)
D. AP humerus (Fig. C5-99)
   1. Distal humerus is not included.
   2. Correct part positioning for AP projection, but centering is off
   3. Evidence of collimation on one side only, indicating incorrect centering; central ray and IR centering too lateral and proximal
   4. Acceptable
   5. Acceptable; anatomic side marker partially seen on radiograph
      Repeatable error(s): 1 (anatomy) and 3 (centering)
      Position: AP projection, external rotation

CHAPTER 6

Review Exercise A: Radiographic Anatomy of the Foot and Ankle

1. A. 14
   B. 5
   C. 7
   D. 26
2. A. Phalanges of the foot are smaller.
   B. The joint movements of the foot are more limited than those of the hand.
3. Tuberosity of base of the fifth metatarsal
4. The plantar surface of the foot near the first metatarsophalangeal joint
5. Calcaneus
6. Subtalar or talocalcaneal
7. A. Posterior facet
   B. Anterior facet
   C. Middle facet
8. Sinus tarsi or tarsal sinus
9. 1. B
   2. F
   3. D
   4. G
   5. E
   6. B
   7. G
   8. A
   9. C
   10. B
10. A. Sinus tarsi (tarsal sinus)
    B. Talus
    C. Navicular
    D. Lateral cuneiform
    E. Base of first metatarsal
    F. Body (shaft) of first metatarsal
    G. Sesamoid bone
    H. Metatarsophalangeal (MTP) joint of first digit
    I. Distal phalanx of first digit
    J. Tuberosity at base of fifth metatarsal
    K. Cuboid
    L. Calcaneal tuberosity
    M. Anteroposterior (AP) 45° medial oblique
    N. Tuberosity of calcaneus
    O. Lateral process of calcaneus
    P. Peroneal trochlea (trochlear process)

Q. Lateral malleolus of fibula
R. Sustentaculum tali
S. Talocalcaneal joint
T. Plantodorsal (axial) projection of calcaneus
11. True
12. B. Cuboid
13. A. Longitudinal arch
   B. Transverse arch
14. A. Talus
   B. Tibia
   C. Fibula
15. Ankle mortise
16. A. Tibial plafond
17. False
18. Sellar
19. A. Tuberosity at base of fifth metatarsal (see fracture on radiograph in Fig. 6-3)
   B. Lateral malleolus of fibula
   C. Distal tibiofibular joint
   D. Medial malleolus
   E. Talus
   F. Calcaneus
   G. Sinus tarsi (tarsal sinus)
   H. Talus
   I. Tibial plafond
   J. Anterior tubercle
   K. Navicular
   L. Cuboid
   M. AP mortise, 15° to 20° medial rotation

Review Exercise B: Radiographic Anatomy of the Lower Leg, Knee, and Distal Femur

1. Tibia
2. Tibial tuberosity
3. Adductor tubercle
4. Fibular notch
5. Tibial plateau
6. D. 10 to 15
7. Apex or styloid process
8. Lateral malleolus
9. Patella
10. A. Intercondylar sulcus
    B. Trochlear groove
11. Intercondylar fossa or notch
12. Because the medial condyle extends lower than the lateral condyle of the femur
13. C. Adductor tubercle
14. A. Medial epicondyle
    B. Lateral epicondyle
15. Popliteal region
16. False
17. True

18. False
19. Quadriceps femoris muscle
20. A. Patellofemoral
    B. Femorotibial
21. A. Fibular (lateral) collateral
    B. Tibial (medial) collateral
    C. Anterior cruciate
    D. Posterior cruciate
22. Medial and lateral menisci
23. A. Suprapatellar bursa
    B. Infrapatellar bursa
24. 1. A
    2. A
    3. C
    4. C
    5. A
    6. A
    7. B
    8. D
    9. A
    10. B
25. 1. C
    2. C
    3. D
    4. D
    5. F
    6. E
26. A. Fibular notch of tibia (also may be identified as distal tibiofibular joint)
    B. Body (shaft) of fibula
    C. Articular facets (or tibial plateau)
    D. Lateral condyle of tibia
    E. Intercondyloid eminence (tibial spine)
    F. Medial condyle of tibia
    G. Tibial tuberosity
    H. Anterior crest of body (shaft of tibia)
    I. Medial malleolus
    J. Lateral malleolus
    K. Body (shaft) of fibula
    L. Neck of fibula
    M. Head of fibula
    N. Apex or styloid process of fibula
    O. 10° to 20°
    P. Tibial tuberosity
    Q. Body (shaft) of tibia
    R. Medial malleolus
    S. Lateral condyle of femur
    T. Patellar surface of femur
    U. Medial condyle of femur
    V. Patellofemoral joint space
    W. Patella
    X. Tangential (patellofemoral joint)

27. A. Base of patella
    B. Apex of patella
    C. Tibial tuberosity
    D. Neck of fibula
    E. Head of fibula
    F. Apex or styloid process of fibula
    G. Superimposed medial and lateral condyles
    H. Patellar surface/intercondylar sulcus or trochlear groove
    I. Adductor tubercle
    J. Lateral femoral condyle
    K. Medial femoral condyle
28. A. 1
    B. 4
    C. 2
    D. 3

Review Exercise C: Positioning of the Foot and Ankle

1. True
2. True
3. False
4. True
5. True
6. False
7. A. 9
   B. 8
   C. 10
   D. 7
   E. 1
   F. 5
   G. 6
   H. 3
   I. 2
   J. 4
8. Chondromalacia patellae
9. Rickets
10. A. 7
    B. 3
    C. 8
    D. 1
    E. 5
    F. 4
    G. 2
    H. 6
11. Opens up the interphalangeal and metatarsophalangeal joints
12. Base of third metatarsal
13. Tangential projection
14. 15° to 20°
15. Opens up metatarsophalangeal and certain intertarsal joints
16. D. None; use perpendicular central ray

17. Second to fifth
18. AP oblique with medial rotation
19. AP oblique with lateral rotation
20. Lateromedial
21. AP and lateral weight-bearing projections
22. 40° cephalad
23. Sustentaculum tali
24. 1 inch (2.5 cm) inferior to medial malleolus
25. C. Lateral surface of joint
26. To demonstrate a possible fracture of the fifth metatarsal tuberosity (a common fracture site)
27. 15° to 20° (medially)
28. 45° AP oblique with medial rotation
29. B. Projected over the posterior aspect of the distal tibia
30. AP stress projections

Review Exercise D: Positioning of the Tibia, Fibula, Knee, and Distal Femur

1. AP and lateral projections
2. A fracture may also be present at the proximal fibula in addition to the distal portion.
3. C. Diagonally
4. B. 3° to 5° cephalad
5. A. ½ inch (1.25 cm) distal to apex of patella
6. C. AP oblique, 45° medial rotation
7. Medial (internal)
8. B. 5° cephalad
9. B. 20° to 30°
10. Improper angle of the central ray or lack of support of the lower leg
11. Over-rotation (toward the IR) or under-rotation of the knee (away from IR)
12. Adductor tubercle on posterolateral aspect of the medial femoral condyle
13. AP or PA weight-bearing knee
14. C. MRI
15. A. Holmblad
16. 40° flexion
17. Distortion caused by central ray angle and increased OID for AP axial projection
18. B. 10° caudad
19. D. 45°
20. C. 60° to 70°
21. D. None. CR is perpendicular to IR

22. True
23. 5° to 10°
24. 30° from horizontal
25. A. 55°
    B. 90°
26. D. None. CR is perpendicular to IR.
27. 1. F
    2. E
    3. D
    4. G
    5. C
    6. A
    7. B
28. A. Rosenberg method
29. True
30. D. None

Review Exercise E: Problem Solving for Technical and Positioning Errors

1. Central ray is not angled correctly; adjust central ray angle to keep it perpendicular to metatarsals.
2. Over-rotation of foot (toward the medial direction)
3. Increase cephalad angle of the central ray to correctly elongate the calcaneus.
4. Possibly a spread of the ankle mortise caused by ruptured ligaments
5. Under-rotation of the ankle (toward the medial direction). The described appearance is that of a true AP ankle with little or no obliquity.
6. Angling the central ray correctly to keep it parallel to the articular facets (tibial plateau)
7. The wrong oblique position of the knee was obtained. This description is that of a laterally or externally oblique position of the knee.
8. Under-rotation of knee (excessive rotation of patella away from the IR)
9. An AP lateral oblique projection with 30° of external rotation will separate the bases of the first and second metatarsals.
10. Repeat the AP projection to ensure the ankle joint is demonstrated.

11. Rotation of the affected limb or incorrect CR angle to match the degree of flexion of the lower limb
12. Decrease the amount of flexion of the knee to only 5° to 10°.
13. An AP or PA weight-bearing bilateral knee projection will best evaluate the joint spaces.
14. AP and lateral weight-bearing foot projections
15. AP and lateral weight-bearing projections
16. Intercondylar fossa projections, including the PA axial projections (Holmblad, Rosenberg, and/or Camp-Coventry methods) demonstrate the entire knee joint and intercondylar fossa region, which may be hiding "joint mice."
17. The lateral knee projection will best demonstrate any separation of the tibial tuberosity from the shaft of the tibia.
18. By angling the central ray 5° to 7° cephalad, the medial femoral condyle will be superimposed with the lateral condyle. If CR angulation was used on the initial projection, increase the amount of angle with the repeat exposure.
19. The superoinferior sitting tangential method is best suited for this patient. While remaining in the wheelchair, the patient's knees can be flexed, the IR can be positioned on a foot stool, and the CR is placed vertically above the knees.
20. The most common error with the tangential (inferosuperior) projection is overflexion of the knee, which will draw the patella into the intercondylar sulcus. Flexion of the lower limb should not exceed 45°. Another possible error is that the CR is not parallel to the joint space.

Review Exercise F: Critique Radiographs of the Distal Lower Limb

A. Bilateral tangential patella (Fig. C6-141)
1. Portion of each patella superimposed over intercondylar sulcus of femur
2. Excessive flexion of knee most likely cause of superimposition of patella over femur
3. Evidence of collimation; correct central ray centering and IR placement; may be an error in central ray angle, which would have contributed to the superimposition
4. Underexposed
5. Anatomic side marker present
   Repeatable error(s): 1 (anatomy demonstrated), 2 (part positioning), and 3 (CR angle) (possibly four-exposure)

B. Plantodorsal (axial) calcaneus (Fig. C6-142)
1. Obvious compound fracture of calcaneus. All pertinent anatomy is seen.
2. Positioning is acceptable but foot is plantar flexed.
3. Off centering of part to IR is too anterior. Better centering would lead to more concise collimation.
4. Acceptable exposure factors
5. Anatomic side marker visible
   Repeatable error(s): None (Note: Centering was incorrect but not repeatable.)

C. AP mortise ankle (Fig. C6-143)
1. Note: Tri-malleolar fracture. All pertinent anatomy demonstrated.
2. Excessive medial rotation superimposes lateral malleolus over lateral aspect of talus.
3. No collimation evident. Centering is correct.
4. Acceptable exposure factors
5. No anatomic side marker visible
   Repeatable error(s): 2 (part positioning). (The ankle must not be rotated and side markers must be used.)

D. AP lower limb (pediatric) (Fig. C6-144)
1. Note fracture of distal femur. All anatomy demonstrated.
2. Positioning is correct for AP projection
3. No collimation nor gonadal shielding is used. Centering is correct for entire lower limb. Unprotected hand used to immobilize the lower limb: Unacceptable practice
4. Acceptable exposure factors
5. Anatomic side marker visible
   Repeatable error(s): 3 (radiation protection issue) (not a repeatable error in this situation)

E. Lateral knee (Fig. C6-145)
1. All pertinent anatomic structures included, but patellofemoral joint not open* (presence of superimposition of patella over lateral condyle because of rotation)
2. Rotation of anterior knee away from cassette (underrotation); almost total superimposition of proximal fibula; visibility of adductor tubercle identifies medial condyle as being posterior; overflexed knee (should be flexed only 15° to 20° rather than the almost 45° used in this radiograph)
3. No evidence of collimation; correct central ray centering and IR placement
4. Acceptable exposure factors
5. Anatomic side marker present
   Repeatable error(s): 1 (anatomy demonstrated) and 2 (part positioning)

F. AP medial oblique knee (Fig. C6-146)
1. Closure of patellofemoral joint space caused by positioning error
2. Excessive rotation of anterior knee toward cassette (overrotation); separation of proximal fibula from tibia; outline of adductor tubercle on medial condyle also anterior to lateral condyle; knee slightly underflexed
3. No evidence of collimation; correct central ray centering and IR placement

4. Acceptable exposure factors
5. Anatomic side marker present
   Repeatable error(s): 1 (anatomy demonstrated) and 2 (rotation)

CHAPTER 7

Review Exercise A: Anatomy of Femur, Hips, and Pelvic Girdle

1. Femur
2. Fovea capitis
3. Medial; posteriorly
4. 15 to 20
5. True
   A. Right and left hip bones, sacrum, and coccyx
   B. Right and left hip bones
   C. Ossa coxae and/or innominate bones
6. A. Ilium
   B. Ischium
   C. Pubis
7. Acetabulum, mid teens
8. A. Crest of ilium (iliac crest)
   B. Anterior superior iliac spine (ASIS)
9. Ischial tuberosity
10. Symphysis pubis
11. Obturator foramen
12. A. 1 inch (2.5 cm)
    B. 1½ to 2 inches (4 to 5 cm)
13. Pelvic brim
14. A. False pelvis
    B. True pelvis
15. A. Supports the lower abdominal organs and fetus
    B. Forms the actual birth canal
16. A. Inlet (superior aperture)
    B. Cavity
    C. Outlet (inferior aperture)
17. 1. B
    2. B
    3. A
    4. A
    5. C
    6. A
    7. C
    8. A
18. Cephalopelvimetry
19. Sonography (ultrasound)
20. 1. F
    2. F
    3. M
    4. M
    5. M
    6. F

21. A. Synovial, diarthrodial, spheroidal
    B. Synovial, amphiarthrodial, limited
    C. Cartilaginous, amphiarthrodial, limited
    D. Cartilaginous, amphiarthrodial, non-movable
22. A. Crest, IL
    B. ASIS, IL
    C. Greater trochanter
    D. Body, IS
    E. Superior ramus, P
    F. Ischial tuberosity, IS
    G. Inferior ramus, P
    H. Obturator foramen
    I. Body, P
    J. Body, IL
    K. Wing (ala), IL
    L. Right sacroiliac (SI) joint
    M. Ischial spine, IS
    N. Sacrum
    O. Body, IL
    P. Posterior superior iliac spine (PSIS), IL
    Q. Posterior inferior iliac spine, IL
    R. Greater sciatic notch, IL
    S. Ischial spine, IS
    T. Lesser sciatic notch, IS
    U. Ischial tuberosity, IS
    V. Ramus, IS
    W. Inferior ramus, P
    X. Acetabulum, IS, IL, P
    Y. Anterior inferior iliac spine, IL
    Z. ASIS, IL

Review Exercise B: Positioning of Femur, Hips, Pelvis, and Sacroiliac Joints

1. A. ASIS
   B. Symphysis pubis (or greater trochanter if palpation of this landmark is not permitted by institution)
2. Approximately 2½ inches (6 to 7 cm) below the midpoint of the line
3. ASIS; 1 to 2 inches (2.5 to 5 cm); symphysis pubis and/or greater trochanter; 3 to 4 inches (8 to 10 cm)
4. 15 to 20
5. Lesser trochanter should not be visible, or should only be slightly visible, on the radiograph.

6. The patient's foot is rotated externally.
7. AP pelvis
8. It covers anatomic structures of primary interest.
9. Yes. Use a shaped ovarian shield with top of shield at level of ASIS and bottom at symphysis pubis.
10. Yes. The top of the shield should be placed at the inferior margin of the symphysis pubis.
11. It reduces patient dose.
12. It reduces radiographic contrast.
13. B. DDH (development dysplasia of hip)
14. True
15. A. Sonography
16. D. Nuclear medicine
17. A. 7
    B. 5
    C. 4
    D. 2
    E. 6
    F. 1
    G. 3
18. C. Compensating filter
19. A. CT
20. True. If an AP and lateral femur study is ordered, both joints must be demonstrated.
21. Midway between ASIS and symphysis pubis
22. 2 inches (5 cm)
23. Rotation toward left side
24. Right rotation
25. A. T
    B. NT
    C. NT
    D. T
    E. T
26. B. PA axial oblique
27. Females (because of location of CR and reproductive organs)
28. 40° to 45°
29. 3 inches (7.5 cm) below level of ASIS (1 inch [2.5 cm] above symphysis pubis)
30. 35 × 43 cm (14 × 17 inches) crosswise
31. Midfemoral neck (see positioning considerations for femoral neck localization in chapter)
32. B. 30° to 45° cephalad
33. A. Acetabular fractures
34. D. 45°
35. D. 12° cephalad

36. C. PA 35° to 40° toward affected side
37. True
38. Traumatic
39. It is flexed and elevated to prevent it from being superimposed over the affected hip.
40. C. Use of gonadal shielding
41. True
42. True
43. 15 to 20
44. A. Posterior oblique projections of acetabulum (Judet method)
    B. 0° (perpendicular)
45. AP axial outlet projection (Taylor method)
46. 1. D
    2. C
    3. F
    4. E
    5. B
    6. A
47. D. 20° to 30° from vertical
48. True
49. 15° from the vertical
50. False

Review Exercise C: Problem Solving for Technical and Positioning Errors

1. Rotate the lower limbs 15° to 20° internally to place the proximal femurs in a true AP position. (With general chronic pain, the lower limbs usually can be rotated safely.)
2. The patient is rotated toward the left—left posterior oblique (LPO).
3. Repeat the exposure and only abduct the femur 20° to 30° from vertical. (It will produce less distortion of the femoral neck.)
4. If possible, elevate the patient at least 2 inches (or 5 cm) by placing sheets or blankets beneath the pelvis.
5. A greater central ray angle is required. Female patients require a central ray angle of 30° to 45°.
6. The PA axial oblique (Teufel method) or posterior oblique (Judet method) can be taken to demonstrate aspects of the acetabulum more completely.

7. When using automatic exposure control (AEC) for an AP pelvis projection, the left and right ionization chambers must be activated. The center chamber is over the less dense pelvic cavity, which may lead to an underexposed image.

8. Ensure that the central ray is centered to near the midline of the grid cassette and the face of the cassette is perpendicular to the central ray.

9. Yes. Any orthopedic appliance or prosthesis must be seen in its entirety in both projections.

10. AP pelvis and axiolateral (inferosuperior) left hip. The AP pelvis radiograph should be taken initially without leg rotation; the radiograph must be reviewed by the physician and checked for fractures or dislocations before attempting an internal rotation of the left leg for the axiolateral (inferosuperior) projection.

11. AP pelvis and modified axiolateral—Clements-Nakayama method

12. Posterior oblique—Judet method. CT is often judged to be superior in detecting pelvic ring fractures.

13. AP axial for pelvic "outlet" (Taylor method) and AP axial for pelvic "inlet" projections and possibly the posterior oblique (Judet method) projections to provide another perspective of the inlet and outlet regions of the pelvis. (If unsure of the request routine, contact the physician for clarification.)

14. Palpate both ASIS and ensure they are equal distance from the tabletop. To verify no rotation is still present, ensure that the iliac wings are symmetric, as seen on the radiograph.

15. AP pelvis and bilateral "frog-leg" (modified Cleaves) projections

Review Exercise D: Critique Radiographs of the Femur and Pelvis

A. AP pelvis (Fig. C7-77)
1. All anatomy of the pelvis is demonstrated.
2. The lesser trochanters are visible, which indicates the

lower limbs were not rotated 15° to 20° medially.
3. No collimation evident (acceptable) and CR centering was slightly off laterally (to the patient's right)
4. Exposure factors are acceptable.
5. Anatomic side marker evident
Repeatable error(s): 2 (Part/ anatomy positioning)
Note: Based on the obtuse angle (>90 degrees) of the pubic arch, flared iliac wings, and round pelvic inlet, this is a **female pelvis**.

B. AP pelvis (Fig. C7-78)
1. All anatomy of pelvis is demonstrated.
2. No rotation of lower limbs evident by presence of lesser trochanters. But because of pelvic ring fracture involving pubis, inadvisable to rotate lower limbs. Fracture may have extended into acetabulum. Slight tilt of pelvis.
3. No collimation evident (acceptable) and CR centering is acceptable.
4. Exposure factors are acceptable.
5. No anatomic side marker visible
Repeatable error(s): 5 (anatomic side marker. Unsure side of fracture)

C. Unilateral "frog-leg" projection (performed cystography) (Fig. C7-79)
1. All pertinent anatomy is demonstrated.
2. Lower limb should not have been rotated into frog-leg position because of the severity of the fracture.
3. No collimation evident and is needed to reduce exposure to abdomen. Note: Patient's right upper limb is in field. Centering is too low.
4. Exposure factors are acceptable.
5. Anatomic side marker is evident.
Repeatable error(s): 2 (part positioning) and 3 (centering—if exposure is to be repeated for other reasons)

D. Bilateral frog-leg (2-year-old) (Fig. C7-80)
1. Left hip (assuming that this is the left side because the side marker is not visible) obscured by artifact (superimposition of patient's hand)
2. Tilted pelvis (and note that the gonadal shield placement is useless for either males *or* females—a serious error for a small child)
3. No visible collimation, which should be visible for this pediatric patient; central ray centering/film placement too high for pelvis centering but acceptable for bilateral hip projection
4. Very low contrast (may have been caused by not using a grid)
5. No visible anatomic side marker
Repeatable error(s): 1 (anatomy demonstrated)

CHAPTER 8

Review Exercise A: Radiographic Anatomy of the Cervical and Thoracic Spine

1. A. 7
   B. 12
   C. 5
   D. 1
   E. 1
   F. 26
2. A. Thoracic
   B. Sacral
3. A. Cervical
   B. Lumbar
4. 1. B and D
   2. A and C
   3. A and C
   4. B and D
   5. A
5. Lordosis
6. Scoliosis
7. Body; vertebral arch
8. Lamina
9. Intervertebral
10. Vertebral (spinal) canal
11. A. Medulla oblongata
    B. Lower border of L1
    C. Conus medullaris

12. Spinal nerves and blood vessels
13. A. Spinous process
    B. Lamina
    C. Transverse process
    D. Facet of superior articular process
    E. Pedicle
    F. Vertebral foramen
    G. Spinous process
    H. Facet of superior articular process
    I. Pedicle
    J. Body
    K. Inferior articular process
    L. Superior articular process
    M. Zygapophyseal joint
    N. Facet for head of rib articulation
    O. Intervertebral foramen
    P. Facet for rib articulation
    Q. Costovertebral joints
    R. Costotransverse joints
14. C. Zygapophyseal joints
15. True
16. False (between C1 and C2 visualized on a frontal or AP projection)
17. A. Annulus fibrosus
    B. Nucleus pulposus
18. Herniated nucleus pulposus (HNP)
19. A. C1: Atlas
    B. C2: Axis
    C. C7: Vertebra prominens
20. A. Transverse foramina
    B. Bifid spinous process
    C. Overlapping vertebral bodies
21. Articular pillar
22. Lateral mass
23. 90; 70 to 75
24. Occipitoatlantal articulation
25. Dens or odontoid process
26. Rotation of the skull
27. Presence of facets for articulation with ribs
28. T5 to T8
29. A. Body, C4
    B. Dens (odontoid), C2
    C. Posterior arch and tubercle, C1
    D. Zygapophyseal joint, C5-C6
    E. Spinous process (vertebra prominens), C7
    F. Posterior arch and tubercle, C1
    G. Pedicle, C4
    H. Intervertebral foramen, C4-C5
30. 15° cephalad

Review Exercise B: Positioning of the Cervical and Thoracic Spine

1. A. Manubrium
   B. Jugular (suprasternal) notch
   C. Body
   D. Sternal angle
   E. Xiphoid process
2. 1. H
   2. E
   3. F
   4. B
   5. D
   6. C
   7. A
   8. G
3. Thyroid, parathyroid glands, and breasts
4. A. Increase in exposure latitude (wider range of densities)
   B. Decrease in patient dose
5. True
6. False (Lead masking should be used even if close collimation is used.)
7. True
8. True
9. A. Keep vertebral column parallel to image receptor (IR)
10. B. Using a small focal spot
    C. Increasing SID
11. A. 9
    B. 10
    C. 4
    D. 8
    E. 2
    F. 6
    G. 1
    H. 7
    I. 5
    J. 3
12. A. Erect (AP/PA) and lateral spine including bending laterals
    B. Lateral cervical
    C. AP open mouth C1-C2, tomography—following lateral projection
    D. Scoliosis series
    E. Lateral cervical spine
    F. Lateral of affected spine
13. Spondylitis is an inflammatory process of the vertebrae. Spondylosis is a condition of the spine characterized by rigidity of a vertebral joint.
14. True

15. Myelography
16. Nuclear medicine
17. Lower margin of upper incisors and base of skull
18. False. The entire dens or odontoid process must be demonstrated. If trauma or injury is ruled out, the technologist could perform the AP or PA projection for odontoid process to demonstrate the tip.
19. To open up the intervertebral disk spaces
20. C. Base of skull
21. True
22. A. Compensates for increased object image receptor distance (OID); reduces magnification
    B. Less divergence of x-ray beam to reduce shoulder superimposition of C7
23. 15° cephalad
24. Right intervertebral foramina (upside)
25. Left intervertebral foramina (downside)
26. Rotate the skull into a near lateral position
27. 60 to 72 inches (152 to 183 cm)
28. Expiration; for maximum shoulder depression
29. Lateral, horizontal beam projection
30. Twining method
31. To T1; 1 inch (2.5 cm) above the jugular notch anteriorly, or level of vertebra prominens posteriorly
32. C5 to T3
33. D. Hyperextension and hyperflexion lateral positions
34. If unable to demonstrate the upper portion of the dens with the AP "open mouth" projection
35. AP "wagging jaw" projection (Ottonello method)
36. Correct use of anode-heel effect; use of compensating (wedge) filter
37. To blur out rib and lung markings that obscure detail of thoracic vertebrae
38. Right (downside)
39. C. Cervicothoracic position
40. True (anterior oblique <5 mrad; posterior oblique <69 mrad)

41. B. Articular pillars (lateral masses of C-spine)
42. C. 20° to 30° caudad
43. Lead mat or masking
44. Mentomeatal line (MML)
45. Right
46. 20° from lateral position

Review Exercise C: Problem Solving for Technical and Positioning Errors

1. Excessive extension of the skull
2. Increase central ray angulation to 15° cephalad.
3. When the lower intervertebral foramina are narrowed while the upper foramina are well demonstrated, the positioning error most often is under rotation of the upper body. The upper body must be rotated 45°.
4. Initiate exposure during suspended expiration and increase SID to 72 inches (183 cm).
5. Reduce mAs and increase exposure time to produce more blurring of the mandible.
6. Use of an orthostatic (breathing) technique to blur lung markings and ribs more effectively
7. Use a compensating (wedge) filter with thicker part of filter placed over the upper thoracic spine to equalize the density along the thoracic spine.
8. Angle CR 3° to 5° caudad.
9. Horizontal beam lateral projection
10. Hyperextension and hyperflexion lateral positions
11. Perform either the (AP) Fuchs or (PA) Judd method.
12. Cervicothoracic (swimmer's) lateral position
13. AP axial—vertebral arch (pillar) projection
14. AP open mouth projection. The patient's mouth must be carefully opened without any movement of the cervical spine.
15. Scoliosis series

Review Exercise D: Critique Radiographs of the Cervical and Thoracic Spine

A. AP open mouth (Fig. C8-91)
  1. Upper aspect of dens obscured by base of skull
  2. Overextension of skull, causing superimposition of base of skull over dens
  3. Collimation is poor, resulting in excessive exposure to face, eyes, and neck region; central ray and IR placement is too high
  4. Acceptable exposure factors
  5. Anatomic side marker
     Repeatable error(s): 1 (anatomy demonstrated), 2 (positioning) and 3 (CR and IR placement)
B. AP open mouth (Fig. C8-92)
  1. Upper aspect of dens and joint space obscured by front incisors
  2. Overflexion of skull causing superimposition of front incisors over top of dens
  3. Collimation too loose, resulting in excessive exposure to face, eyes, and neck region; slightly low central ray and IR
  4. Acceptable exposure factors
  5. No evidence of anatomic side marker
     Repeatable error(s): 1 (anatomy demonstrated) and 2 (positioning)
C. AP axial projection (Fig. C8-93)
  1. Distorted vertebral bodies and intervertebral joint spaces; base of skull superimposed over upper cervical spine
  2. Overextension of skull and/or excessive central ray cephalic angle, which probably led to poor definition of vertebral bodies and joint spaces
  3. Evidence of collimation; slightly low central ray centering but correct IR placement
  4. Acceptable exposure factors
  5. Evidence of anatomic side marker
     Repeatable error(s): 1 (anatomy demonstrated) and 2 (positioning)

Note: Unsure of the origin of the artifact seen on lower, left cervical spine region
D. Right posterior oblique (Fig. C8-94)
  1. Lower intervertebral joint spaces and foramina not clearly demonstrated
  2. Appears that body is underrotated from AP position (with appearance of upper rib cage suggesting underrotation rather than overrotation), an error that led to narrowing and obscuring of the lower intervertebral foramina.
  3. Collimation is evident. CR is centered too low.
  4. Acceptable exposure factors
  5. Anatomic side marker is evident
     Repeatable error(s): 1 (anatomy demonstrated), 2 (positioning), and 3 (CR centering)
E. Lateral (trauma) (Fig. C8-95)
  1. Aspect of C1 and dens cut off; C7-T1 not demonstrated
  2. Need to depress shoulders (because chin cannot be adjusted as a result of the trauma)
  3. No evidence of collimation except along anterior, upper margin; central ray centered too posterior, causing upper cervical spine to be cut off; IR placement centered too low
  4. Acceptable exposure factors (poor contrast resulting from using a nongrid technique)
  5. No evidence of anatomic side marker
     Repeatable error(s): 1 (anatomy demonstrated), 2 (positioning), and 3 (CR centering)
F. AP for odontoid process—Fuchs method (Fig. C8-96)
  1. Upper part of odontoid process is not demonstrated.
  2. The skull and neck is underextended, which produces a poor image of the dens within the foramen magnum. There is slight rotation of the skull.

3. The CR is centered too high and collimation is absent.
4. Slightly underexposed
5. No evidence of anatomic side marker
   Repeatable errors: 1 (anatomy demonstrated), 2 (positioning), 3 (CR centering), and 5 (no side marker)

G. AP thoracic spine (Fig. C8-97)
   1. Necklace is obscuring T1/2 region
   2. Positioning is acceptable
   3. CR is centered slightly high but acceptable
   4. Overexposed near the region of T1 to T3
   5. Anatomic side marker is visible but placement may be obscuring costotransverse joint
      Repeatable errors: 1 (anatomy demonstrated), 4 (exposure), and 5 (anatomic side marker placement)

CHAPTER 9

Review Exercise A: Anatomy of the Lumbar Spine, Sacrum, and Coccyx

1. Pars interarticularis
2. B. Intervertebral foramina
3. Lateral position
4. A. Pedicle
   B. Transverse process
   C. Superior articular process and facet
   D. Lamina
   E. Spinous process
   F. Zygapophyseal joints
   G. Intervertebral foramina
5. 50° for upper and 30° for lower vertebrae to the midsagittal plane
6. Pelvic sacral foramina
7. Promontory
8. Cornua
9. 30°
10. Coccyx
11. Base
12. A. Synovial, diarthrodial, plane, or gliding
    B. Cartilaginous, amphiarthrodial (slightly movable), none

13. A. Intervertebral disk space, L1-L2
    B. Spinous process, L2
    C. Transverse process, L3
    D. Region of lamina (body), L4
    E. Left ala of sacrum
    F. Left sacroiliac (joint)
    G. Body of L1
    H. Pedicles of L2
    I. Intervertebral foramina, L3-L4
    J. Intervertebral disk space, L5-S1
    K. Sacrum
    L. Inferior articular process, L3 (leg)
    M. Zygapophyseal joint, L4-L5
    N. Pars interarticularis, L3 (neck)
    O. Pedicle, L3 (eye)
    P. Transverse process, L3 (nose)
    Q. Superior articular process, L3 (ear)
14. A. Left zygapophyseal joints
    B. Left zygapophyseal joints
    C. Intervertebral foramina
    D. Right zygapophyseal joints
    E. Right zygapophyseal joints
15. 50°, 30°, 45°

Review Exercise B: Topographic Landmarks and Positioning of the Lumbar Spine, Sacrum, and Coccyx

1. 1. C
   2. E
   3. A
   4. B
   5. D
2. False
3. True
4. False (not used for females if the shield would obscure essential anatomy)
5. False (PA would open intervertebral joint spaces better.)
6. False (should be flexed)
7. True
8. False
9. A. 4
   B. 1
   C. 1
   D. 5
   E. 2
10. A. 8
    B. 3

C. 1
D. 2
E. 4
F. 7
G. 6
H. 5
11. Iliac crest
12. A. Sacroiliac (SI) joints are equidistant from the spine.
    B. Spinous process should be midline to the vertebral column (transverse processes are equal length)
13. 30°
14. Right (upside)
15. Pedicle
16. Excessive rotation
17. Lateral
18. 5° to 8°, caudad
19. With the sag or convexity of the spine closest to the IR
20. Reduces lumbar curvature, which opens the intervertebral disk space
21. True
22. 1½ inches (4 cm) inferior to iliac crest and 2 inches (5 cm) posterior to ASIS
23. 30° cephalad
24. True
25. False (lower margin 1 to 2 inches [3 to 5 cm] below iliac crest)
26. True
27. D. Compensating filter
28. The convex side of the spine
29. Pelvis
30. Hyperextension and hyperflexion projections
31. 15° cephalad
32. A PA (prone) with 15° caudad central ray angle
33. 2 inches (5 cm) superior to the symphysis pubis
34. False (need different central ray angles for AP projections; can combine lateral but not AP projections)
35. AP of sacrum and coccyx
36. Place lead blocker on tabletop behind patient.
37. Left
38. 25° to 30°
39. D. 35° cephalad
40. 1 inch (2.5 cm) medial from upside ASIS

Review Exercise C: Problem Solving for Technical and Positioning Errors

1. Rotation of the spine
2. Insufficient rotation of the spine (pedicle "eye" should be to midvertebral bodies)
3. If the patient has a wide pelvis, the central ray can be angled 5° to 8° caudad.
4. Place additional support beneath the spine, or use a 5° to 8° caudad angle.
5. An increase in central ray angle is required to separate the coccyx from the symphysis pubis.
6. Decrease rotation of the body and spine.
7. AP or PA and collimated lateral projections would provide the best view of the L3 region. The central ray should be about 2 inches (5 cm) above the iliac crest.
8. A. Use high kV technique.
   B. Perform a PA rather than an AP projection.
   C. Use breast shields.
9. Perform a PA rather than an AP projection and reverse the direction of the central ray from caudad to cephalad.
10. A lateral L5-S1 position would demonstrate the degree of forward displacement of L5 onto S1.
11. The CR should be angled 15° to 20° cephalad.
12. Although AP and lateral projections of the lumbar spine are helpful, posterior or anterior oblique positions best demonstrate advanced signs of spondylolysis.
13. B. MRI
14. Hyperflexion and hyperextension lateral positions
15. Routine lumbar spine projections should be performed erect.

Review Exercise D: Critique Radiographs of the Lumbar Spine, Sacrum, and Coccyx

A. Lateral lumbar spine (Fig. C9-83)
   1. Posterior elements of upper lumbar spine cut off
   2. Patient too far posterior
   3. Evident and acceptable collimation (could be collimated a little more tightly if centering were correct); central ray centering too anterior, causing posterior elements to become cut off
   4. Acceptable but slightly underexposed exposure factors
   5. Anatomic side marker cut off
      Repeatable errors: 1 (anatomy demonstrated), 2 (part positioning), and 3 (CR centering)
B. Lateral lumbar spine (Fig. C9-84)
   1. All structures demonstrated. Note: This patient has a transitional vertebra, which produces six lumbar vertebrae. Also, there is calcification of the abdominal aorta.
   2. Poor visibility of upper intervertebral joint spaces caused by poor positioning of upper thoracic. Often if the shoulders are not superimposed, there is closure of the upper joint spaces.
   3. Collimation not evident; acceptable central ray centering and IR placement
   4. Overexposed exposure factors
   5. No evidence of anatomic side marker (it may have been placed too low on IR)
      Repeatable errors: 2 (part positioning) and 5 (no side marker)
C. Lateral L5-S1 (Fig. C9-85)
   1. All pertinent anatomic structures included
   2. Excellent part and central ray centering
   3. Additional collimation needed; S1 joint space not open; may need waist support or central ray caudal angle
   4. Underexposed L5-S1 joint space region
   5. Evidence of anatomic side marker (better to place up and posterior to spine)
      Repeatable errors: 3 (collimation and part positioning) and 4 (exposure)
D. RPO lumbar spine (Fig. C9-86)
   1. Posterior elements of upper lumbar spine cut off
   2. Over-rotated upper aspect of lumbar spine (eye of "Scottie dog" [pedicles] posterior and not centered to body)
   3. Evidence of collimation; central ray centered too anterior; posterior elements of lumbar spine to become cut off
   4. Acceptable exposure factors
   5. Evidence of anatomic side marker
      Repeatable errors: 1 (anatomy demonstrated), 2 (part positioning), and 3 (centering of CR and anatomy)
E. AP lumbar spine (Fig. C9-87)
   1. Entire lumbar spine demonstrated
   2. Under-rotated lumbar spine (eye of "Scottie dog" [pedicles] too anterior)
   3. Collimation too loose and not evident (should be visible on sides); central ray centering and IR placement correct
   4. Acceptable but slightly overexposed exposure factors
   5. No evidence of anatomic side marker
      Repeatable error: 2 (part positioning)
F. LPO lumbar spine (Fig. C9-88)
   1. Entire lumbar spine demonstrated but over-rotation of spine obscures essential anatomy and joints
   2. Excessive rotation
   3. No evidence of collimation and incorrect centering of anatomy to IR
   4. Acceptable
   5. Right side marker is barely visible by distorted. May have been placed on sheet on table.
      Repeatable error(s): 2 (part positioning) and 3 (collimation and centering)
G. AP lumbar spine (Fig. C9-89)
   1. All lumbosacral spine anatomy demonstrated*
   2. Slight tilt of hips

---

*Note underwire of bra and clasp visible. Although not obscuring critical anatomy, indicates improper patient preparation for procedure.

3. No collimation evident. CR centered too high
4. Exposure factors acceptable
5. Anatomic side markers evident
   Repeatable error(s): None (although centering and positioning are not ideal)

CHAPTER 10

Review Exercise A: Anatomy of the Bony Thorax, Sternum, and Ribs

1. A. Sternum
   B. Thoracic vertebra
   C. 12 pairs of ribs
2. A. Jugular (suprasternal) notch
   B. Facet for sternoclavicular joint
   C. Facet for first rib
   D. Manubrium
   E. Sternal angle
   F. Xiphoid process
   G. Costicartilage of seventh rib (last of "true" ribs)
   H. Tenth rib
   I. Costicartilage of second rib
   J. Clavicle
3. Body
4. 40
5. 6 inches (15 cm)
6. A. T9 to 10
   B. T4 to 5
   C. Manubriosternal joint
7. Sternoclavicular joint
8. Costicartilage
9. True ribs connect to the sternum by their own costicartilage. False ribs are connected to the sternum via the costicartilage of the seventh rib.
10. True
11. False (called the sternal end)
12. D. Tubercle
13. A. Artery
    B. Vein
    C. Nerve
14. A. Posterior vertebral ends
    B. 3 to 5 inches (7.5 to 12.5 cm)
    C. First (anterior sternal end)
    D. Eighth or ninth
    E. 11
15. 1. B
    2. A
    3. B
    4. A
    5. A

6. A
7. C
16. Synovial
17. A. True ribs, 1 through 7
    B. False ribs, 8 through 12
    C. Floating ribs, 11 through 12
18. Each rib attaches to the sternum by its own costicartilage.
19. They do not connect to anything anteriorly (thus the term "floating" ribs).
20. A. Vertebral end (posterior)
    B. Tubercles (for articulation with vertebrae)
    C. Axillary or angle portion of rib
    D. Costal groove
    E. Sternal end (anterior)
    F. Neck
    G. Head

Review Exercise B: Positioning of the Ribs and Sternum

1. True
2. False (less obliquity)
3. Approximately 15°
4. A. 65 to 70 kV (5 to 10 kV higher typically for digital systems)
   B. Low
   C. High (2 to 3 seconds) with orthostatic breathing technique
5. It blurs lung markings and ribs, which improves the visibility of the sternum.
6. Increase in patient dose, especially skin dose
7. CT or nuclear medicine
8. A. Recumbent
   B. Expiration
   C. Medium kV range—70 to 80 kV and 80 to 90 kV for digital systems
9. Above
10. Away from
11. PA and anterior obliques (Placing the area of interest closest to the IR is one recommended routine.)
12. AP and RPO (to shift spine away from area of interest)
13. By taping a small, metallic "BB" or other opaque marker over the site of the injury
14. Erect PA and lateral chest
15. B. Pulmonary injury caused by blunt trauma to two or more ribs.

16. A. Irregular bony margins
17. C. Depressed sternum due to congenital defect
18. A. Osteoblastic
19. False
20. True
21. RAO; it places the sternum over the heart to provide a uniform background for added visibility of the sternum.
22. Midsternum (midway between jugular notch and xiphoid process)
23. LPO (oblique supine position)
24. 60 to 72 inches (152 to 183 cm); reduces magnification created by the long object image receptor distance (OID)
25. B. The entire sternum should lie over the heart shadow adjacent to the spine.
26. B. Level of T2-T3
27. A. Suspend respiration on inspiration.
28. 10° to 15° from PA position
29. LAO
30. A. The nature of the trauma or patient complaint
    B. The location of the rib pain or injury
    C. Whether or not the patient has been coughing up blood
31. 3 to 4 inches (8 to 10 cm) below the jugular notch, level of T7
32. RAO or LPO elongates the left axillary ribs (and shifts the spine away from the injury site)
33. PA and LAO (to elongate the right axillary rib region)
34. 45°
35. 72 inches (183 cm)
36. 70 to 80 kV
37. True
38. False. The right SC joint is projected closest to the spine with an RAO projection.
39. C. 38 inches (97 cm)
40. B. Hemothorax

Review Exercise C: Problem Solving for Technical and Positioning Errors

1. Under-rotation of the patient
2. Lower the kV to 65 for higher contrast and to prevent overpenetration of the sternum.

3. Increase the exposure time (and lower the mA) to allow for greater blurring of the lung markings.
4. Have the patient bring the breasts to the side; hold them in this position with a wide bandage.
5. CT
6. 15° to 20° RAO sternum with orthostatic (breathing) technique; lateral sternum on inspiration; and 10° to 15° LAO of sternoclavicular joint with suspended inspiration
7. Suspend respiration during inspiration to move the diaphragm below the eighth ribs.
8. LPO and horizontal beam lateral projections (may use 15° to 20° mediolateral central angle if patient cannot be in oblique position)
9. Erect PA and LAO (or RPO) position with suspended inspiration
10. Recumbent PA (or AP if the patient cannot assume prone position) and RAO (or LPO) positions with suspended expiration
11. Because of patient condition, it is best to perform all positions erect and initiate exposure on full inspiration for upper ribs and full expiration for lower ribs. AP projections and both oblique positions (RPO and LPO) must be performed. It is recommended that kV (manual technique employed) for all projections be lowered because of the advanced osteoporosis.
12. A limited rib series will indicate which ribs are fractured (and whether this has led to flail chest). Because the patient is restricted to a backboard, the oblique positions may not be possible.

Review Exercise D: Critique Radiographs of the Bony Thorax

A. Bilateral ribs above diaphragm (Fig. C10-46)
   1. Ninth through eleventh ribs are cut off at left lateral margin.

   2. Tilt of body toward projected ribs nos. 9 and 10 below collimation field
   3. CR centering is acceptable.
   4. Acceptable exposure factors
   5. Anatomic side marker is evident.
      Repeatable errors: 1 (anatomy demonstrated) and 2 (positioning)

B. Oblique sternum (Fig. C10-47)
   1. All pertinent anatomic structures included
   2. Sternum is over-rotated; sternum away from the spine and rotated beyond heart shadow and distorted (Note: Because of additional patient dose, some departments may choose not to repeat this projection given that the outline of the sternum is visible.)
   3. Collimation not completely evident; central ray centering and IR placement correct
   4. Acceptable exposure factors and processing
   5. No evidence of anatomic side marker
      Repeatable errors: 2 (positioning)

C. AP ribs below diaphragm (Fig. C10-48)
   1. Right lower ribs cut off; only lower three pair of ribs demonstrated, indicating diaphragm is too low from poor expiration
   2. No elevation of diaphragm; need to take exposure during expiration with the patient in a recumbent position to raise the diaphragm to the highest level
   3. No evidence of collimation; acceptable central ray centering, but IR should have been placed crosswise to prevent lateral margins of ribs from being cut off
   4. Acceptable exposure factors and processing
   5. Anatomic side marker evident but placed a little low and almost off the radiograph
      Repeatable errors: 1 (anatomy demonstrated) and 3 (IR placement)

D. Lateral sternum (Fig. C10-49)
   1. Lower aspect of sternum cut off
   2. Acceptable part positioning
   3. No evidence of collimation; central ray centering and IR placement too high, causing lower sternum to be cut off
   4. Acceptable exposure factors
   5. No evidence of markers
      Repeatable errors: 1 (anatomy demonstrated) and 3 (CR centering and IR placement)

CHAPTER 11

Part I: Radiographic Anatomy

Review Exercise A: Anatomy of the Cranium

1. A. 8
   B. 14
2. A. Frontal
   B. Right parietal
   C. Left parietal
   D. Occipital
3. A. Right temporal
   B. Left temporal
   C. Sphenoid
   D. Ethmoid
4. A. Frontal
   B. Right parietal
   C. Right temporal
   D. Sphenoid
   E. Ethmoid
   F. Left temporal
   G. Left parietal
   H. Occipital
5. A. Frontal
   B. Ethmoid
   C. Sphenoid
   D. Left temporal
   E. Left parietal
   F. Occipital
   G. Right parietal
   H. Right temporal
6. A. Crista galli
   B. Cribriform plate
   C. Perpendicular plate
   D. Lateral labyrinth (mass)
   E. Middle nasal conchae (turbinate)
7. Cribriform plate
8. Perpendicular plate
9. A. Anterior clinoid processes
   B. Lesser wing

C. Greater wing
D. Sella turcica
E. Dorsum sellae
F. Posterior clinoid process
G. Clivis
H. Foramen rotundum
I. Foramen ovale
J. Foramen spinosum
K. Foramen magnum
L. Optic foramen
M. Lateral pterygoid process (plate)
N. Pterygoid hamulus
O. Medial pterygoid process (plate)
P. Superior orbital fissure
Q. Body of sphenoid (sinus)
10. Sella turcica
11. Dorsum sellae
12. Optic foramen
13. Medial and lateral pterygoid processes
14. Lateral
15. Orbital or horizontal portion
16. A. Coronal
B. Squamosal
C. Lambdoidal
D. Sagittal
E. Bregma
F. Lambda
G. Pterion
H. Asterion
I. Anterior (bregma)
J. Posterior (lambda)
K. Sphenoid (pterion)
L. Mastoid (asterion)
17. Fibrous or synarthrodial
18. Sutural or wormian; lambdoidal
19. Supraorbital margin (SOM)
20. Ethmoidal notch
21. Right and left parietals
22. Occipital
23. External occipital protuberance, or inion
24. Occipital condyles, or lateral condylar portions
25. A. Squamous
B. Mastoid
C. Petrous
26. False (petrous portion)
27. Top of the ear attachment (TEA)
28. Internal acoustic meatus
29. Fig. 11-15
A. Supraorbital margins of right orbit
B. Crista galli of ethmoid
C. Sagittal suture—posterior skull

D. Lambdoidal suture— posterior skull
E. Petrous ridge
Fig. 11-16
A. External acoustic meatus (EAM)
B. Mastoid portion of temporal bone
C. Occipital bone
D. Lambdoidal suture
E. Clivus
F. Dorsum sellae
G. Posterior clinoid processes
H. Anterior clinoid processes
I. Vertex of skull
J. Coronal suture
K. Frontal bone
L. Orbital plates of frontal bone
M. Cribriform plate
N. Sella turcica
O. Body of sphenoid bone: sphenoid sinus

Review Exercise B: Specific Anatomy and Pathology of the Temporal Bone

1. A. Squamous
B. Mastoid
C. Petrous
2. Petrous portion
3. Auricle or pinna
4. 1 inch (or 2.5 cm)
5. Tympanic membrane (eardrum)
6. Auditory ossicles
7. Eustachian or auditory tube
8. To equalize the atmospheric pressure within the middle ear
9. Aditus
10. Tegmen tympani
11. Malleus
12. Stapes
13. Incus
14. Oval or vestibular window
15. A. Hearing
B. Equilibrium
16. Round or cochlear window
17. True
18. A. Malleus
B. Incus
C. Stapes
D. Oval window
E. Cochlea
F. Round window
G. Eustachian tube
H. Tympanic cavity
I. Tympanic membrane
J. EAM or canal

19. A. 5
B. 3
C. 1
D. 6
E. 2
F. 4
20. A. Expansion of the internal acoustic canal
21. B. CT

Review Exercise C: Radiographic Anatomy of the Facial Bones

1. A. Middle nasal conchae
2. Maxilla
3. A. Frontal process
B. Zygomatic process
C. Alveolar process
D. Palatine process
4. Frontal process
5. Acanthion
6. Horizontal portion of the palatine bones
7. Frontal and ethmoid
8. Zygomatic or malar bones
9. D. Sphenoid
10. Lacrimal bones
11. Conchae, turbinates
12. False (Most of the nose is made up of cartilage.)
13. Septal cartilage, vomer (pushed laterally to one side)
14. A. 3
B. 8
C. 6
D. 7
E. 5
F. 1
G. 2
H. 4
15. A. Nasal bones
B. Lacrimal bones
C. Zygomatic bones
D. Maxillary bones
E. Inferior nasal conchae
F. Mandible
16. Vomer and palatine bones
17. A. Pterygoid hamulus, sphenoid
B. Right palatine process, right maxilla
C. Left palatine process, left maxilla
D. Horizontal portions, right and left palatine bones
18. A. Perpendicular plate of ethmoid
B. Vomer
C. Septal cartilage

19. A. Condyle
    B. Neck
    C. Ramus
    D. Gonion or mandibular angle
    E. Body
    F. Mental foramen
    G. Mentum or mental protuberance
    H. Alveolar process
    I. Coronoid process
    J. Mandibular notch
    K. Temporal bone
    L. Temporomandibular joint (TMJ)
    M. External auditory meatus (EAM)
    N. Mastoid process
20. A. Lacrimal (facial)
    B. Ethmoid (cranial)
    C. Frontal (cranial)
    D. Sphenoid (cranial)
    E. Palatine (facial)
    F. Zygomatic (facial)
    G. Maxilla (facial)
21. H. Optic foramen
    I. Superior orbital fissure
    J. Inferior orbital fissure
    K. Sphenoid strut
22. 30°, 37°
23. Inferior orbital fissure
24. A. Superior orbital fissure
25. B. Optic nerve

Review Exercise D: Radiographic Anatomy of the Paranasal Sinuses

1. Antrum of Highmore
2. Maxillary
3. Between the inner and outer tables of the skull, posterior to the glabella
4. 6 years
5. Lateral masses or labyrinths
6. B. Ostiomeatal complex
7. Sphenoid sinus
8. A. Nasal cavity (fossae)
    B. Maxillary sinuses
    C. Right temporal bone (squamous portion)
    D. Frontal sinuses
    E. Ethmoid sinuses
    F. Sphenoid sinuses
    G. Maxillary sinuses
    H. Ethmoid sinuses
    I. Frontal sinuses
    J. Squamous portion of left temporal bone

K. Mastoid portion of left temporal bone
    L. Sphenoid sinus
    M. Roots of upper teeth (alveolar process)
9. A. Sphenoid sinus
    B. Maxillary sinuses
    C. Ethmoid sinuses
    D. Frontal sinus
    E. Frontal sinuses
    F. Sphenoid sinus
    G. Ethmoid sinuses
    H. Maxillary sinuses
10. Infundibulum
11. True
12. B. Prone

Part II: Radiographic Positioning of Cranium

Review Exercise A: Skull Morphology, Topography, and Positioning of the Cranium

1. A. Mesocephalic (c)
    B. Brachycephalic (b)
    C. Dolichocephalic (a)
2. Mesocephalic, 47
3. ±40
4. False (These are other terms for the infraorbitomeatal line.)
5. 7° to 8°; 7° to 8° (same degrees of difference)
6. 1. G
    2. E
    3. J
    4. N
    5. H
    6. K
    7. D
    8. F
    9. B
    10. I
    11. O
    12. L
    13. C
    14. A
    15. M
7. 65 to 85 kV (analog) and 75 to 90 kV (digital systems)
8. A. Rotation
    B. Tilt
    C. Excessive neck flexion
    D. Excessive neck extension
    E. Incorrect central ray angulation
9. A. Rotation
    B. Tilt

10. A. LeFort
11. A. Computed tomography (CT)
12. B. Ultrasound
13. D. Nuclear medicine
14. A. 3
    B. 5
    C. 6
    D. 1
    E. 2
    F. 4
    G. 7
15. A. Advanced Paget's disease
16. Occipital
17. A. OML
18. C. Foramen magnum
19. D. Rotation
20. IOML; 37
21. Dorsum sellae and posterior clinoids should be projected into the foramen magnum.
22. 25° cephalad
23. 2 inches (5 cm) above the EAM
24. B. Rotation
25. In the lower ⅓ of the orbits
26. Excessive flexion or insufficient central ray angle
27. 0° posteroanterior (PA)
28. Rule out any possible cervical fractures or subluxation.
29. Tilt of the skull
30. B. IOML
31. D. Lateral
32. C. 25° to 30° PA axial
33. C. Lateral
34. A. 1½ inches (4 cm) superior to the nasion
35. A. CT

Review Exercise B: Problem Solving for Technical and Positioning Errors

1. Rotation of skull present; rotation of patient's face toward left
2. Excessive extension or excessive caudad central ray angle— projects the petrous ridges lower than expected (should be in the lower third of the orbit)
3. Rotation of the patient's face (skull) to the left
4. Insufficient extension of the skull, or central ray was not perpendicular to IOML
5. Skull tilt
6. Skull rotation
7. Central ray angled <37° to the IOML, or <30° to the OML

(would be caused by 30° angle to IOML). This error can be addressed with more flexion of the neck as well.

8. Collimated, lateral projection of the sella turcica
9. Right lateral projection of the skull
10. Should perform the PA axial projection (Haas method)
11. Horizontal beam (dorsal decubitus) lateral position—will demonstrate a possible air-fluid level in the sphenoid sinus
12. Ultrasound (sonography)—a noninvasive means of evaluating the newborn's cranium
13. Either MRI or CT can be performed.
14. Overangulation of the CR or excessive flexion of neck
15. No repeat exposure is required. Because of elongation of the facial mass with the AP axial projection for the skull, cutting off aspects of the mandible is acceptable.

Part III: Radiographic Positioning of Facial Bones, Mandible, and Paranasal Sinuses

Review Exercise A: Positioning of the Facial Bones

1. False (Best to perform erect)
2. True
3. False
4. True
5. False (It is used for this.)
6. False (Strong magnets in MRI prohibit this.)
7. Blow-out fracture
8. Tripod
9. Dense petrous pyramids superimpose the orbits, obscuring facial bone structures.
10. C. Zygoma
11. Waters method
12. Orbits including infraorbital rims, bony nasal septum, maxillae, zygomatic bones, and arches
13. B. 30°
14. Orbital rims and orbital floors
15. A. Reduces OID of facial bones
    B. Reduces exposure to anterior facial bones and neck

structures such as thyroid glands
16. A. IR is placed lengthwise for facial bones but crosswise for the cranium.
    B. CR is centered to the zygoma for facial bones and 2 inches (5 cm) above the EAM for the cranium.
17. Mentomeatal; 37°
18. Acanthion
19. Nasion
20. Lips—meatal; 55°
21. True
22. False (toward the affected side)
23. True
24. Maxillary sinuses; inferior orbital rims
25. Glabelloalveolar (GAL)
26. Zygomatic arches
27. 1 inch (2.5 cm) superior to glabella to pass through midarches
28. A. Rhese method
    B. Three-point landing
29. A. Cheek, nose, chin
    B. 53°
    C. Acanthiomeatal
    D. Lower outer
30. 1. E
    2. C
    3. F
    4. A
    5. D
    6. B

Review Exercise B: Positioning of the Mandible and Temporomandibular Joints (TMJ)

1. True
2. Axiolateral oblique
3. Extend the chin
4. A. 30°
    B. 45°
    C. 0°, true lateral
    D. 10° to 15°
    E. 25° cephalad
5. Insufficient cephalic CR angle or skull tilt
6. Acanthion (at lips for PA projection)
7. Orbitomeatal line (OML)
8. True
9. False (cephalad)
10. Condyloid process
11. A. 35° caudad
    B. 42° caudad

12. Glabella
13. SMV projection
14. Orthopantomography (panoramic tomography)
15. Narrow, vertical slit diaphragm
16. Infraorbitomeatal line (IOML)
17. Curved, nongrid cassette
18. True
19. True
20. B. Schuller
21. 25° to 30°; caudad
22. A. Modified Law
    B. 15°
    C. 15°
23. 40° caudad
24. Midsagittal

Review Exercise C: Positioning of the Paranasal Sinuses

1. 65 to 80 kV (analog); 75 to 85 kV (digital systems)
2. A. Perform positions erect when possible
    B. Use horizontal x-ray beam
3. True
4. True
5. False
6. A. Lateral
    B. PA Caldwell
    C. Parietoacanthial (Waters method)
    D. SMV
7. Lateral
8. Horizontal x-ray beam
9. Frontal and anterior ethmoid
10. 15°
11. A. Maxillary
    B. 37°
12. Mentomeatal line (MML)
13. Just below the maxillary sinuses
14. Sphenoid, ethmoid, and maxillary sinuses
15. Level of the acanthion
16. The mouth (oral cavity) is open with the PA transoral projection.
17. Sphenoid sinuses
18. 1. C
    2. D
    3. E
    4. A
    5. B

Review Exercise D: Problem Solving for Technical and Positioning Errors

1. Rotation of the skull
2. No. The petrous ridges should be projected just below the maxillary sinuses. The patient's head needs to be extended more.
3. Rotation of the skull
4. Yes, this image meets the evaluation criteria for a 30° PA axial projection.
5. Excessive flexion of the head and neck or incorrect CR angle will project the glabella into the nasal bones. The CR must be parallel to the glabelloalveolar line.
6. The head was tilted. Ensure that the MSP is parallel to the image receptor.
7. No. Increase extension of the head and neck. The AML should be placed perpendicular to the IR to ensure that the optic foramen is open and is projected into the lower outer quadrant of the orbit (skull rotation is correct).
8. Insufficient rotation of the skull toward the IR. The skull should be rotated 30° (from lateral position) toward the IR to prevent foreshortening of the body.
9. Parietoacanthial and R and L lateral projections. The parietoacanthial (Waters method) or the optional PA axial projections would demonstrate any possible septal deviation. The lateral projections would demonstrate any possible fracture of the nasal bones or anterior nasal spine. (The superoinferior tangential projection would provide an axial perspective but is considered an optional projection in most departments and not part of the routine unless specifically requested.)
10. Modified parietoacanthial (modified Waters method) projection
11. Perform the oblique inferosuperior (tangential) projections. These projections are ideal to demonstrate a depressed fracture of the zygomatic arch. (Bilateral projections are generally taken for comparison.)
12. Angle CR to place it perpendicular to the IOML. Angle the image receptor to maintain a perpendicular relationship between the CR and the image receptor. This will prevent distortion of the anatomy.
13. The head and neck need to be extended more to project the petrous ridges below the ethmoid sinuses.
14. Rotation of the skull
15. Tilt of the skull
16. Increase extension of the head and neck to project the entire sphenoid sinus through the oral cavity.
17. None. The petrous ridges should be below the floors of the maxillary sinuses on a well-positioned parietoacanthial projection.
18. The most diagnostic projection is the horizontal beam lateral projection to demonstrate any air-fluid levels.
19. The PA transoral special projection in addition to the routine four sinuses projection series (the lateral, PA Caldwell, parietoacanthial, and SMV)
20. PA, PA axial, and parietoacanthial projections will demonstrate a possible bony nasal septal deviation.

Part IV: Learning Exercises

Review Exercise A: Critique Radiographs of the Cranium

A. Lateral skull: 4-year-old (Fig. C11-198)
1. Foreign bodies (earrings) obscuring essential anatomic structures
2. Correct part positioning, but patient's hand seen supporting mandible; can use positioning sponge if needed to support skull
3. No evidence of collimation; correct central ray and IR placement
4. Appears underexposed on this printed copy (may be a repeatable error if actual radiograph also appears this underexposed)
5. No evidence of anatomic side marker
   Repeatable errors: 1 (anatomy demonstrated) and possibly 4 (slightly underexposed)

B. Lateral skull: 54-year-old, post-traumatic injury (Fig. C11-199)
1. Vertex of the skull just slightly cut off (may be repeatable error because of proximity to the site of trauma)
2. Tilted and rotated skull (separation of the orbital plates from the tilt; separation of the greater wings of the sphenoid, the rami of the mandible, and the EAMs—all indicating rotation)
3. No evidence of collimation; slightly high central ray centering if the photo borders are also the collimation borders, which would add to the tilt appearance
4. Acceptable exposure factors
5. No evidence of anatomic side marker
   Repeatable errors: 1 (anatomy demonstrated) and 2 (part positioning)

C. AP axial (Towne) skull: (Fig. C11-200)
1. Entire occipital bone and foramen magnum demonstrated
2. Correct part positioning
3. No evidence of collimation; overangled central ray; anterior arch of C1 projected into the foramen magnum rather than the dorsum sellae
4. Acceptable but slightly underexposed exposure factors
5. No evidence of anatomic side marker
   Repeatable errors: 3 (part positioning)

D. AP or PA skull (Fig. C11-201) AP 15° cephalad projection, as indicated by the large size of the orbits, which was caused by magnification from increased OID (can compare with radiograph that follows)
1. All pertinent anatomic structures demonstrated but with some foreshortening of frontal bone
2. Petrous ridges not in the lower third of orbits; position requires more flexion or less central ray angle as an AP; skull slightly rotated (note distance between orbits and lateral margins of skull)
3. No evidence of collimation; less central ray angle needed (can also compare with correctly angled central ray on PA radiograph in Fig. C11-202)
4. Acceptable exposure factors
5. No evidence of anatomic side marker
Repeatable errors: 2 (part positioning) and 3 (collimation and CR angle)

E. AP or PA skull (Fig. C11-202) PA 15° Caldwell projection
1. All pertinent anatomic structures not demonstrated; patient ID marker and side marker obscuring skull
2. Correct part positioning
3. Evidence of collimation (circular cone); size of IR too small for the skull; correct central ray placement and angle (petrous ridges in lower third of orbit)
4. Acceptable exposure factors
5. Evidence of anatomic side marker, but placed over skull; patient ID marker over upper right cranium—both repeatable errors
Repeatable errors: 1 (anatomy demonstrated) and 5 (incorrect placement of ID marker)

Review Exercise B: Critique Radiographs of the Facial Bones

A. Parietoacanthial (Waters) projection (Fig. C11-203)
1. Pertinent anatomy is all included but not well demonstrated because of positioning and exposure errors.
2. Skull is underextended. This led to the petrous ridges being projected into the lower maxillary sinuses. Also, skull appears to be rotated.
3. Collimation is not evident. CR and image receptor appears correct.
4. Acceptable exposure factors
5. Anatomic side marker is not evident.
Repeatable error(s): 2 (part positioning)

B. SMV mandible (Fig. C11-204)
1. Pertinent anatomy is included but not well demonstrated because of positioning error.
2. Skull is underextended and/or CR angle is incorrect. (IOML was not parallel to IR and not perpendicular to CR.) Mandible is foreshortened and rami projected into temporal bone.
3. Collimation is not evident. CR centering and IR placement are correct.
4. Image appears to be slightly underexposed.
5. Anatomic side marker is not evident.
Repeatable error(s): 2 (part positioning) (possibly 4—underexposed)

C. Optic foramina, Parieto-orbital oblique—Rhese method (Fig. C11-205)
1. Optic foramen is included but is slightly distorted.
2. Skull is rotated excessively toward a PA. (The skull is rotated >53° from the lateral position. This led to the optic foramen being projected into the middle lower aspect of the orbit.)
3. Collimation is not evident. CR and IR placement are correct.

4. Exposure factors are acceptable.
5. Anatomic side marker is not evident.
Repeatable error(s): 2 (The foramen is demonstrated; therefore, this may not be a repeatable error.)

D. Optic foramina, Parieto-orbital oblique—Rhese method (Fig. C11-206)
1. Optic foramen is distorted and totally obscured.
2. Skull appears to be overextended. (The AML was not perpendicular.) This projects the optic foramina into the infraorbital rim structure. Skull also appears to be under-rotated toward a lateral position. (If the skull is rotated <53° from the lateral position, the optic foramen will be projected into the lateral margin of the orbit.)
3. Collimation is evident and appears satisfactory. CR and IR placement are correct.
4. Exposure factors are acceptable.
5. Anatomic side marker is not evident.
Repeatable error(s): 1 (anatomy demonstrated) and 2 (part positioning)

E. Lateral facial bones (Fig. C11-207)
1. Very distal end of mandible is cut off. Probably would not justify repeat exposure unless this was a specific area of interest.
2. Skull is rotated. (Note the separation of rami of mandible, greater wings of sphenoid, and orbits.)
3. Collimation is evident and acceptable (except for cutoff of lower tip of mandible). CR and IR placement are acceptable.
4. Exposure factors appear to be satisfactory.
5. Anatomic side marker is not evident.
Repeatable error(s): 2 (part positioning) (possibly 1—anatomy demonstrated)

537

Review Exercise C: Critique Radiographs of the Paranasal Sinuses

A. Parietoacanthial transoral (open mouth Waters) (Fig. C11-208)
   1. Sphenoid and maxillary sinuses not well demonstrated. Petrous ridges are projected into lower aspect of maxillary sinuses. The base of the skull is superimposed over the sphenoid sinus.
   2. Skull is underextended, leading to errors previously described. (Chin is not elevated sufficiently.)
   3. Collimation is not centered to film. CR is centered too low (inferior) according to circular collimation on top, but this is not a repeatable error by itself. Film appears centered high, not aligned with CR.
   4. Exposure factors are acceptable.
   5. Anatomic side marker is not evident.
      Repeatable errors: 1 (anatomy demonstrated) and 2 (part positioning)
B. Parietoacanthial (Waters) (Fig. C11-209)
   1. Maxillary sinuses not well demonstrated. Petrous ridges are projected into lower aspect of maxillary sinuses. Artifacts appear to be either surgical clips and devices or external hair pins or clips.
   2. Skull is underextended and severely rotated.
   3. Collimation is not evident. CR centering and film placement are slightly low.
   4. Exposure factors are acceptable.
   5. Anatomic side marker is not evident.
      Repeatable errors: 1 (anatomy demonstrated) and 2 (part positioning)
C. Submentovertex (SMV) (Fig. C11-210)
   1. Maxillary and ethmoid sinuses not well demonstrated and partially cut off. Mandible is superimposed over sinuses.

   2. Skull is grossly underextended and tilted. (Also some rotation.)
   3. Collimation would have been OK if centering would have been correct. CR centering is off laterally. This led to cutoff of the anatomy.
   4. Exposure factors are acceptable.
   5. Anatomic side marker is not evident.
      Repeatable errors: 1 (anatomy demonstrated), 2 (part positioning), and 3 (CR centering)
D. Lateral projection (Fig. C11-211)
   1. Part of ethmoid and maxillary sinuses not well demonstrated because of superimposed mandible. Earrings were not removed.
   2. Skull is underextended and slightly rotated to the right.
   3. Collimation is acceptable. CR centering and film placement are acceptable but slightly anterior.
   4. Exposure factors are acceptable for the sphenoid/ethmoid sinuses.
   5. Anatomic side marker is not evident.
      Repeatable errors: 1 (anatomy demonstrated) and 2 (part positioning)

CHAPTER 12

Review Exercise A: Radiographic Anatomy and Pathology of the Gallbladder and Biliary System

1. 3 to 4 pounds (1. 5 kg), or 1/36 of total body weight
2. Right upper quadrant (RUQ)
3. Falciform ligament
4. Right
5. A. Quadrate
   B. Caudate
6. True
7. False (1 quart, or 800 to 1000 mL)
8. A. Store bile
   B. Concentrate bile
   C. Contracts to release bile into duodenum
9. True
10. Duodenal papilla

11. True
12. False (duct of Wirsung)
13. Anteriorly
14. 1. C
    2. A
    3. C
    4. C
15. A. Left hepatic duct
    B. Common hepatic duct
    C. Common bile duct
    D. Pancreatic duct
    E. Hepatopancreatic ampulla (ampulla of Vater)
    F. Duodenal papilla
    G. Duodenum
    H. Fundus of gallbladder
    I. Body of gallbladder
    J. Neck of gallbladder
    K. Cystic duct
    L. Right hepatic duct
16. A. No ionizing radiation
    B. Better detection of small calculi
    C. No contrast media required
    D. Less patient preparation
17. Study of both the gallbladder and biliary ducts
18. D. Nuclear medicine
19. True
20. 1. C
    2. D
    3. F
    4. A
    5. E
    6. B

Review Exercise B: Radiographic Anatomy of the Upper Gastrointestinal System

1. A. Mouth
   B. Pharynx
   C. Esophagus
   D. Stomach
   E. Small intestine
   F. Large intestine
   G. Anus
2. A. Salivary glands
   B. Pancreas
   C. Liver
   D. Gallbladder
3. A. Intake and digestion of food
   B. Absorption of digested food particles
   C. Elimination of solid waste products
4. Esophagram or barium swallow

5. Upper gastrointestinal (UGI) series or upper GI
6. A. Parotid
   B. Sublingual
   C. Submandibular
7. Deglutition
8. A. Nasopharynx
   B. Oropharynx
   C. Laryngopharynx
9. A. Aortic arch
   B. Left primary bronchus
10. A. Esophagus
    B. Inferior vena cava
    C. Aorta
11. Duodenal bulb or cap
12. Duodenojejunal flexure (suspensory muscle of the duodenum or ligament of Treitz)
13. Retroperitoneal (or "behind peritoneum")
14. A. Tongue
    B. Oral cavity (mouth)
    C. Hard palate
    D. Soft palate
    E. Uvula
    F. Nasopharynx
    G. Oropharynx
    H. Epiglottis
    I. Laryngopharynx
    J. Larynx
    K. Esophagus
    L. Trachea
15. False (inferiorly and anteriorly)
16. A. Fundus
    B. Greater curvature
    C. Body
    D. Gastric canal
    E. Pyloric portion (pylorus)
    F. Pyloric orifice (or just pylorus)
    G. Angular notch (incisura angularis)
    H. Lesser curvature
    I. Esophagogastric junction (cardiac orifice)
    J. Cardiac antrum
    K. Cardiac notch (incisura cardiaca)
17. A. Fundus (labeled A on Fig. 12-3)
    B. Body (labeled C)
    C. Pylorus (labeled E)
18. Pyloric antrum and pyloric canal
19. Rugae
20. A. Supine
    B. Prone
    C. Erect

21. A. Pylorus (pyloric sphincter)
    B. Bulb or cap of duodenum
    C. First (superior) portion of duodenum
    D. Second (descending) portion of duodenum
    E. Third (horizontal) portion of duodenum
    F. Fourth (ascending) portion of duodenum
    G. Head of pancreas
    H. Suspensory muscle of duodenum or ligament of Treitz
22. A. Head of pancreas
    B. C-loop of duodenum
23. A. Distal esophagus
    B. Area of esophagogastric junction
    C. Lesser curve of stomach
    D. Angular notch (incisura angularis)
    E. Pyloric region of stomach
    F. Pyloric valve or sphincter
    G. Duodenal bulb
    H. Second descending portion of duodenum
    I. Body of stomach
    J. Greater curvature of stomach
    K. Mucosal folds or rugae of stomach
    L. Fundus of stomach

Review Exercise C: Mechanical and Chemical Digestion and Body Habitus

1. True
2. A. Pharynx
3. Chyme
4. Rhythmic segmentation
5. A. Carbohydrates
   B. Proteins
   C. Lipids (fats)
6. Enzymes
7. A. Simple sugars
   B. Fatty acids and glycerol
   C. Amino acids
8. Bile
9. Large fat droplets are broken down to small fat droplets, which have greater surface area (to volume) and give enzymes greater access for the breakdown of lipids
10. A. Small intestine
    B. Stomach
11. Carbohydrates
12. Large intestine

13. Mechanical
14. Chyme
15. A. Hypersthenic
16. C. Hyposthenic/asthenic
17. 1 to 2 inches (2.5 to 5 cm)
18. A. Stomach
    B. Gallbladder
19. Inferior, because of its proximity to the diaphragm
20. 1. A, B
    2. B
    3. B, C
    4. C, D
    5. C, E

Review Exercise D: Contrast Media, Fluoroscopy, and Clinical Indications and Contraindications for Upper Gastrointestinal Studies

1. True
2. Radiolucent contrast medium
3. Calcium or magnesium citrate
4. Barium sulfate
5. Suspension (colloidal)
6. True
7. True
8. One part water to one part barium sulfate (1:1 ratio)
9. $BaSO_4$
10. When the mixture may escape into the peritoneal cavity
11. Sensitivity to iodine
12. Better coating and visibility of the mucosa. Polyps, diverticula, and ulcers are better demonstrated.
13. Motility
14. It forces the barium sulfate against the mucosa for better coating.
15. C. CCD (charge-coupled device)
16. C. Bucky slot shield
17. By moving the Bucky tray all the way to the end of the table
18. B. 0.5 mm Pb/eq apron
19. C. Reduces exposure to arms and hands of radiologist
20. 1. $7 - 3.3 \times 5 = 8.5 - 16.5$ mrad
21. A. Time
    B. Distance
    C. Shielding
22. Distance
23. A. Optional postfluoroscopy overhead images

B. Multiple frames formatting and multiple original images
C. Cine loop capability
D. Image enhancement and manipulation
24. Cine loop capability
25. A. 7
 B. 5
 C. 6
 D. 3
 E. 2
 F. 1
 G. 4
26. A. 4
 B. 5
 C. 8
 D. 3
 E. 7
 F. 1
 G. 6
 H. 2
27. A. 5
 B. 6
 C. 7
 D. 3
 E. 2
 F. 8
 G. 4
 H. 1
28. Endoscopy
29. Antral muscle at the orifice of the pylorus
30. Ultrasound (sonography)

Review Exercise E: Patient Preparation and Positioning for Esophagram and Upper Gastrointestinal Study

1. Literally stands for *non per os*, a Latin phrase meaning "nothing by mouth"
2. False (8 hours NPO for upper GI but not for an esophagram)
3. True
4. Barium-soaked cotton balls, barium pills, or marshmallows followed by thin barium
5. A. Breathing exercises
 B. Water test
 C. Compression (paddle) technique
 D. Toe-touch maneuver
6. Valsalva maneuver
7. LPO (slight)
8. Esophagogastric junction
9. Oral, water-soluble iodinated contrast media

10. 8 hours
11. Both activities tend to increase gastric secretions
12. D. All of the above
13. Left hand
14. Newborn to 1 year: 2 to 4 ounces
 1 to 3 years: 4 to 6 ounces
 3 to 10 years: 6 to 12 ounces
 >10 years: 12 to 16 ounces
15. Pulsed, grid-controlled fluoroscopy (to reduce dose for all patients, but especially children)
16. D. Endoscopy
17. B. Radionuclides
18. Places the esophagus between the vertebral column and heart
19. 35° to 40°
20. Optional swimmer's lateral
21. A. RAO
 B. Left lateral
 C. AP
22. B. Pylorus of stomach and C-loop
23. C. 40° to 70°
24. 100 to 125 kV
25. Body and pylorus of stomach and duodenal bulb
26. To prevent superimposition of the pylorus over the duodenal bulb, and better visualize the lesser and greater curvatures of the stomach
27. C. 35° to 45° cephalad
28. B. Lateral
29. 90 to 100 kV range
30. Upright (erect)
31. A. RAO
 B. PA
 C. Right lateral
 D. LPO
 E. AP
32. Left upper quadrant (LUQ)
33. Right
34. False (expiration)

Review Exercise F: Problem Solving for Technical and Positioning Errors

1. When using thin barium, have the patient drink continuously during the exposure. With thick barium, have the patient hold two or three spoonfuls in the mouth and make the exposure immediately after swallowing.

2. When using barium sulfate as a contrast medium, 100 to 125 kV should be used to ensure proper penetration of the contrast-filled stomach and visualize the mucosa; 90 to 100 kV would be adequate for a double-contrast study.
3. AP. Because the fundus is more posterior than the body or pylorus, it will fill with barium when the patient is in a supine (AP) position.
4. With a hypersthenic patient, more rotation (up to 70°) may be required to better profile the duodenal bulb. (Note: The radiologist under fluoroscopic guidance will frequently move the patient as needed for the overhead oblique to best profile the duodenal region. Observe the degree of rotation of the body required to profile the stomach during fluoroscopy.)
5. The LPO position (recumbent) produces an image in which the fundus and body are filled with barium but the duodenal bulb is air filled.
6. Upper GI series
7. An oral, water-soluble contrast media should be used for an upper GI when ruptured viscus or bowel is suspected (not barium sulfate, which is not water soluble).
8. With radiolucent foreign bodies in the esophagus, shredded cotton soaked in barium sulfate may be used to help locate it. But today, most foreign body studies of the esophagus are located and removed through endoscopy.
9. Would center lower than usual, to the mid-L3 to L4 region or about 1½ to 2 inches (4 to 5 cm) above the level of the iliac crest
10. A mass of undigested material that gets trapped in the stomach; a rare condition that can be diagnosed with an upper GI study
11. Under-rotation of the body into the RAO position led to the esophagus being superimposed

over the vertebral column. An increase in rotation of the body during the repeat exposure will separate the esophagus from the spine.

12. Angle the CR 20° to 25° cephalad to open up the body and pylorus of the stomach.

13. The lateral position best demonstrates a gastric diverticulum located in the posterior region of the stomach.

14. Nuclear medicine is an effective modality in detecting Barrett's esophagus.

15. Hemochromatosis is a condition of abnormal iron deposits in the liver parenchyma. Magnetic resonance imaging (MRI) is an effective imaging modality in diagnosing this condition.

CHAPTER 13

Review Exercise A: Radiographic Anatomy and Function of the Lower Gastrointestinal System

1. A. 23 feet, or 7 m
   B. 15 to 18 feet, or 4.5 to 5.5 m
   C. 5 feet, or 1.5 m
2. A. Duodenum
   B. Jejunum
   C. Ileum
3. Duodenum
4. LUQ and LLQ
5. Jejunum
6. Ileum
7. Cecum and rectum
8. Four sections; two flexures
9. A. Prevents contents of the ileum from passing too quickly into cecum
   B. Prevents reflux back into the ileum
10. Vermiform appendix
11. 1. H, 2. F, 3. D, 4. B, 5. C, 6. I, 7. E, 8. A, 9. G
12. A. *Taeniae coli*
    B. Haustra
13. Plicae circulares
14. A. Vermiform appendix (appendix)
    B. Cecum
    C. Ileocecal valve (sphincter)
    D. Ascending colon
    E. Right colic (hepatic) flexure

F. Transverse colon
G. Left colic (splenic) flexure
H. Descending colon
I. Sigmoid colon
J. Rectum
K. Anal canal
L. Anus
M. Sacrum
N. Coccyx
O. Anal canal
P. Anus
Q. Rectal ampulla
R. Rectum
15. Jejunum
16. Ileum
17. Ileum
18. Duodenojejunal junction
19. Right lower quadrant (RLQ)
20. Suspensory muscle of the duodenum or ligament of Treitz (This site is a reference point for certain small bowel exams because it remains in a relatively fixed position.)
21. Cecum
22. Left colic (splenic)
23. Appendicitis
24. B. Transverse colon
    D. Sigmoid colon
25. A. Small intestine
26. C. Large intestine
27. A. Peristalsis
28. A. Duodenum
    B. Region of suspensory muscle of duodenum/duodenojejunal flexure
    C. Jejunum
    D. Ileum
    E. Region of ileocecal valve
29. A. Cecum
    B. Ascending colon
    C. Right colic (hepatic) flexure
    D. Transverse colon
    E. Left colic (splenic) flexure
    F. Descending colon
    G. Sigmoid colon
    H. Rectum
30. 1. A
    2. B
    3. A
    4. B
    5. A
    6. B
    7. C
    8. B
    9. A
    10. A

Review Exercise B: Clinical Indications and Radiographic Procedures for the Small Bowel Series and Barium Enema

1. D. All of the above
2. A. Possible perforated hollow viscus
   B. Large bowel obstruction
3. Young and dehydrated
4. A. 3
   B. 8
   C. 1
   D. 4
   E. 2
   F. 6
   G. 5
   H. 7
5. A. 3
   B. 5
   C. 1
   D. 4
   E. 2
   F. 6
6. D. All of the above
7. D. Nuclear medicine
8. B. Proximal small intestine
9. 2 cups or 16 ounces
10. When the contrast medium passes through the ileocecal valve
11. 2 hours
12. 15 to 30 minutes after ingesting the contrast medium
13. True
14. Double-contrast method
15. High-density barium sulfate and air or methylcellulose
16. Regional enteritis (Crohn's disease) and malabsorption syndromes
17. False (24 hours)
18. A. Duodenojejunal flexure (suspensory muscle of duodenum)
19. It dilates the intestinal lumen to produce a more diagnostic study.
20. C. Therapeutic intubation
21. NPO for at least 8 hours before procedure; no smoking or gum chewing
22. Prone. To separate the loops of intestine
23. A. 4
    B. 2
    C. 6
    D. 5
    E. 3
    F. 1

24. Infant
25. Diverticulosis
26. C. Volvulus
27. A. Ulcerative colitis
28. C. Annular carcinoma
29. False
30. True
31. False
32. True
33. A. Gross bleeding
    B. Severe diarrhea
    C. Obstruction
    D. Inflammatory lesions
34. False (castor oil is an irritant cathartic)
35. A. Plastic disposable
    B. Rectal retention
    C. Air-contrast retention
36. True
37. Room temperature (85° to 90°)
38. B. Lidocaine
39. Sims' position
40. C. Umbilicus
41. B. Double-contrast barium enema
42. C. Anorectal angle
43. C. Rectal prolapse
44. C. Evacuative proctogram
45. D. Lateral
46. True
47. False (not more than 24 inches [60 cm] above tabletop when beginning the procedure)
48. True
49. True
50. False
51. B. 0.1% barium sulfate suspension is instilled before the procedure
52. Virtual colonoscopy
53. False
54. C. To mark or "tag" fecal matter
55. A. Cannot remove polyps discovered during CTC

Review Exercise C: Positioning of the Lower Gastrointestinal System

1. False
2. D. Prone PA
3. False
4. Every 20 to 30 minutes
5. False (generally should not be removed until after overhead projections are completed unless directed to do so by the radiologist)
6. Ventral decubitus
7. 100 to 125 kV
8. C. 2 inches (5 cm) above iliac crest
9. Make exposure on expiration
10. Ileocecal valve—large intestine
11. A. Hypersthenic
12. RAO or LPO
13. 35° to 45°
14. RPO
15. Left lateral decubitus
16. Level of ASIS at the midcoronal plane
17. Right lateral decubitus (left side up)
18. Rectosigmoid region
19. Creates less superimposition of the rectosigmoid segments
20. A. Butterfly projections
    B. AP: CR angled 30° to 40° cephalad
    C. PA: CR 30° to 40° caudad
21. A. PA prone
22. 90 to 100 kV
23. A. 100 to 125 kV
    B. 90 to 100 kV
24. Glucagon (review patient history to ensure not diabetic before given)

Review Exercise D: Problem Solving for Technical and Positioning Errors

1. PA prone. Because the transverse colon is an intraperitoneal aspect of the large intestine located more anteriorly, it will fill with barium in the PA prone position.
2. Even with the use of a wedge compensating filter, a reduction in kV is required. Because less barium sulfate is used during an air-contrast procedure, the kV range should be 90 to 100.
3. The CR was angled in the wrong direction. The AP axial projection requires a 30° to 40° cephalad angle.
4. Use two 35- × 43-cm (14- × 17-inch) crosswise IRs for the AP/PA and oblique projections, one centered higher and one lower. Because hypersthenic patients have a wider distribution of the large intestine, two crosswise-placed cassettes will ensure that all of the pertinent anatomy is demonstrated.
5. Retention catheters should be fully inflated only by the radiologist under fluoroscopic guidance.
6. Lay on left side and flex head and upper body forward, drawing the right leg up above the partially flexed left leg.
7. Enteroclysis, a double-contrast small bowel procedure. A routine small bowel series may also demonstrate this condition, but the enteroclysis with double contrast is more effective in demonstrating mucosal changes. A CT enteroclysis may provide further evidence of obstruction or narrowing of the small intestine.
8. Because the patient is having surgery soon after the small bowel series, a water-soluble, iodinated contrast medium should be used. Barium sulfate should not be given to presurgical patients.
9. A diagnostic intubation small bowel series is preferred. A nasogastric tube is passed into the small intestine, allowing the contrast medium to be instilled. This procedure is effective for patients who cannot swallow.
10. A barium enema or air enema often leads to re-expansion of the telescoped aspect of the large intestine.
11. Inform the radiologist and have him or her insert it under fluoroscopic guidance.
12. RAO or LPO projections
13. A small bowel series (Enteritis is an inflammation or infection of the small intestine.)
14. A small bowel series (Giardiasis is a parasitic infection of the small intestine.)
15. The patient should undergo a cleansing bowel preparation. The morning of the procedure, food intake should be limited to clear liquids. The patient should wear loose-fitting clothing without any metal snaps or clips.

CHAPTER 14

Review Exercise A: Radiographic Anatomy of the Urinary System

1. D. Retroperitoneal
2. Suprarenal (adrenal) glands
3. Psoas major muscles
4. Perirenal fat or adipose capsule
5. 30°
6. Xiphoid process and iliac crest
7. Nephroptosis
8. A. Remove nitrogenous waste
   B. Regulate water levels
   C. Regulate acid-base balance
9. B. Uremia
10. Hilum
11. Cortex
12. Renal parenchyma
13. Nephron
14. False (afferent)
15. Bowman capsule
16. False (located in the cortex)
17. Renal pyramids
18. A. Renal pelvis
    B. Major calyx
    C. Minor calyx
    D. Renal sinuses
    E. Cortex
    F. Medulla
    G. Ureter
19. A. Loop of Henle, medulla
    B. Distal convoluted tubule, cortex
    C. Afferent arteriole, cortex
    D. Efferent arteriole, cortex
    E. Glomerular capsule, cortex
    F. Proximal convoluted tubule, cortex
    G. Descending limb, medulla
    H. Ascending limb, medulla
    I. Collecting tubule, medulla
20. A. Peristalsis
    B. Gravity
21. C. Urinary bladder
22. Ureterovesical junction
23. Trigone
24. Prostate gland
25. C. 350 to 500 mL
26. D. Kidneys
27. A. Minor calyces
    B. Major calyces
    C. Renal pelvis
    D. Ureteropelvic junction (UPJ)
    E. Proximal ureter
    F. Distal ureter
    G. Urinary bladder

Review Exercise B: Venipuncture

1. A. Bolus injection
   B. Drip infusion
2. True
3. D. Antecubital fossa
4. C. 18 to 22 gauge
5. Butterfly and over-the-needle catheter
6. 1. Wash hands and put on gloves.
   2. Select site, apply tourniquet, and cleanse the site.
   3. Initiate puncture.
   4. Confirm entry and secure needle.
   5. Prepare and proceed with injection.
   6. Remove needle or catheter.
7. False (facing upward)
8. False (The needle should be withdrawn and pressure applied.)
9. True
10. False (The technologist or person performing the venipuncture is responsible.)

Review Exercise C: Contrast Media and Urography

1. A. I
   B. N
   C. I
   D. I
   E. N
   F. N
   G. N
   H. I
   I. N
   J. I
2. A. Diatrizoate or iothalamate
3. D. Chemotoxic theory
4. Side effect
5. 0.6 to 1.5 mg/dL
6. 8 to 25 mg/100 mL
7. A. Diabetes mellitus
   B. 48 hours
8. Extravasation (infiltration)
9. A. Local
   B. Systemic
10. Anaphylactic reaction
11. Vasovagal reaction
12. False
13. A. 3
    B. 2
    C. 2
    D. 1
    E. 3
    F. 3
    G. 3
    H. 3
    I. 1
14. True
15. False (the term for hives)
16. C. Severe
17. A. 4
    B. 1
    C. 3
    D. 4
    E. 2
    F. 2
    G. 1
    H. 4
    I. 5
    J. 4
    K. 3
18. Call for medical assistance
19. To reduce the severity of contrast media reactions
20. C. Combination of Benadryl and prednisone
21. B. Asthmatic patient
22. Elevate the affected extremity or use a cold compress followed by a warm compress
23. False—peaks 24 to 48 hours after extravasation
24. True
25. A. Hypersensitivity to iodinated contrast media
    B. Anuria
    C. Multiple myeloma
    D. Diabetes mellitus
    E. Severe hepatic or renal disease
    F. Congestive heart failure
    G. Pheochromocytoma
    H. Sickle cell anemia
    I. Patients taking metformin or similar medication
    J. Renal failure, acute or chronic

Review Exercise D: Radiographic Procedures and Pathologic Terms and Indications

1. Lasix
2. A. An IVP (intravenous pyelogram) is a study of the renal pelvis (hence, *pyelo-*).
   B. Intravenous urogram (IVU)
3. The collecting system of the kidney
4. C. Hematuria
5. A. Pheochromocytoma
6. A. 5

B. 8
C. 3
D. 10
E. 1
F. 11
G. 12
H. 4
I. 2
J. 7
K. 9
L. 6
7. A. 7
B. 4
C. 8
D. 1
E. 5
F. 2
G. 3
H. 6
8. A. 5
B. 7
C. 8
D. 3
E. 2
F. 1
G. 4
H. 6
9. Angioedema
10. Bronchospasm
11. Syncope
12. Urticaria
13. Staghorn calculi
14. True
15. To enhance filling of the pelvi-caliceal system with contrast media
16. A. Possible ureteric stones
B. Abdominal mass
C. Abdominal aortic aneurysm
D. Recent abdominal surgery
E. Severe abdominal pain
F. Acute abdominal trauma
17. At start of injection of contrast media
18. A. 1-minute nephrogram or nephrotomography
B. 5-minute full KUB
C. 10- to 15-minute full KUB
D. 20-minute posterior R and L oblique positions
E. Postvoid (prone PA or erect AP)
19. A hypertensive IVU requires a shorter span of time between projections.
20. Surgery (inpatient or outpatient facility)

21. False (nonfunctional exam)
22. False (used for males only)
23. D. All of the above
24. C. Magnetic resonance imaging
25. True
26. True
27. Height and weight
28. True
29. A. MRI
30. True

Review Exercise E: Radiographic Positioning of the Urinary System

1. The prostate gland will indent the floor of the bladder.
2. Just medial to the ASIS and lateral to the spine (placed over the outer pelvic brim)
3. Place the patient in a 15° Trendelenburg position.
4. Renal pelvis, major and minor calyces of the kidneys
5. A. Verify patient preparation
B. Determine whether exposure factors are acceptable
C. Verify positioning
D. Detect any abnormal calcifications
6. A. Primarily the ureters
7. 30° RPO
8. 70 to 75 kV analog; 75 to 80 kV digital
9. False (both an AP erect and supine IVU image have a recommended 40-inch SID)
10. False (not female; would obscure essential anatomy)
11. True
12. Three
13. D. Within 1 minute after injection
14. B. Midway between xiphoid process and iliac crest
15. RPO
16. 30°
17. Erect position
18. C. 10° to 15° caudad
19. True

Review Exercise F: Problem Solving for Technical and Positioning Errors

1. A second projection of the bladder should be taken, using a smaller IR placed crosswise to

include this region. The larger IR should be centered 1 or 2 inches (2 to 5 cm) higher to include the upper abdomen.
2. Too long of a delay between the injection of contrast media and the imaging of the nephrogram. The nephrogram needs to be taken no later than 60 seconds after injection.
3. Decrease the obliquity of the RPO to no more than 30°.
4. Place the pneumatic paddles just medial to the ASIS to allow for compression of the distal ureters against the pelvic brim.
5. Increase caudad angulation of the central ray to project the symphysis pubis below the bladder. The typical CR angle is 10° to 15° caudad.
6. Decrease the span of time between projections to capture all phases of the urinary system. (Take images at 1, 2, and 3 minutes rather than 1, 5, and 15 minutes.)
7. The technologist should not perform the compression phase of the study. Ureteric compression is contraindicated when an abdominal aortic aneurysm is suspected. (The technologist should consult with the radiologist or physician.)
8. The erect prevoid AP projection will best demonstrate an enlarged prostate gland.
9. Ultrasound, CT, or nuclear medicine scan
10. CT is preferred, but a nuclear medicine procedure could also be performed.
11. The patient should be asked whether he is taking metformin or similar medication to control diabetes. If the response is yes, document and inform the radiologist of the patient's condition and medication history before injection. The referring physician may be asked to check kidney function before the patient resumes this medication.
12. These are expected side effects, and the technologist should reassure the patient. No medical treatment is required.

13. Although the technologist should inform the radiologist or injecting technologist of the blood chemistry levels, both BUN and creatinine levels are within the range of normal.

CHAPTER 15

Review Exercise A: Mobile X-Ray Equipment and Radiation Protection

1. A. Battery-powered, battery-driven type
   B. Standard AC power source, nonmotor drive
2. True
3. 8 hours
4. Standard power source, nonmotor drive
5. C-arm
6. A. X-ray tube
   B. Image intensifier
7. Because it results in a significant increase in exposure to the head and neck region of the operator
8. A. Intensifier side
   B. The radiation field pattern extends out farther on the x-ray tube side.
9. Left monitor
10. True
11. True
12. Four
13. False (can be used)
14. Roadmapping
15. C. 50 to 100 mR/h
16. A. 5 mR (60 mR ÷ 60 min = 1 mR × 5 min = 5)
17. B. 25 mR/h
18. 67 mR (400 ÷ 60 × 10 = 67)
19. C. 100 to 300 mR/h
20. False (reduces exposure to patient)

Review Exercise B: Trauma Positioning Principles and Fracture Terminology

1. Adaptation
2. Move the CR and IR around the patient to produce similar projections rather than moving the patient.
3. Two. Two projections should be taken 90° to each other.
4. Two. Both joints must be included on the initial study.
5. False (must include at least one joint nearest injury)
6. True
7. True
8. False (It is important to rotate the x-ray tube and image receptor around patients if they are unable to move.)
9. A. Dislocation
   B. Luxation
10. A. Shoulder
    B. Fingers or thumb
    C. Patella
    D. Hip
11. Subluxation
12. Sprain
13. Contusion
14. Apposition
15. Bayonet apposition
16. A. Varus (deformity) angulation
    B. Lateral apex
17. A simple fracture does not break through the skin, but a compound fracture protrudes through the skin.
18. A. Torus fracture
    B. Greenstick fracture
19. Butterfly fracture
20. Impacted fracture
21. A. Chauffeur's
    B. Mallet
    C. Open
    D. Ping-pong
    E. Closed
22. False. (A chip fracture involves an isolated fracture not associated with a tendon or ligament.)
23. Closed reduction
24. 1. G
    2. H
    3. A
    4. I
    5. D
    6. J
    7. B
    8. M
    9. L
    10. N
    11. F
    12. O
    13. E
    14. K
    15. C
25. A. Colles' fracture
    B. Distal radius, posterior displacement of distal fragment

C. Fall on outstretched arm
26. A. Pott's fracture
    B. Distal fibula and occasionally the distal tibia or medial malleolus

Review Exercise C: Trauma and Mobile Positioning and Procedures

1. Centered 3 to 4 inches (8 to 10 cm) below jugular notch, angled caudad so as to be perpendicular to sternum
2. A. Crosswise
   B. To prevent side cutoff of the right or left lateral margins of the chest. More important with portable chests because of increased divergence of x-ray beam at the shorter SID.
3. False (not recommended because of probable grid cutoff)
4. 15° to 20° LPO
5. Crosswise
6. 30° to 40° cross-angled mediolateral projection (Note: This results in image distortion and should be done as a last resort.)
7. A. Left lateral decubitus
8. D. Dorsal decubitus
9. Increased OID of the thumb (increases distortion)
10. PA and lateral projections
11. C. 65 kV and 10 mAs
12. True
13. True
14. AP and horizontal beam, transthoracic lateral or scapular Y projection
15. A horizontal beam transthoracic lateral
16. A. 25 to 30
17. B. 15°
18. C. 10° posteriorly from perpendicular to plantar surface (Note: This would also be 10° posteriorly from plane of IR.)
19. Angle the CR 15° to 20° lateromedially to the long axis of the foot.
20. AP and horizontal beam lateral with no flexion of knee
21. 45° lateromedial cross-angle AP projection of the knee and proximal tibia/fibula
22. A. Danelius-Miller method

23. Direct horizontal CR perpendicular to the femoral neck and to the plane of the IR
24. D. Fuchs method (Review Chapter 8 for details)
25. Swimmer's lateral using a horizontal beam CR
26. D. 35° to 40° cephalad axial projection (CR parallel to MML)
27. AP axial trauma oblique projections
28. A. 45° lateromedial
    B. 15° cephalad
29. False. A grid can be used for this projection because of the double angulation
30. C. Horizontal beam lateral skull
31. C. AP skull, CR 15° cephalad to OML
32. False (should not exceed 45°)
33. True
34. Parallel to the mentomeatal line, centered to acanthion
35. 25° to 30° cephalad and possibly 5° to 10° posterior to clear the shoulder
36. D. PA or AP and horizontal beam lateral forearm
37. A. Pediatric
38. A. AP and horizontal beam lateral lower leg
39. C. Stellate fracture

Review Exercise D: Surgical Radiography

1. A. Confidence
   B. Mastery
   C. Problem-solving skills
   D. Communication
2. 1. E
   2. A
   3. B
   4. D
   5. F
   6. C
3. False
4. False (The technologist is responsible to ensure radiation safety in the OR.)
5. True
6. Asepsis
7. D. Surgical asepsis
8. C. The shoulders to the level of the sterile field
9. False

10. A. Drape the image intensifier, x-ray tube, and C-arm using a sterile cloth and/or bags.
    B. Drape the patient or surgery site with an additional sterile cloth before the undraped C-arm is positioned over the anatomy.
    C. Maintain the sterile area by using a "shower curtain."
11. False
12. True
13. True
14. False
15. Aerosol
16. Added patient dose
17. Brighter image
18. Distance
19. A. Time
    B. Distance
    C. Shielding
20. C. Use intermittent or "foot-tapping" fluoroscopy
21. Biliary ductal system
22. "Pizza pan"
23. Crosswise to prevent grid cutoff
24. 6 to 8 mL
25. A. Can be performed as an outpatient procedure
    B. Less invasive procedure
    C. Reduced hospital time and cost
26. A. Left hepatic duct
    B. Right hepatic duct
    C. Common hepatic duct
    D. Common bile duct
    E. Duodenum
27. D
28. B
29. C
30. D
31. A
32. A
33. Modular bipolar hip prostheses
34. Laminectomy
35. Interbody fusion cages
36. Supine
37. A. Harrington rods
    B. Luque rods
38. A. 4
    B. 5
    C. 3
    D. 8
    E. 9
    F. 10
    G. 7
    H. 2

I. 1
J. 6
39. A. Compression fracture of the vertebral body

CHAPTER 16

Review Exercise A: Introduction, Immobilization, Ossification, Radiation Protection, Pre-exam Preparation, and Clinical Indications

1. A. Technologist's attitude and approach to a child
   B. Technical preparation of the room
2. A. Serve as an observer in the room to lend support and comfort to their child.
   B. Serve as a participator to assist with immobilization.
   C. Remain in the waiting room, and do not accompany the child into the room.
3. False (may be permissible with proper lead shielding if not pregnant)
4. True
5. True
6. Pigg-O-Stat
7. Erect chest and abdomen studies
8. It can damage the skin.
9. A. Twisting the tape so that the adhesive surface is not against the skin
   B. Placing a gauze pad between the tape and the skin
10. 1. Place the sheet on the table folded in half or thirds lengthwise.
    2. Place patient in middle of sheet with the right arm down to the side. Fold sheet across the patient's body and pull sheet across the body, keeping the arm against the body.
    3. Place the patient's left arm along the side of the body and on top of the sheet. Bring the free sheet over the left arm to the right side of the body. Wrap the sheet around the body as needed.
    4. Pull the sheet tightly so that the patient cannot free arms.

11. Diaphysis
12. Epiphyses
13. Metaphysis
14. C. 25 years old
15. D. 12 years old
16. False (correct term is *nonaccidental trauma, NAT*)
17. False (The technologist should report to the radiologist or supervising technologist.)
18. 1. Neglect
    2. Physical abuse
    3. Sexual abuse
    4. Psychological maltreatment
    5. Medical neglect
19. Multiple and posterior fractures are an indication of a child being held up and shaken.
20. A. Proper immobilization
    B. Short exposure times
    C. Accurate manual technique charts
21. A. Close collimation
    B. Low-dosage techniques
    C. Minimum number of exposures
22. 1. B, 2. A, 3. B, 4. A, 5. B, 6. A
23. False (These items may cause artifacts and should be removed.)
24. True
25. D. Pitch ratio
26. False
27. A. Sonography
28. A. Sonography
29. C. Hydrocephalus
30. A. 4
    B. 2
    C. 7
    D. 1
    E. 3
    F. 5
    G. 6
31. A. 6
    B. 7
    C. 4
    D. 8
    E. 2
    F. 1
    G. 3
    H. 5
32. A. 5
    B. 1
    C. 6
    D. 3
    E. 7
    F. 2
    G. 4

33. A. (−)
    B. (−)
    C. (−)
34. C. Dark green secretion of the liver and intestinal glands mixed with amniotic fluid
35. True

Review Exercise B: Pediatric Positioning of the Chest, Skeletal System, and Skull

1. True
2. A. Nongrid
   B. Analog: 70 to 80 kV; Digital: 75 to 85 kV
   C. Crosswise
   D. 50 to 60 inches (127 to 153 cm)
   E. 72 inches (183 cm)
3. Analog: 75 to 80 kV; Digital: 80 to 90 kV
4. No
5. Two to four
6. As the child fully inhales and holds his or her breath
7. The sternoclavicular joints and lateral rib margins should be equidistant from the vertebral column.
8. Horizontally
9. False (9 to 10)
10. True
11. True
12. A. 1
    B. 2
    C. 1
    D. 2
    E. 1
13. Bilateral frog-leg
14. AP and lateral feet, Kite method
15. False (Take two projections 90° from each other.)
16. True (if correctly placed)
17. Base selection on the size of the anatomy be selected (10 × 12 or 24 × 30 cm if the skull is near adult size)
18. A. 15° cephalad to OML
19. C. Craniostenosis
20. B. OML
21. False
22. True
23. A. Mamillary (nipple) line
    B. 1 inch (2. 5 cm) above umbilicus

C. At level of iliac crest
D. Glabella

Review Exercise C: Positioning of the Pediatric Abdomen and Contrast Media Procedures

1. Vesicoureteral reflux
2. False (Retention tips should not be used on small children.)
3. Air for the pneumatic reduction of intussusception
4. 3 feet (1 meter) (for pediatric patients)
5. True
6. False (Most bony landmarks are nonexistent in infants.)
7. True
8. False (Contrast is low.)
9. A. 4 hours
   B. 3 hours
   C. No prep required
   D. 4 hours (solid food)
10. A. Hirschsprung's disease
    B. Extensive diarrhea
    C. Appendicitis
    D. Obstruction
    E. Dehydration (patients who cannot withstand fluid loss)
11. The following indicators apply: B, C, D, F, G
12. 1 inch (2.5 cm) above the umbilicus
13. A. Analog: 65; Digital: 70
    B. 10 cm
14. C. Dorsal decubitus abdomen
15. A. Wilms' tumor
16. Urinary tract infection (UTI)
17. A. NEC
18. D. AP erect abdomen
19. True
20. A. 2 to 4 ounces
    B. 4 to 6 ounces
    C. 6 to 12 ounces
    D. 12 to 16 ounces
21. Insert a nasogastric tube into the stomach.
22. False (usually 1 hour)
23. False (Latex tips should not be used because of possible allergic response to latex.)
24. AP and oblique positions (LPO and RPO)
25. True

1. C. Have another health professional (nonradiology) hold the child and have the guardian wait outside of the room.
2. B. Pigg-O-Stat
3. A. AP and lateral upper airway
4. D. Chest
5. C. AP and lateral hip
6. A. Foot
7. C. Kite method
8. D. Barium enema
9. D. Upper GI
10. A. fMRI

CHAPTER 17

Review Exercise A: Anatomy of Cardiovascular System, Pulmonary and Systemic Circulation, and Cerebral Arteries and Veins

1. A. Cardiovascular
   B. Lymphatic
2. A. Heart
   B. Blood vessels
   C. Heart to lungs
   D. Throughout the body
3. A. Transportation of oxygen, nutrients, hormones, and chemicals
   B. Removal of waste products
   C. Maintenance of body temperature, water, and electrolyte balance
4. A. Heart
   B. Artery
   C. Arteriole
   D. Capillary
   E. Venule
   F. Vein
5. B. (artery) and C. (arteriole)
6. E. (venule) and F. (vein)
7. 1. A. Red blood cells
      B. Transports oxygen
   2. A. White blood cells
      B. Defends against infection and disease
   3. A. (no other term given)
      B. Repairs tears in blood vessels and promotes blood clotting
8. A. 92
   B. 7

9. A. Right ventricle
   B. Left ventricle
   C. Left atrium
   D. Capillaries of left lung
   E. Pulmonary arteries
   F. Aorta (arch)
   G. Superior vena cava
   H. Capillaries of right lung
   I. Pulmonary veins
   J. Right atrium
   K. Inferior vena cava
10. A. Pulmonary arteries
    B. Pulmonary veins
11. A. Superior vena cava
    B. Inferior vena cava
    C. Right atrium
12. A. Tricuspid (right atrioventricular) valve
    B. Pulmonary (pulmonary semilunar) valve
    C. Mitral (left atrioventricular or bicuspid) valve
    D. Aortic (aortic semilunar) valve
13. A. Right and left coronary arteries
    B. Aortic bulb
14. A. Great cardiac vein
    B. Middle cardiac vein
    C. Small cardiac vein
15. A. Left subclavian
    B. Left common carotid
    C. Left vertebra
    D. Left internal carotid
    E. Right and left external carotid
    F. Right internal carotid
    G. Right vertebra
    H. Right common carotid
    I. Right subclavia
    J. Brachiocephalic
16. A. Right common carotid artery
    B. Left common carotid artery
    C. Right vertebral artery
    D. Left vertebral artery
17. A. Brachiocephalic artery
    B. Left common carotid artery
    C. Left subclavian artery
18. False (right common carotid and right subclavian)
19. True
20. Internal and external carotid
21. D. Carotid siphon
22. A. Anterior cerebral artery
    B. Middle cerebral artery
23. Anterior cerebral
24. Vertebrobasilar arteries

25. Basilar
26. Middle cerebral arteries
27. Lateral
28. 1. A
    2. D
29. 1. Posterior cerebral arteries
    2. Posterior communicating arteries
    3. Internal cerebral arteries
    4. Anterior cerebral arteries
    5. Anterior communicating arteries
    6. A. Hypophysis (pituitary) gland
       B. Vertebral arteries
       C. Basilar
30. A. Right and left internal jugular veins
    B. Right and left external jugular veins
    C. Right and left vertebral veins
31. A. Brachiocephalic
    B. Superior vena cava; right atrium
32. True
33. True
34. B. Inferior sagittal sinus
35. C. Internal occipital protuberance

Review Exercise B: Anatomy of Thoracic and Abdominal Arteries and Veins, Hepatic Portal System, Upper and Lower Arteries and Veins, and Lymphatic System

1. A. Aortic bulb (root)
   B. Ascending aorta
   C. Aortic arch
   D. Descending aorta
2. A. Left circumflex
   B. Inverse aorta
   C. Pseudocoarctation
3. B. Azygos vein
4. 1. Celiac artery
   2. Superior mesenteric arteries
   3. Right renal arteries
   4. Left renal artery
   5. Inferior mesenteric artery
5. B. T12
6. A. Liver
   B. Spleen
   C. Stomach
   D. Left common iliac artery
   E. Left external iliac artery
   F. Left internal iliac artery
7. L4

8. A. Left external iliac vein
   B. Left internal iliac vein
   C. Inferior mesenteric vein
   D. Splenic vein
   E. (Inferior vena cava)
   F. Hepatic vein
   G. Hepatic portal vein
   H. Right renal vein
   I. Superior mesenteric vein
   J. Right common iliac vein
9. A. Superior mesenteric vein
   B. Splenic vein
   C. Hepatic portal vein
   D. Hepatic veins
   E. Inferior vena cava
10. A. Brachiocephalic
    B. Subclavian
    C. Axillary
    D. Brachial
    E. Radial
    F. Ulnar
11. A. Superficial palmar arch vein
    B. Deep palmar arch vein
    C. Median cubital
    D. Brachial
    E. Superior vena cava
    F. Subclavian
    G. Cephalic
12. Median cubital vein
13. A. External iliac
    B. Femoral
    C. Deep artery of thigh (profunda femoris)
    D. Lateral circumflex femoral
    E. Popliteal
    F. Dorsalis pedis
14. A. Dorsalis pedis (dorsal venous arch)
    B. Anterior tibial
    C. Great (long) saphenous
    D. Deep femoral (profunda femoris)
    E. Femoral
    F. External iliac
    G. Internal iliac
    H. Inferior vena cava
15. Great (long) saphenous vein
16. Thoracic duct
17. A. Fights diseases by producing lymphocytes and microphages
    B. Returns proteins and other substances to the blood
    C. Filters lymph in the lymph nodes
    D. Transfers fats from the intestine to the blood

18. False (one direction—away from tissues)
19. True
20. Lymphography
21. Computed tomography

Review Exercise C: Angiographic Procedures, Equipment, and Supplies

1. B. Respiratory therapist
2. Seldinger technique
3. A. Insertion of compound (Seldinger) needle
   B. Placement of needle in lumen of vessel
   C. Insertion of guide wire
   D. Removal of needle
   E. Threading of catheter to area of interest
   F. Removal of guide wire
4. Cutdown procedure
5. C. Hypertension
6. A. Femoral artery
7. C. Help the patient relax
8. Water-soluble, nonionic contrast media
9. 1. Bleeding at the puncture site
   2. Thrombus formation
   3. Embolus formation
   4. Dissection of a vessel
   5. Infection of puncture site
   6. Contrast media reaction
10. B. Just inferior to inguinal ligament
11. C. 4 hours
12. D. 30°
13. True
14. True
15. Oxygen and suction
16. A. Analog-to-digital conversion
    B. Flat detector—direct digital conversion
17. False
18. True
19. A. Pixel-shifting or remasking
    B. Magnified or zooming
    C. Quantitative analysis of image to measure distances and calculate stenosis
20. Length and diameter
21. A. To maintain temperature of contrast media at body temperature
    B. Reduce viscosity of the contrast media
22. True
23. False (does require contrast media)

24. True
25. False
26. True
27. False (does not require contrast media)
28. False (up to 180°)
29. False
30. False

Review Exercise D: Angiography and Interventional Procedures

1. A. Vascular stenosis and occlusions
   B. Aneurysms
   C. Trauma
   D. Arteriovenous malformations
   E. Neoplastic disease
2. Lateral
3. A. Common carotid arteries
   B. Internal carotid arteries
   C. External carotid arteries
   D. Vertebral arteries
4. A. Arterial
   B. Capillary
   C. Venous
5. A. Aneurysm
   B. Congenital abnormalities
   C. Vessel stenosis
   D. Embolus
   E. Trauma
6. False. (CT has become the modality of choice for pulmonary emboli.)
7. A. Femoral vein
8. D. Femoral artery
9. A. Femoral vein
10. D. 30 to 50 mL
11. C. 45
12. A. Coronary arteries
13. Femoral vein
14. C. 15 to 30 frames per second
15. A. Ejection fraction
16. Venacavography
17. A. Aneurysm
    B. Congenital abnormality
    C. GI bleed
    D. Stenosis or occlusion
    E. Trauma
18. Femoral artery
19. A. Renal arteries
    B. Celiac artery
    C. Superior and inferior mesenteric arteries
20. True
21. D. Left subclavian artery
22. True

23. Radiologic procedures that intervene in disease process, providing a therapeutic outcome
24. B. Shorter hospital stays
25. False (primarily for treatment of disease)
26. False (performed primarily in angiographic suite)
27. Embolization of the uterine artery can shrink fibroids and eliminate associated pain and bleeding.
28. B. Enteric stenting
29. 1. A
    2. A
    3. B
    4. B
    5. A
    6. A
    7. B
    8. B
    9. A
    10. B
    11. B
    12. A
30. Through the right jugular vein
31. Vasoconstrictor
32. Basket catheter or loop snare
33. Kyphoplasty
34. Kyphoplasty balloon
35. Balloon catheter
36. Thrombolysis
37. D. Unresectable malignant disease
38. False (>80%)
39. True
40. D. Heating

CHAPTER 18

Review Exercise A: Brain and Spinal Cord Anatomy

1. A. Brain (encephalon)
   B. Spinal cord (medulla spinalis)
2. A. L1
   B. Conus medullaris
3. A. Neurons
   B. Dendrites
4. A. Dura mater
   B. Arachnoid mater
   C. Pia mater
   D. Epidural space
   E. Subdural space
   F. Subarachnoid space
5. Venous sinuses
6. A. Frontal lobe
   B. Parietal lobe

C. Occipital lobe
   D. Temporal lobe
   E. Insula or central lobe
7. A. Cerebrum
   B. Thalamus
   C. Hypothalamus
   D. Cerebellum
   E. Pons
   F. Medulla (medulla oblongata)
8. A. Occipital lobe
   B. Parietal lobe
   C. Frontal lobe
   D. Longitudinal fissure
9. E. Anterior (precentral) central gyrus
   F. Central sulcus
   G. Posterior (post central) central gyrus
10. D. Corpus callosum
11. B. Longitudinal fissure
12. A. Cerebrospinal fluid
    B. CSF
    C. Subarachnoid
    D. Hydrocephalus
13. A. Cisterns
    B. Cistern cerebellomedullaris (Cisterna magna)
14. Brainstem
15. A. Hypothalamus
    B. Pituitary (hypophysis) gland
16. Pineal gland
17. A. Tracts of myelinated axons of nerve cells
    B. Primarily dendrites and cell bodies
18. A. Gray
    B. White
19. A. Infundibulum
    B. Posterior pituitary gland
    C. Optic chiasma
20. A. Midbrain
    B. Pons
    C. Medulla
21. C. Thalamus
22. B. Cerebellum
23. D. Hypothalamus
24. B. Pituitary gland
25. A. Caudate nucleus
    B. Lentiform nucleus
    C. Claustrum
    D. Amygdaloid nucleus
26. A. Lateral
    B. Third
    C. Fourth
       1. Posterior horn
       2. Body
       3. Anterior horn
       4. Interventricular foramen
       5. Cerebral aqueduct

6. Inferior horn
       7. Lateral recess
       8. Pineal gland
27. A. Olfactory
    B. Optic
    C. Oculomotor
    D. Trochlear
    E. Trigeminal
    F. Abducens
    G. Facial
    H. Acoustic
    I. Glossopharyngeal
    J. Vagus
    K. Spinal accessory
    L. Hypoglossal

Review Exercise B: Basic Principles of Computed Tomography (CT)

1. 1. B
   2. A
   3. E
   4. C
   5. C and D
   6. D and E
   7. C
   8. A
   9. D
   10. C and D
   11. D
   12. E
   13. C
2. False (number and arrangement of the detectors)
3. True
4. False (multiple rotations possible)
5. C. Slip rings
6. True
7. D. Low-cost system to operate
8. C. Multiplanar reconstruction
9. A. Gantry
   B. Operator control console
   C. Computer
10. Gantry
11. Aperture
12. Cadmium tungstate or rare earth oxide ceramic crystals
13. A. Size of detector row
14. D. 262,144
15. A. PACS
16. Attenuation of radiation by a given tissue
17. Volume element
18. Three, two
19. A. Slice thickness
20. B. Isotropic
21. C. Attenuation
22. Lower

23. Attenuation
24. A. Cortical bone: +1000 to +3000
    B. White brain matter: +45
    C. Blood: +20
    D. Fat: −100
    E. Lung tissue: −200
    F. Air: −1000
    G. Water: 0
25. Water
26. A. 1
    B. 2
    C. 3
    D. 1
27. B. Displayed image contrast
28. A. Image brightness
29. Amount of anatomy examined during a particular scan
30. Table speed; slice thickness
31. 2:1 pitch
32. A. Undersampling
33. C. 10-mm couch movement and 20-mm slice thickness
34. True
35. B. Electromechanical injector
36. A. Saline
37. A. 1% or less
38. D. Dose modulation
39. B. Bismuth
40. To strive to reduce dose to children during CT procedures through the application of accepted protocols, safety measures, and open dialogue with patients and health care team.

Review Exercise C: Clinical Applications of CT and Imaging of the Brain

1. A. Visualization of anatomic structures with no superimposition
   B. Increased contrast resolution between various types of soft tissue
   C. MPR (multiplanar reconstruction)
   D. Manipulation of attenuation data
2. B. Scout view
3. 50% to 90%
4. False (4 minutes)
5. False (not able to pass through)
6. True
7. A. Proteins
8. True
9. False (lower pitch ratio leads to higher dose)

10. A. Narrow window (brain tissue visualized)
    B. Wide window (bony detail visualized)
11. Rotation; tilt
12. Subdural hematoma
13. A. Anterior corpus callosum-genu
    B. Anterior horn of left lateral ventricle
    C. Head of caudate nucleus
    D. Region of thalamus
    E. Third ventricle
    F. Pineal gland or body
    G. Posterior horn of left lateral ventricle
14. A. Anterior corpus callosum-genu
    B. Anterior horn of left lateral ventricle (CT only)
    C. Third ventricle
    D. Region of pineal gland
    E. Internal occipital protuberance (CT only)

Review Exercise D: Additional and Specialized CT Procedures and CT Terminology

1. A. 2 to 3 mm
2. True
3. C. Spinal cord deformity
4. False
5. True
6. Air
7. Prone and supine
8. Carbon dioxide
9. False
10. D. Up to 2000 mL
11. To ensure heart is scanned only during the times of the least motion in the cardiac cycle
12. True
13. True
14. C. 8 to 12 images per second
15. D. Biopsies
16. D. Special needle holders
17. True
18. D. 85%
19. Gantry
20. Matrix
21. Scanogram, topogram, or scout
22. Slip rings
23. Window level (WL)
24. Window width (WW)
25. Maximum intensity projection (MIP)

CHAPTER 19

Review Exercise A: Arthrography

1. Synovial joints
2. Magnetic resonance imaging (MRI) or computed tomography (CT)
3. A. Tears of the joint capsule
   B. Tears of the menisci
   C. Tears of ligaments
4. Baker's cyst
5. Allergic reactions to iodine-based contrast media and allergic reactions to local anesthetics
6. True
7. False (needs to be flexed to distribute contrast media)
8. Clear and tinged yellow
9. A. Positive or radiopaque media such as iodinated, water-soluble contrast agent
   B. Negative or radiolucent contrast agents, such as room air, oxygen, or carbon dioxide
10. A. AP
    B. Lateral
11. A. Six views per meniscus
    B. 30°
12. A. Joint capsule
    B. Rotator cuff
    C. Long tendon of biceps muscle
    D. Articular cartilage
13. Rotator cuff
14. 2¾- to 3½-inch spinal needle
15. A. Chronic pain
    B. General weakness
    C. Suspected tear in the rotator cuff
16. A. AP scout
    B. AP internal rotation
    C. AP external rotation
    D. Glenoid fossa (Grashey) projection
    E. Transaxillary (inferosuperior axial) projection
    F. Intertubercular (bicipital) groove projection

Review Exercise B: Biliary Procedures

1. B. Biliary stones
2. False
3. BUN and creatinine
4. Too concentrated contrast media may obscure small stones in the biliary ducts

551

5. False
6. RPO position
7. In the radiology department
8. C. Remove a biliary stone
9. A. Endoscopic retrograde chol-
angiopancreatogram
   B. ERCP
   C. Duodenoscope or video
endoscope
   D. Gastroenterologist
   E. Prevent aspiration of food or
liquid into the lungs
10. Pseudocyst

Review Exercise C: Hysterosalpingography

1. Uterus; uterine tubes
2. Rectosigmoid colon; urinary
bladder
3. A. Fundus
   B. Corpus (or body)
   C. Isthmus
   D. Cervix
4. Corpus (or body)
5. Cervix
6. A. Endometrium
   B. Myometrium
   C. Serosa
7. A. Cornu
8. True
9. True
10. B. Patency
11. Assessment of female infertility
12. A. Demonstrate intrauterine
pathology
   B. Evaluation of the uterine
tubes after tubal ligation or
reconstructive surgery
13. A. Endometrial polyps
   B. Uterine fibroids
   C. Intrauterine adhesions
14. A. Water-soluble, iodinated
15. Tenaculum
16. Slight Trendelenburg
17. A. LPO
   B. RPO
18. D. 2 inches (5 cm) superior to
symphysis pubis

Review Exercise D: Myelography

1. A. Spinal cord
   B. Nerve root branches
2. A. Herniated nucleus pulposus
(HNP)
   B. Cancerous or benign tumors
   C. Cysts
   D. Possible bone fragments

3. Herniated nucleus pulposus
(HNP)
4. False (Most common are cervical and lumbar regions.)
5. A. Blood in the cerebrospinal
fluid
   B. Arachnoiditis
   C. Increased intracranial
pressure
   D. Recent lumbar puncture
(within 2 weeks)
6. 1 hour
7. 90°/45° or 90°/90° tilting table
8. Subarachnoid space
9. A. Lumbar (L3-L4)
   B. Cervical (C1-C2)
10. Lumbar (L3-L4)
11. A. Prone or left lateral
   B. Erect or prone
12. For spinal flexion to widen the
interspinous spaces to facilitate
needle placement
13. Nonionic, water-soluble, iodine-
based
14. C. 1 hour
15. C. 9 to 15 mL
16. A. 4
   B. 5
   C. 8
   D. 1
   E. 6
   F. 2
   G. 7
   H. 3
17. Swimmer's lateral using a horizontal x-ray beam
18. To keep the contrast media from
entering the cranial subarachnoid
space
19. True (Right and left lateral
decubitus positions are taken.)
20. 1. A. Horizontal beam lateral
(prone), C5
   B. Horizontal beam lateral
(swimmer's), C7
2. A. R lateral decubitus
(AP or PA), T7
   B. L lateral decubitus
(AP or PA), T7
   C. R or L lateral, vertical
beam, T7
3. A. Semierect horizontal
beam lateral (prone), L3
21. True
22. Excreted by kidneys

Review Exercise E: Orthoroentgenography

1. CT is more costly and requires
specialized equipment.
2. A straight or right angle
radiograph
3. To prevent elongation (magnification) of the limb as a result of
the divergence of the x-ray beam
4. A special metallic (Bell-
Thompson) ruler to measure
bone length from one joint to
another
5. Epiphysiodeses
6. Hip, knee, and ankle
7. True
8. True
9. A single center-placed ruler
makes it difficult or impossible
to shield the gonads without
obscuring the upper part of the
ruler.
10. True
11. False (PA would cross radius
and ulna.)
12. False (Patient is supine, arm
extended, and hand supinated.)

Review Exercise F: Conventional Tomography

1. A. The radiograph produced during a tomographic procedure
   B. The pivot point of the connecting rod between tube
and IR
   C. The distance from tabletop
to fulcrum
   D. The plane or section of the
object that is clear and in
relative focus
   E. The thickness of the objective or focal plane
   F. The total distance the x-ray
tube travels during the *actual*
exposure.
   G. The total distance the x-ray
tube travels (including exposure and nonexposure time).
   H. The area of distortion of
objects outside the objective
plane
2. Longitudinal tube, Bucky tray,
and angle locks
3. False
4. False

5. A. Tube travel speed
   B. Objective plane
   C. Tube center
   D. Fulcrum
6. False (Objects away from objective plane have greatest blurring.)
7. Objects farther from the fulcrum level or objective plane will be blurred by the movement of the tube and IR. Objects closer to this fulcrum level and those that are parallel to tube travel will remain almost stationary and experience little or no blurring.
8. A. Distance the object is from the objective plane
   B. Exposure angle or amplitude
   C. Distance the object is from the IR (OID)
   D. Alignment of anatomic part to tube movement
9. False (increases)
10. True
11. B. Perpendicular
12. C. 5°
13. D. 20°
14. 10° or less
15. True
16. Orthostatic breathing technique
17. B. 2 seconds

CHAPTER 20

Review Exercise A: Nuclear Medicine and PET

1. Radiopharmaceuticals
2. True
3. D. All of the above
4. C. Technetium 99m (Tc-99m)
5. 6 hours
6. Single photon emission computed tomography
7. 200 microcuries (μCi) and 30 millicuries (mCi)
8. 2 years
9. A. Kidney transplants
10. B. Gastric emptying
11. C. Sodium iodide 123 (^{123}I)
12. A. 1
    B. 3
    C. 1
    D. 1
    E. 2
    F. 3
    G. 2

H. 4
I. 3
J. 1
13. A. 3
    B. 6
    C. 2
    D. 8
    E. 1
    F. 5
    G. 4
    H. 7
14. D. 48 hours
15. B. 140 keV
16. Positron emission tomography
17. C. Biochemical function of the body's organs and tissue
18. False (The PET scanner itself does not produce radiation.)
19. B. Positrons
20. Annihilation radiation
21. A. Emitted photons
22. Coincidence
23. D. Carbon and fluorine
24. C. Cellular reproduction
25. A. 2
    B. 1
    C. 4
    D. 3
26. Cyclotron
27. A. 120 seconds to 110 minutes
28. False
29. True
30. C. Staging
31. False
32. True
33. A. ^{82}Rbn chloride
34. True
35. True
36. D. Identify the location of key motor and sensory regions of the brain
37. Decreased
38. D. Fusion technology
39. EEG
40. True

Review Exercise B: Radiation Oncology (Therapy)

1. True
2. Palliative or palliation
3. A. External beam irradiation (teletherapy)
   B. Brachytherapy
4. Brachytherapy
5. A. Cobalt—60 units
   B. Linear accelerator

6. A. 1. 25 MeV
7. D. High-speed electrons striking tungsten target
8. Breathing and other bodily
9. Stereotactic body radiation therapy
10. Intraoperative radiation therapy (IORT)
11. A. 3
    B. 1
    C. 1
    D. 4
    E. 2
    F. 3
    G. 1
12. Short-distance therapy

Review Exercise C: Ultrasound Imaging (Sonography)

1. A. Sonography
   B. Ultrasonography
   C. Echosonography
   D. Sonography
2. 1 to 20 MHz
3. False (not ideal for ileus)
4. False (not used for bone cyst)
5. True
6. Converts electrical energy to waves of (sound) energy
7. B. Ceramic
8. True
9. True
10. A. General
    B. Echocardiography
    C. Vascular
11. No ionizing radiation
12. Bats
13. B. B-mode (patient mode)
14. D. Doppler
15. True
16. False
17. True
18. False
19. True
20. The lowest MI and TI settings
21. False
22. A. 2
    B. 1
    C. 3
23. True
24. B. Stomach
25. Sonomammography
26. True
27. C. Gel
28. False
29. A. 8
    B. 3

C. 9
D. 1
E. 7
F. 5
G. 10
H. 4
I. 2
J. 6
30. D. Normal from abnormal breast tissue

MAMMOGRAPHY

Review Exercise A: Breast Cancer, Anatomy of the Breast, and Mammography Quality Standards Act

1. Mammography
2. B. 40
3. C. 1994
4. 1 million
5. Between 1% and 2%
6. 2 cm
7. C. 32%
8. Canadian Association of Radiologists
9. B. VA facilities
10. Inframammary fold
11. Areola
12. Axillary prolongation
13. Mediolateral
14. Lower inner quadrant (LIQ)
15. 10 o'clock
16. Pectoralis major muscle
17. Retromammary
18. Lactation or secretion of milk
19. A. Glandular
    B. Fibrous or connective
    C. Adipose (fatty)
20. Trabeculae
21. Cooper's (suspensory) ligaments
22. 1. FG
    2. FG
    3. FF
    4. FG
    5. F
    6. F
    7. FG
    8. F
23. Adipose
24. A. Skin
    B. Pectoralis major muscle
    C. Retromammary space
    D. Adipose (fatty) tissue
    E. Glandular tissue
    F. Nipple

G. Inframammary crease
H. Sixth rib (lower breast margin-varies among individuals)
I. Second rib (upper breast margin)
J. Clavicle
25. A. Areola
    B. Nipple
    C. Ampulla
    D. Ducts
    E. Alveoli
    F. Mammary fat
    G. Lobe
    H. Cooper's ligament
26. 15 to 20
27. Base
28. Apex
29. Base
30. C. 800 to 900 mrad
31. B. 5%
32. False (mean glandular dose)
33. True (Ensure shield does not obscure the chest wall anatomy.)

Review Exercise B: Patient Preparation, Technical Considerations, Alternative Modalities, and Radiographic Positioning

1. Talcum powder and antiperspirant deodorant
2. True
3. A. Number of pregnancies? Are you currently pregnant?
   B. Is there a family history of cancer, including breast cancer?
   C. Medications currently taking?
   D. Previous breast surgery?
   E. Had previous mammogram? When and where?
   F. Reason for current examination? Screening mammogram? Any changes in breast, including lumps, pain, or discharge?
4. True
5. False
6. 25 to 28 kV
7. Molybdenum
8. 0.1 to 0.3 mm
9. 25 to 45
10. A. Decreases the thickness of the breast
    B. Brings the breast structures as close to the IR as possible

C. Decreases dose and scattered radiation
D. Decreases motion and geometric unsharpness
E. Increases radiographic contrast
F. Separates breast structure
11. A. Reduces scatter radiation
    B. Separation of superimposed structures in breast
12. D. 75 to 85
13. A. Fine detail
    B. Edge sharpness
    C. Soft tissue visibility
14. True
15. False
16. B. Magnify specific regions of interest
17. A. 130 to 150 mrad
18. A. Lower operating costs
    B. Can send images to remote locations via telemammography
    C. Archiving and PACS options (Images can be archived and stored electronically in a PACS.)
    D. Image manipulation, which can reduce the number of repeat exposures
19. Flat Panel Detector (Also termed Thin Film Transistor [FPD-TFT] technology in Chapter 1)
20. True
21. B. 15%
22. Distinguishing a cyst from a solid mass
23. True
24. True
25. D. Technetium-99m-sestamibi
26. B. Detect metastasis to a lymph node surrounding the breast
27. A. Sulfur colloid
28. C. Glucose (sugar) metabolism
29. Gamma camera is much smaller therefore in closer proximity to the patient's breast
30. A. Higher cost
    B. Radiation exposure to the patient
31. False
32. A. High false-positive rate
    B. Higher cost
    C. Length of the exam time
33. B. DBT (digital breast tomosynthesis)
34. A. Fibroadenoma

35. C. Infiltrating ductal carcinoma
36. C. Fibroadenoma
37. True
38. A. Craniocaudal (CC)
    B. Mediolateral oblique (MLO)
39. Inframammary fold
40. Axillary
41. Nipple
42. Away from
43. Mediolateral oblique (MLO)
44. 45° from vertical (Note: CR is perpendicular to the patient's pectoral muscle.)
45. False
46. B. Forward, toward the front of the body
47. Exaggerated craniocaudal (lateral), or XCCL
48. Base
49. Exaggerated craniocaudal (lateral), or XCCL
50. Exaggerated craniocaudal (lateral), or XCCL
51. 90° from vertical
52. A. True
    B. False
    C. False
    D. True
    E. False
    F. False (overexposed)
    G. True
    H. True
    I. False
    J. True
53. Eklund method
54. The breast implant needs to be "pinched" or pushed posterior carefully toward the chest wall out of the exposure field.
55. D. Axillary tail
56. A. Mediolateral oblique
    B. Superolateral-inferomedial oblique
    C. Axillary tail
    D. Craniocaudal
    E. Rolled lateral
    F. Lateromedial
    G. Exaggerated craniocaudal (laterally)
    H. Lateromedial oblique
    I. Implant displaced

Review Exercise C: Critique Radiographs of the Breast

A. CC projection (Fig. C20-79)
   1. *Folds of fatty tissue superimpose breast tissue.
   2. *Breast is not pulled away from chest wall; folds of tissue are not pulled back.
   3. Collimation is not applicable for mammography. CR centering is acceptable.
   4. Exposure factors are acceptable.
   5. Anatomic side marker is visible.
      Repeatable error(s): 1 (anatomy demonstrated) and 2 (part positioning)
B. MLO projection (Fig. C20-80)
   1. *Pertinent muscle is not seen to nipple level, and outer tissue is not compressed.
   2. *Lower part of breast not pulled away from chest wall onto IR sufficiently.
   3. Collimation not applicable for mammography. CR centering is acceptable.
   4. Exposure factors are acceptable.
   5. Anatomic side marker is visible.
      Repeatable error(s): 1 (anatomy demonstrated) and 2 (part positioning)
C. CC projection (Fig. C20-81)
   1. *Part of lateral posterior breast is cut off.
   2. *Medial posterior breast is not included, and shoulder is superimposed over the lateral posterior tissue.
   3. Collimation is not applicable for mammography. CR centering is acceptable.
   4. Exposure factors are acceptable
   5. Anatomic side marker is visible.
      Repeatable error(s): 1 (anatomy demonstrated) and 2 (part positioning)
D. MLO projection (Fig. C20-82)
   1. *Posterior medial breast is cut off; no pectoral muscle is visible. (White specks are calcifications; they are not dust artifacts.)
   2. *Breast is not pulled out away from chest wall.
   3. Collimation is not applicable for mammography. CR centering is acceptable.
   4. Exposure factors are acceptable.
   5. Anatomic side marker is visible.
      Repeatable error(s): 1 (anatomy demonstrated) and 2 (part positioning)
E. CC projection (Fig. C20-83)
   1. *Motion is present, which obliterates all detail.
   2. Acceptable—dark half-circle indicates posterior breast is included
   3. Collimation is not applicable for mammography. CR centering is acceptable.
   4. Exposure factors are acceptable.
   5. Anatomic side marker is visible.
      Repeatable error(s): 1 (anatomy demonstrated)
F. CC projection (Fig. C20-84)
   1. *Hair artifacts are evident on posterior breast tissue, obscuring breast tissue detail.
   2. Acceptable.
   3. Collimation is not applicable for mammography. CR is slightly off-centered toward medial side.
   4. Exposure factors are acceptable.
   5. Anatomic side marker is visible.
      Repeatable error(s): 1 (anatomy demonstrated)

Review Exercise: Bone Densitometry

1. 44
2. A. Bone density
   B. Bone quality
3. 30% to 50%
4. Osteoblasts; osteoclasts
5. 35 years
6. 90% collagen and 10% other proteins
7. Bone mineral content (BMC)
8. D. All of the above
9. D. Polycystic kidney disease
10. True
11. B, C, G, I
12. False (less risk)
13. True
14. True

15. D. 2.5 standard deviations below the average young normal population
16. The number of standard deviations an individual's BMD is from the mean BMD of an average, young individual of the same sex and ethnicity
17. A. Normal bone
18. Z scores
19. B. Parathyroid hormone
20. True
21. A. Dual-energy x-ray absorptiometry (DXA)
    B. Quantitative computed tomography (QCT)
    C. Quantitative ultrasound (QUS)
22. A. Quantitative computed tomography (QCT)
23. False (Fan-beam)
24. Micro-Sieverts (μSv)
25. <5 μSv
26. B. An average individual of the same sex and age
27. C. T12 to L5
28. True
29. False
30. Trabecular and cortical
31. 30 μSv
32. C. Os calcis (calcaneus)
33. C. QUS
34. A. Lumbar spine
    B. Hip (proximal femur)
35. True
36. True
37. True
38. False
39. False
40. B. Reproducibility
41. A. Patient positioning
42. 10%
43. 70 years
44. A. Thoraco-lumbar spine
45. D. 66%

MAGNETIC RESONANCE IMAGING (MRI)

Review Exercise A: Physical Principles of MRI

1. Magnetic fields and radio waves
2. Nuclei
3. 2. A. 10^3 to 10^{-2} meters
      B. 10^5 to 10^{10} hertz
      C. 10^{-7} electron volts (eV)

4. A. Hydrogen (single-proton nucleus)
   B. The large amount of hydrogen present in any organism (Hydrogen atoms are present in each water molecule, and the body is roughly 85% water.)
5. Proton
6. A. 1022
7. Is similar to the wobble of a slowly spinning top
8. Increases
9. An outside force (the magnetic field)
10. Radio waves
11. Increase in time increases the angle of precession
12. Resonance
13. Nucleus or proton
14. Radio; precessing or rotating
15. T1 relaxation and T2 relaxation
16. Longitudinal
17. Transverse
18. Spin (or proton) density; minor
19. So that the returning signal can be located (because only the precessing nuclei within these regions or slice transmit signals)
20. A. Spin density
    B. T1 relaxation rate
    C. T2 relaxation rate

Review Exercise B: Clinical Applications, Safety Considerations, and Appearance of Anatomy

1. A. Potential hazards of projectiles
   B. Electrical interference with implants
   C. Torquing of ferromagnetic objects
2. Greater; directly
3. Danger of ferromagnetic objects used in emergency situations becoming projectiles
4. 5
5. 50
6. 10
7. Ferromagnetic intracranial aneurysm clips (unless the exact type is known and has been proved to be nonferromagnetic)
8. W/kg (watts per kilogram)
9. Specific absorption ratio (SAR)

10. Whole-body averaged SAR should not exceed 3.5 W/kg for 15 minutes of scanning
11. False. MR should be avoided in the first 3 months of pregnancy unless diagnosis crucial for conditions such as acute appendicitis or other emergencies as determined by a physician.
12. True
13. Contrast resolution
14. Normal; abnormal
15. A. Surgical history
    B. Occupational history
    C. Accidental history
16. GFR (glomerular filtration rate)
17. Metastasis, infection, inflammatory processes, subacute cerebral infarcts, and scarring versus recurrent disk disease
18. 0. 2; 10
19. A. Internal pacemakers
    B. Ferromagnetic aneurysm clips
    C. Metallic fragments in the eye
    D. Cochlear implants
    E. Starr-Edwards pre-6000 model prosthetic heart valve
    F. Internal drug infusion pumps
    G. Internal pain pumps (unless certified as MRI safe)
    H. Neurostimulators
    I. Bone growth stimulators
    J. Ferromagnetic gastrointestinal surgical clips
20. A. 1
    B. 2
21. *T1 T2*
    B. Light gray; Dark gray
    C. Bright; Dark
    D. Light gray; Dark gray
    E. Dark; Bright
    F. Dark gray; Dark gray
    G. Dark; Dark
22. True
23. False (appear black)

Review Exercise C: MRI Examinations

1. B. White matter
   C. Nerve tissue
   D. Ventricles
2. A. White matter disease (multiple sclerosis or demyelinating disease)
   B. Ischemic disorders

C. Neoplasm
D. Infectious diseases (such as AIDS and herpes)
3. A. Posterior fossa
B. Brainstem
C. Detecting small changes in tissue water content
4. D. All of the above
5. A. Cysts
B. Syrinx
C. Lipomas
6. A. MRI does not require the use of intrathecal ("within a sheath") contrast media.
B. MRI covers a large area of the spine in a single sagittal view.
7. True
8. A. Meniscal abnormalities

B. Avascular necrosis of the hip and other bony regions
C. Soft tissue masses
D. Bone marrow abnormalities
9. Fat and hemorrhage
10. Water content in tissues (associated with tumors and other abnormalities)
11. True
12. False
13. True
14. B. ECG
15. True
16. C. Blood oxygen level-dependent (BOLD) signal
17. True
18. False
19. False

20. A. 8
B. 7
C. 9
D. 3
E. 10
F. 2
G. 5
H. 6
I. 4
J. 1
21. A. 5
B. 7
C. 4
D. 10
E. 8
F. 9
G. 3
H. 2
I. 6
J. 1